071-566-7800

THE PRESCRIBER

by the same author

A DICTIONARY OF PRACTICAL
MATERIA MEDICA (3 *vols.*)
A CLINICAL REPERTORY TO THE
DICTIONARY OF MATERIA MEDICA

THE
PRESCRIBER

by

JOHN HENRY CLARKE, M.D.

HEALTH SCIENCE PRESS
1 Church Path, Saffron Walden
Essex, England

Ninth edition (completely
revised and reset) 1972
Reprinted 1977
Reprinted 1980
Reprinted 1981

ISBN 0 85032 088 7

Printed and bound in Great Britain
at The Pitman Press, Bath

PREFACE

THE PRESCRIBER was first published by the firm of Messrs. Keene & Ashwell. Mr. Ashwell was himself the author of the invaluable *Companion to the British and American Homœopathic Pharmacopeias*, a volume of about the same size as THE PRESCRIBER. It may interest readers to know how I came to compile the book. I had been at the time some nine years in homœopathic practice, and the only work of reference of the kind put into my hands by my instructors was the *Clinical Index* of Dr. Ruddock's well-known *Vade Mecum*. Excellent as this is, it is of necessity limited, and although I had my copy interleaved this soon became overloaded, and so I set about compiling a work which should more or less completely cover the whole ground. In this instance, as in that of most of my other works, my own necessities led to its compilation. I needed it for my own use, so that I might find instantly, without reference to long treatises or dissertations, the points needed for present application in the cure of the sick.

The prompt acceptance of the work by the homœopathic profession proved that I had not been wrong in believing that others had felt the need of a work of the kind as well as myself. And there has been no slackening in the demand for it ever since. A large edition has appeared in America, and it has been translated into Spanish for the benefit of the great Spanish-speaking population of both hemispheres.

The exhaustion of the last English edition has given me an

opportunity of putting it through a complete revision, and very few are the pages on which I have not seen cause to make some addition. For the sake of Indian readers and those Britons whose lives are spent largely in tropical countries I have added items on diseases which are mostly met with in those parts. In compiling these the admirable work by Drs. E. A. Neatby and T. Miller Neatby, *A Manual of Tropical Disease and Hygiene for Missionaries*, has been of great assistance. Another acknowledgment I have to make is to my friend Mr. W. H. Knight, the literary executor of the late Dr. Leopold Salzer of Calcutta, who, when he heard there was to be a new edition of THE PRESCRIBER, sent me his own annotated copy. In this he has collated therapeutic items from many sources, including my own *Materia Medica*. A large number of these will be found fitted into their own appropriate niches in the present edition.

The position of THE PRESCRIBER in medical literature is unique. There are books in abundance which tell all there is to tell about diseases, their history, etiology, course, progress, pathology, histology and all the rest. But the weak point of them all is when they come to tell of the treatment. The directions these works give for treatment are couched in generalities as a rule. THE PRESCRIBER deals with nothing else but treatment, and the directions, instead of dealing with generalities, go into minute particulars for ready application to any case of any disease. The descriptions of disease I leave to its describers, and thank them for doing that part of the work. My part is to tell the practitioner what he can do when he has learned all the others can teach him.

That there are many in old school ranks who are anxious to learn I have good reason to know. The *Lancet* has quite recently acknowledged that the homœopathic doctrine is true; but after delivering itself of the admission it stops there, and does not proceed to take the action which the admission would seem to require. It says "if the proof of the pudding is in the eating," it is impossible to deny that likes cure likes. But it declines to eat of the pudding or to invite its readers to the feast. So the task of providing the banquet is still left to the homœopathic body, and as long as healers of the sick can find in THE PRESCRIBER the nourishment they require, it shall be served up for them as well and as daintily as its author and publishers can effect.

Before concluding this preface I wish to say a word to my readers on behalf of that most important and essential person the homœopathic chemist. It is impossible for anyone to practise homœopathy properly without the aid of a skilful and conscientious chemist. No medical man can collect, prepare and dispense all the remedies of the homœopathic pharmacopeia by himself. He must have a pharmacist to do this for him, if not in the same locality as himself, yet somewhere within the reach of the post, even if it is a thousand miles away. It is nothing short of a calamity to homœopathy that of late years many homœopathic pharmacies have had to close down. The spread of "stores" has had a good deal to say to that, but not all. If homœopathic doctors had made more use of homœopathic chemists and done less dispensing themselves it would have been better for both. As for homœopathic medicines dispensed at "stores," I take no responsibility for them. They may be quite genuine and of proper dilutions, but at best they are second-hand. The "stores" do not keep skilled homœopathic chemists who know all about the characters of the drugs used by homœopaths, and that is what the homœopathic practitioner needs. When the right chemist is found, let him have all his share of the work. In localities where there is no chemist the practitioner must perforce be his own dispenser.

Trusting I may be pardoned for this lengthy preface to THE PRESCRIBER'S new edition on its fortieth birthday, I herewith make my bow to my readers and hope they will find in it all they expect.

JOHN H. CLARKE

CONTENTS

INTRODUCTION TO *THE PRESCRIBER*

Part I.—HOW TO PRACTISE HOMŒOPATHY

1. Necessary Implements.

The completion of my *Dictionary of Practical Materia Medica* and of its *Clinical Repertory* since the sixth edition of *The Prescriber* appeared, enables me to give more full directions to my readers than I could before as to the best way to approach the study and practice of homœopathy. I have therefore decided to add to the former introductory portion of *The Prescriber* a separate essay, which I think will prove useful alike to the student who is desirous of acquiring the homœopathic art and to the practitioner who has had to be content hitherto with fragmentary implements.

The Prescriber was originally designed to put into convenient and accessible shape all the more salient indications for the use of homœopathic remedies from the *clinical point of view*. This is the approach which naturally first invites those who have been drilled in the practice of the ordinary schools. But homœopathy can never be properly practised by means of a clinical Index or Repertory (such as *The Prescriber* is in essence) unaided by other works. The homœopath must have his foundation authority always ready for instant reference. This authority is the Homœopathic Materia Medica.

It is of the greatest importance that a clear conception should be formed at the outset as to what the Homœopathic Materia Medica is. It is so unlike anything known as Materia Medica in the old school, that it is a pity, as I have pointed out below, that a different name could not have been found for it. The homœopathic materia medica consists of a *Register of Symptoms*. It is the *Semiology of Drugs*. For the practice of homœopathy we must know the symptoms which each drug has produced, and we must have these so arranged that they can be found instantly for any required region of the body. Hahnemann arranged them, for each of the remedies he tested, in a definite anatomical order, and this arrangement is the foundation of the order in which the symptoms are given in all works on the subject compiled since his day. This is named technically in homœopathy "The Hahnemannian *Schema*."

The homœopathic materia medica thus consists of a *schematic arrangement of the symptoms produced by each drug*, together with amplifications from the observed action of remedies in practice.

When I commenced the practice of homœopathy I found no little difficulty in the fact that the works on Materia Medica were too numerous and too scattered to be readily accessible. The only book which gave a comprehensive idea of the remedies contained in the homœopathic materia medica was Dr. Hughes's *Pharmacodynamics;* but this work, whilst giving much information *about* homœopathic remedies, is in no real sense a homœopathic materia medica at all: it contains no *Symptom Register* of the remedies it speaks about, and yet, for better or worse, it has had to do duty for a materia medica for many practitioners; and as its form is like that of the materia medicas of the old school, it has appealed very strongly to new converts.

It was the consciousness that something more was needed that impelled me to undertake the compilation of my *Dictionary of Practical Materia Medica*, which after sixteen years of labour saw the light. In this work I have given, as Hahnemann has done, the Symptom Register (or Schema) of each drug, which is the foundation of the work. In addition, I have given an introductory essay on each drug which enables the reader to apprehend its main characteristics. At the head of each remedy, under the heading, "CLINICAL," I have given a list of the principal diseases in which it has been used in practice. At this point I have linked the work to *The Prescriber*. Among the names of diseases given under this heading in the *Dictionary*, I have printed in italics those under which, in *The Prescriber*, the indications for this remedy will be found.

In the introductory article prefixed to the Symptom Register, or Schema, of each remedy, I have been able to condense the history of the work it has accomplished. In this way the *Dictionary* illustrates and illuminates the Schema and makes the study of the individual symptoms much more easy and interesting than it otherwise might be. Thus it comes about that the *Dictionary* comprises a whole library of clinical experiences which could only be reached otherwise by the expenditure of much time, labour, and research. Moreover, a great deal of it could not be found at all; since it was gathered by myself in conversations from the great clinicians whom it was my privilege to know.

It has been a source of very great satisfaction to me that the work was immediately recognised on its appearance, by those best able to judge, as filling a place that had long remained unoccupied. On the other hand, the force of old habit is so strong that many who had contentedly settled down within the limits of older works have not seen the necessity of enlarging their borders and accepting the liberty which is within their reach. This is one reason why at this juncture I think it essential to draw attention to the way in which the study and practice of homœopathy may and should be approached.

There are many ways in which the practice of homœopathy may be approached; some find one way more suited to their genius, some another. But I am writing now primarily for those who use *The Prescriber*, and will therefore take the approach by way of a Clinical Repertory.

I will suppose that my reader is one who has become convinced of the truth of Hahnemann's law, and of the efficacy of his method, and who wishes to avail himself of the power it puts into the hands of one who can use it; and I will suppose, further, that *The Prescriber* has been put into his hands as a ready instrument by means of which he can put its precepts to the test. With this book at his elbow he will be able to find, in a case of any disease, the remedies that are most generally appropriate, with their differential indications. In most cases he will be able to find a remedy which fits with tolerable closeness of similarity the case in question, and will thus be enabled to prescribe. But it will sometimes happen that the differential symptoms named in *The Prescriber* are not sufficient to enable a choice to be made with due certainty. In that case if reference is made to the Materia Medica, the actual symptoms of the different remedies can be studied in full, and compared with each other.

At this point it is necessary to mention the *Clinical Repertory to the Dictionary of Materia Medica*. This is a "Clinical" Repertory and much more besides, as I shall explain later. But it is different from *The Prescriber* in two respects: it names far more remedies under each heading, and it gives no differential indications. In the *Clinical Repertory*, under each rubric, the remedies mentioned in *The Prescriber* will be found printed in italics, and those not mentioned therein, in Roman type. It is thus a complement of *The Prescriber*, giving a greatly extended list of remedies under each rubric, and reference to the *Dictionary of Materia Medica* will supply the necessary information to enable the practitioner to make a choice among them. *The Prescriber* and the *Clinical Repertory* together provide as complete an approach as is possible, I think, to homœopathic practice, from the clinical aspect.

But, after all, this is only a limited approach—that is, it is an approach to a limited area of the field. It is the glory of Hahnemann that he liberated medical practice from its bondage to the names of diseases. Every case of disease is a problem in itself—presenting a new combination of morbid phenomena; the symptom-lists of the homœopathic materia medica presenting the possibility of finding similar combinations under one or other of the remedies named. Clinical repertories form one out of many of the means of fitting the remedy to the case.

2. THE COMPARATIVE VALUE OF SYMPTOMS. "THE PRESCRIBER" AND THE "CLINICAL REPERTORY." CASES IN POINT.

Before proceeding farther it will be well to make clear that some symptoms or disease-manifestations are of much more value than others from the point of view of selecting the remedy; and it often happens that those symptoms which are of the greatest value in correctly naming the disease, are of the smallest value in diagnosing the remedy. It will be noted throughout *The Prescriber* that in distinguishing one remedy from another great attention is paid to the *Times* and *Conditions* under which the various symptoms are better or worse—ameliorated or aggravated. (The sign ">" is used to indicate amelioration, and the sign "<" aggravation.) This point is often of more consequence than the actual symptom itself. And yet these characteristics would give little or no help in the diagnosis of the *disease*.

Perhaps it may help in understanding the differential value of symptoms and their Conditions or modalities if I instance a case. Miss T., 60, consulted me on October 7, 1908, about a pain which had troubled her more or less for twenty-five years. It affects the *right side* of the head and right cheek. In the temple are violent sharp shoots of pain. In the cheek it is a sudden pain, burning as if on fire. It is *worse* while eating; *worse* by touch; *better* after eating. It is *worse* if the patient is chilled; and is sometimes *worse* at night.

In dealing with a case like this it does not assist us much whether we name the affection "neuralgia", "neuritis," or "Tic douloureux"—we must deal with it on the strength of its characteristic symptoms.

The first point of importance to note is the *locality* of the pain—it is *one-sided*, the side affected being the *right*.

The next point is—it is a *sudden* pain—violent, sharp, shooting, and burning. In this instance the nature of the pain is of importance on account of the peculiarity of *suddenness*.

The next point is the *condition*—aggravation *by chewing*, by the least *movement* or *touch; and the last* point—aggravated *at night*.

If this patient had applied to an old-school practitioner all these details would have been useless to him; all he would have needed to base his prescription on would have been the word "neuralgia." It would have signified nothing, so far as his prescription went, whether it was right side, left side, or both sides. It would not have mattered what made it better or what made it worse, or at what time of day it came on. To the homœopath these are everything.

Turning to *The Prescriber*, under the heading of "Neuralgia" will be found a number of remedies affecting the right side of the head and face, and among them this: "Sudden pains, especially of right side of the head and face, < by the least movement or touch, eating or speaking; < 4 to 8 p.m., *Lyc.*" *Lycopodium* 200 was prescribed, and two months later the patient wrote to say "the pain was relieved in a most wonderful way."

There are other ways in which this remedy might have been found besides consulting *The Prescriber*: it could have been found by the ordinary symptom repertories, and it could have been found by reference to the Materia Medica itself. The fact that the pain was on the *right side* of the head and face was enough to make any one but slightly acquainted with the homœopathic Materia Medica look up *Lycopodium;* and a reference to the headings HEAD, FACE and TEETH would quickly reveal its appropriateness. It is impossible to carry all the symptoms of the Materia in one's head, but it is quite possible to remember a very large number of the characteristic symptoms and modalities (or Conditions) of the chief remedies. And after all, the best repertory any one can have is in his own memory. Only it must be possible to supplement it whenever required. Every remedy has a number of symptoms and modalities which are GENERAL in respect to it. That is to say, they qualify a very large proportion of its manifestations. So that when the practitioner meets with them in a patient he will be able to select the remedy even if the *particular* symptoms are not in precise correspondence.

And it is the same with patients. Many patients have GENERAL conditions which belong rather to themselves than to the particular complaint they may be suffering from, and when these are present they are often of greater importance from the prescribing standpoint than the actual symptoms of the disease. For instance, if the cardinal symptoms of *Sulphur* crop up in a patient—sinking at the pit of the stomach at 11 a.m.; aggravation of the symptoms at night in bed; hot hands and feet, burning on the soles, must put them out of bed to find a cool place— *Sulphur* will be the remedy for the patient, no matter what the nature of the disease may be.

Under the heading "CHRONIC DISEASES" in *The Prescriber*, I have indicated how this knowledge may be made use of in selecting remedies. In this way *The Prescriber* is something more than a *mere* clinical repertory—it is a repertory of *localities*. Under the different organs and parts of the body named will be found the remedies which have a specific relationship to them. Further, under the heading MIND will be found some leading *mental* symptoms and states, the presence of which, complicating bodily diseases—or, "concomitant" with them, as it is technically called in homœopathy—will point to the remedy to be selected.

I will now relate another case in illustration. J. P., 58, a coachman, was sent to me by his master on May 10, 1910. He had had severe domestic trouble, and was suffering from great mental depression, and, in addition, there was pain in the head. The pain was situated in the vertex, and was greatly aggravated if he was in the least worried.

The second of the five sections into which the *Clinical Repertory to the Dictionary of Materia Medica* is divided is a repertory of CAUSATION. It is often of great importance to know the *cause* in which every state has originated. The effects of a chill, physical injury or mental shock correspond to different remedies, and the knowledge of the *cause* is often an important guide in finding the remedy. On turning to this part of the *Clinical Repertory*, under the heading "Worry" will be found among the remedies *Ignatia*. As this patient had had much worry and as his complaint was aggravated by worry, *Ignatia* 30 was given. But it did no good. The reason of this failure was this—although worry was an exciting factor in the case it was not the fundamental cause. The complaint belonged to the patient himself. The condition now was; head bad; pain at vertex; comes any time; feels it for a time after getting into bed; very low spirited. Hands and feet warm and moist.

On referring to the description of different constitutions under CHRONIC DISEASES in *The Prescriber*, it will be found that this patient corresponds to *Sulphur* in some of these characteristics: hot, perspiring hands and feet; low spirits; night aggravation. On referring to *Sulphur* in the Materia Medica, under section HEAD it will be found that *Sulphur* has numerous pains referred to the vertex. On these indications *Sulphur* 30 was prescribed, with very speedy relief to all the symptoms.

But the improvement only went a certain way and then ceased. What next? There is a section of the CLINICAL REPERTORY which I think I use more than any other, and which I fear most of my readers have not learned to use, or feel the want of—it is the section of CLINICAL RELATIONSHIPS.

In the olden days when homœopaths had fewer remedies to commit to memory, each remedy was known much more intimately than it is at present. It was not only known as an entity in itself—it was known in its relations to its friends. For example, if *Belladonna* had relieved a case of inflammatory or congestive trouble and then ceased to help, the old homœopaths would know that one of the nearest relations to *Bell.*, and one of its best friends, is *Mercurius*. And they would naturally think of

Mercurius before any other to prescribe in the case. In my Repertory of CLINICAL RELATIONSHIPS I have given in tabular form a list of all the relations of remedies so far as recorded. This shows at a glance which remedy follows any remedy well— which are followed well by it, which are compatible, which are complementary, which inimical, and which antidotal. These lists are not to be regarded as complete or exclusive, but as far as they go I find them most helpful and suggestive. And whenever I meet an instance in which one remedy helps out the action of another in a marked way I enter it on my list for future use, and this I advise my readers to do likewise.

This by the way. My patient now remarked that although he was much better in himself, he still had the pain in his head and it was *worse when he had his hat on*.

Referring now to *The Prescriber* under HEADACHE, it will be found that *Lycopodium* has a headache at the vertex which is *worse when covered*. Turning now to the CLINICAL RELATIONSHIPS of the CLINICAL REPERTORY it will be found that *Lycopodium* is one of the remedies which is compatible with *Sulphur*. *Lycopodium* 30 was now given, with complete relief of these symptoms. The patient's livery hat was heavy, so it was particularly trying in his employment.

The relief in this case continued for several months, when an attack of influenza brought back the old trouble. When the influenza was cured, the old head pain remained and *Lycopodium* only partially relieved it. What was next to be done? Turn once more to the Repertory of CLINICAL RELATIONSHIPS under the reference, LYCOPODIUM. Among the remedies given as "complementary"—that is to say most closely related in action and helping out each other—is *Chelidonium*. A reference to the Materia Medica will show a close similarity between the two remedies in their symptoms and Conditions. *Chelid* 30 was given, and this completely relieved the patient.

Returning now to the former patient, Miss T., who suffered from neuralgia. In her case also *Lycopodium* failed on one occasion to control the pain, and here again the complementary remedy, *Chelidonium*, came to its aid and removed the whole trouble, and further illustrated the use of a repertory of Clinical Relationships.

In each of these cases *pressure* was a condition of aggravation. It is necessary to be able to reduce to its common denomination on the instant any symptom which a patient presents to you. Patients must not be expected to describe their sensations in the bald language of the repertories. A patient will be more likely to say "The pain is much worse when my hat is on," than he will to say "The pain is aggravated by pressure." In the same way a patient with right-sided sciatica will be more likely to say, "I can't bear to lie on my right side," than he will say "The pain is aggravated by pressure." But it comes to the same thing, and many a case of right-sided sciatica with this modality have I cured with *Lycopodium*.

When *The Prescriber* fails to indicate the remedy required for any case, on turning to the same heading in the *Clinical Repertory* a large number of remedies not mentioned in *The Prescriber* will in most instances be found. For their special indications it will be necessary to turn to the Materia Medica and compare them one with another. In compiling the Materia Medica I was able to save much space, and consequently save my readers much trouble, by placing at the head of each article a list of the diseases to whose symptoms the drug corresponds. The necessity for much repetition was thus avoided, since the leading indications for any remedy are available in any disease, whatever may be its name, when these are prominent in a patient. But the list, nevertheless, gives a good idea of the range of the drug's action; and when the whole of these lists came to be indexed, as it is in the *Clinical Repertory*, it afforded at once a valuable approach to the Materia Medica from the clinical side and a greatly enlarged clinical instrument as compared with *The Prescriber*. It would be beyond the scope of the work to attempt to give the differential indications for each remedy in the *Clinical Repertory* as is done in *The Prescriber*; just as it would be beyond the scope of *The Prescriber* to have included all the remedies named in the *Clinical Repertory*. But the lack of differential indications in the latter is no real loss, since the Materia Medica supplies them for ready reference and the study of the Materia Medica entailed in the use of it is pure gain. *There is no road to the practice of homœopathy*—whether it is the clinical road or the symptomatic road—*which does not entail close and constant study of the Materia Medica.*

I have already referred to the CLINICAL RELATIONSHIPS section of the *Repertory* and some of its uses. In homœopathic practice it is often necessary to modify or arrest the action of a remedy which has been administered. The means of doing this will be found in the *Antidote* column of this section. When more antidotes than one are given, the one which corresponds most closely to the symptoms of the case which it is desired to put an end to will be selected.

The late Dr. R. T. Cooper found great assistance in his practice from utilising the natural relationship of remedies. For instance, when he had given with good effect a remedy belonging to a certain botanical species and the good action came to an end, his next choice was often a remedy from an allied species, which would carry on the action. In the *Repertory* these will be found for instant reference under the section of *Natural Relationships*.

The Repertory of *Causation* I have already mentioned; this may be also used as a limited Repertory of Aggravation. Causation and Aggravation are not identical, but they frequently overlap.

The other section of the *Clinical Repertory* is the Repertory of *Temperaments*, *Age*, and *Sex*. In the selection of a remedy it often makes a great difference whether a patient is young or old, stout or spare, male or female, fair or dark, nervous or lymphatic. In this section of the Repertory all these points will be found indexed for ready reference.

I may mention a practical point which I have found a great time-saver. Wherever possible I block out on the front edges of my Repertories the different sections. In this way I am able to find with great ease the part I want to refer to without great turning over of pages.

3. THE DICTIONARY OF PRACTICAL MATERIA MEDICA.

I should like to add here a few words in regard to my *Dictionary of Practical Materia Medica*. I do not offer it to the exclusion of any other author's work, but I do offer it as the most complete and perfect presentment of the homœopathic Materia Medica for the student and practitioner. It is the fruit of years of labour to combine within the compass of a single work the material needed for daily practice, arranged in such a form that all the sections of the information included are readily accessible and do not obscure each other. In my work it will not be found that one "cannot see the forest on account of the trees." The introductory part of each article gives the reader in the shortest compass possible, a picture of the whole drug with the history of the work it has done. So that the work is just as useful for the student as it is for the practitioner. I have seen it stated in lists of works recommended for students that my Materia Medica is a valuable book of "reference"—meaning by this that it is a book to be referred to now and then. It is more than that: it is a book for reference every hour of the working day; it is a book for the study and the prescribing desk. It was compiled, first and foremost, for my own personal needs in practice—just as *The Prescriber* was—and I offer it as the greatest labour-saving and labour-rewarding materia medica for student and practitioner which we possess at the present day. With the *Dictionary of Materia Medica*, the *Clinical Repertory*, and *The Prescriber* it is possible to practise homœopathy—with works which only *describe* remedies without giving their actual symptoms this is not possible.

4. BŒNNINGHAUSEN'S "POCKET BOOK."

The above-named three works I offer as a *minimum* stock in trade for the practitioner who wishes to do justice to his work. But I no less strongly urge on him to obtain other works as soon as ever he is able to introduce them into his armamentarium. And first among these is von Bœnninghausen's famous *Pocket Book*. The full title of this work is *Therapeutic Pocket Book for Homœopathic Physicians to use at the Bedside and in the Study of the Materia Medica*. This is, in a sense, the parent of all our Repertories and an analysis of the Materia Medica. The most convenient edition is Dr. T. F. Allen's, for it is in reality a "pocket" book.* This work carries analysis and generalisation

---

* Dr. Boger's large work, *Bœnninghausen's Characteristics and Repertory*, contains Bœnninghausen's characteristic Materia Medica as well as the repertories of all his works combined into one. It is a most valuable compilation, but it has not the portability and compactness of the *Pocket Book*.

as far as these can be carried, and forms a symptom index of
the Materia Medica that is beyond price. My work has been to
approach practice from the clinical side. Bœnninghausen's work
approaches it from the symptomatic side. His Repertories of
"Sensations" and of Aggravations and Ameliorations have been
of enormous service to many generations of homœopathic
practitioners and will be to many yet to be born. I urgently
advise every reader to procure a copy and to read and reread
Bœnninghausen's *Preface*—and, incidentally, I may say the
same in respect to the prefaces of my own works to those who
possess them. I will take the liberty of quoting here a passage of
Bœnninghausen's Preface, which may give my readers a stimulus
in their study of the Materia Medica;—

"In using the *Pocket Book* at the bedside," says Bœnninghausen, "much depends upon whether one is entirely a beginner,
or is already somewhat skilled in homœopathy. But he who
knows nothing whatever must, indeed, make a most careful
search for everything without exception. The more he knows,
the less he has to look for, and, finally only to use it here and
there to help his memory. This may be best shown by an example:
this I have taken for the purpose from my most recent practice,
wherein the choice of the remedy was not difficult, and at first
seemed very easy, though, through lack of attention a mistake
might very easily have been made. This case may serve for a
beginner in homœopathy to try his own skill.

"E. N. of L., a man of about 50 years, of a blooming, almost
florid complexion, usually cheerful, but during his more violent
paroxysms inclined to outbreaks of anger with decided nervous
excitement, had suffered for a few months with a peculiar kind
of violent pain in the right leg after the previous dispersion
allopathically of a so-called rheumatic pain in the right orbit by

external remedies, which could not be found out; this last pain attacked the muscles of the posterior part of the leg, especially from the calf down to the heel, but did not involve the knee or ankle-joint. The pain itself he described as extremely acute, cramping, jerking, tearing, frequently interrupted by stitches extending from within outward; but in the morning hours, when the pain was generally more endurable, it was a dull burrowing with a bruised feeling. The pain became worse towards evening and during rest, especially after previous motion, while sitting or standing, particularly if he did it during a walk in the open air. While walking the pain jumped suddenly from the right calf into the left upper arm, if he put his hand into his coat-pocket or his breast and kept the arm quiet, which was relieved by moving the arm, and then the pain suddenly jumped back again into the right calf. The greatest relief was experienced while walking up and down the room and rubbing the affected part. The concomitant symptoms were sleeplessness before midnight, frequently recurring attacks in the evening of sudden flushes of heat with thirst without previous chill, a disagreeable fatty taste in the mouth, with nausea in the throat, and an almost constant pressing pain in the lower part of the chest and pit of the stomach as if something there was forcing itself outward.

"No skilful homœopathist who is perfectly familiar with the action of his remedies will long remain in doubt as to the correct remedy in this case, with so complete and accurate a picture of the disease, for all these symptoms together correspond to a single one, which is thoroughly homœopathic; but the beginner will be obliged to look for nearly every symptom and only after long search will he find the one most fit among the concurrent remedies. Between these two extremes of knowing and not knowing, lie many degrees of partial knowledge, which require a more or less frequent consultation of the book.

"One person, for example, knows that the pains repeatedly changing from place to place, with the fatty taste in the mouth, the sleeplessness before midnight, and others of the symptoms mentioned belong especially to the action of *Pulsatilla*, but he is not sure whether the remaining symptoms also belong to it, and he will not, if he acts conscientiously, spare the trouble to compare these latter; but he will soon see that *Pulsatilla* is not the correct homœopathic remedy, because, in addition to the mental symptoms there are others which are not similar, but, indeed, are directly contradictory to it.

"Another person who has studied more the peculiarities of the pains distinctly remembers that *China* corresponds to the paralytic and bruised pains as well as to the jerking tearings, and the stitches from within outward and to the pains jumping from place to place. In addition, he believes that also symptoms like sleeplessness before midnight, the aggravation during rest, as well as the relief from motion and rubbing, together with the flushes of heat with thirst, correspond to this drug, but because he does not know, he also must consult the books; and he will soon meet with contradictions, just as the previous one did, and he will see clearly the unfitness of *China* for the case.

"Neither of these two, however, ever think of administering to the patient a remedy whose curative power in this case is so improbable; but as conscientious homœopathic physicians they will look further and compare, and by the help of this book they will soon find, without great difficulty, the only really indicated homœopathic remedy.

"But even a third physician, educated in homœopathy, one who recognises the contra-indications of *Pulsatilla*, *China*, and other concurrent remedies, does not know sufficiently that *Valeriana* corresponds to the chief symptoms, and in order to be perfectly sure about this rather infrequently used remedy, he will quickly look up the few doubtful symptoms, and convince himself that this drug among all the known medicines, is the best adapted to this case, as was proved by the result; for after a single very small dose exhibited in a high potency in water, the whole trouble, with all the concomitant symptoms, was completely removed in three days."

I leave my readers, after perusing this case, to make up their minds as to which of Bœnninghausen's degrees of knowing and not knowing they consider that they belong.

In conclusion, I will repeat that there is only one road by which success in homœopathic practice may be attained, and the name of this road is—WORK. It is only hard application, intelligent and unremitting, that can ensure success in the mastery of the infinity of details comprised in the homœopathic materia medica. The result is worth all the labour and very much more besides; but I would seriously warn off at the outset all who think they will find in homœopathy an easy road to the cure of the sick. It is possible by the improvement of our instruments to make the practice of homœopathy less arduous than it is at present, but like every other great and good work it can never be made easy.

5. The Scope of Clinical Repertories.

The Prescriber was designed primarily for the beginner in homœopathic practice by one who had felt the need of a work of the kind when he became convinced of the truth of the

homœopathic law. As all British homœopaths receive their
training in allopathic schools, it is inevitable that allopathic ways
of looking at things should to a large extent prevail for some
time after their graduation or conversion. In the old-school text-
books remedies are considered in relation to *diseases:* in homœopathy remedies are considered first and foremost in relation to
individuals. In homœopathy when the cardinal symptoms of a
remedy are marked in any case, the name of the disease the
patient may be suffering from is of no weight whatever in
determining either for or against the selection; the remedy
which corresponds to the symptoms of the patient must be
given, and if the case is curable it will cure. To give an example,
I may relate a case as it was told to me. A patient suffering from
pneumonia had gone from bad to worse under homœopathic
treatment based on nosological lines, when it was decided to call
in further help. The consultant on entering the room observed
the patient shrink away from him in great fear. He found him
collapsed and cold, with cold sweat on his forehead. He said to
the other attendants that he would take their word for all the
rest of the patients symptoms; there was one medicine that
would cure the patient and one only, and that was *Veratrum
album;* and *Veratrum album* very speedily did. *Veratrum* had
not been given in the case before because it was not recognised
by those in attendance as a pneumonia remedy. In a very severe
case of pleuro-pneumonia of my own I rapidly cleared up all the
dangerous symptoms with *Stramonium*, to which I was led by
the delirium of the patient, in which he saw animals about his
bed, and especially a large black dog. The patient was a youth
and there was no question of alcoholism in the case. One of the
best cures of rheumatic fever I ever made was with *Ignatia*,
which was given because of the mental concomitants in the case.

I mention these instances to show that however valuable a clinical repertory may be, it can never be paramount in homœopathy; and whilst *The Prescriber* may seem to justify the allopathic arrangement of medicines as remedies for diseases, I only offer it as one, and that the most elementary, of the methods by which the similar, that is to say, the homœopathic remedy may be found. For a clinical or nosological repertory is perfectly justifiable from a homœopathic point of view, provided its limits are clearly understood. Names of diseases correspond to well-defined groups on the symptom-record of various medicines. *The Prescriber* shows at a glance what these medicines are, and how they are to be distinguished from each other. Thus in a very large number of cases a closely similar, if not the most similar remedy may be found.

But whilst offering *The Prescriber* as the most natural step in homœopathic practice to an allopathically trained mind, and as a convenient remembrancer to older homœopaths, I wish most strongly to insist that readers shall make themselves superior to it and independent of it by a thorough acquaintance with the materia medica and by making themselves proficient in the use of symptom repertories. Classical works like those of Bell on *Diarrhœa*, H. C. Allen on *Intermittent Fever*, Minton on *Uterine Therapeutics*, all give elaborate and detailed repertories of symptoms compiled on a clinical basis, enabling the reader to find by their means the most similar remedy. The scope of *The Prescriber* does not permit of my doing this in respect to all diseases, but I have adapted from Hering his excellent repertory to *Toothache* (which has often enabled me to find the remedy), and I give this in its proper place as an example of the kind, and as an exercise for junior homœopaths in the use of the more advanced methods. Although primarily arranged as a repertory for

Toothache it is equally available for neuralgic pains affecting the face and head whether connected with diseases of the teeth or not.

6. KINDS AND DEGREES OF SIMILARITY.

A homœopathic practitioner must perforce be original if he is to achieve any great measure of success. No two cases are exactly alike, and he must be prepared to adapt his means to any case that may arise, and happily there is in homœopathy scope for the exercise of a great variety of talent. In most cases there are more remedies than one that will benefit; and if the exact simillimum is not found, the next or the next to that will give a measure of help; so the beginner need not abandon the ideal as too difficult of attainment. Then there are many different *kinds* of similarity, as well as of *degrees*, and every kind is available for the prescriber's use. There is similarity between drug and disease in organ-affinity; in tissue-affinity; there is similarity of diathesis; similarity of sensations and conditions—all these and other kinds of *like-ness* are available for the prescriber to find his correspondence in: and he is no friend of Hahnemann, or of Hahnemann's system who would tie up practitioners to any one of them.

7. HAHNEMANN'S DOCTRINE OF CHRONIC DISEASES.

Hahnemann's discovery of the nature of chronic diseases is evidence that his mind was not closed to further progress, as it well might have been, by the transcendent importance of his discovery of the homœopathic law. Finding that certain cases were only temporarily benefited by remedies which seemed to correspond accurately with the apparent symptoms, he was led to note that there were points of importance in the cases to which they failed to correspond. In the cases referred to there was the fact that the disease manifestations, though taking the form, it might be, of an ordinary acute illness, were really only one event in a series; and it was necessary to find remedies corresponding to the *series*, if a cure was to be affected. For instance, an attack of asthma may look, and generally does look, like an isolated event in a patient's history. But inquiry will probably discover that the same patient has at a former period suffered from a skin eruption, a diarrhœa, or some other affection. All these are not many diseases, but varied expressions of one morbid taint. In the case of syphilis a sequence of disease-manifestations was known to exist. Hahnemann added to this two others—"sycosis," or the "miasm" whose keynote manifestation is the appearance of fig-warts, and the origin of which is often traceable to constitutional gonorrhœa; and, chiefly, the "miasm" which he called "Psora," whose keynote is the appearance at some period of the patient's history of an itch-like eruption. Without going into the question of how far Hahnemann was right or wrong in his explanation of the genesis of this miasm, there can be little doubt (in my mind there is none whatever) that he was right in the main fact. Old-school medicine has confirmed his observation in respect to the constitutional nature of gonorrhœa, and the "herpetic diathesis" of French writers is only Psora doctrine in another form.

And I may here point out that it is necessary to bear in mind the particular meaning attached to the word "chronic" by Hahnemann in the phrase "chronic diseases." He did not use it in the ordinary sense of "long-lasting"; he meant a disease which was due to a poison (or "miasm," as he called it) which had a *chronic evolution*, just as the poison of scarlatina, for example, has an *acute evolution*. Syphilis is a "chronic disease," in his sense whether the manifestations are acute or whether they are long-lasting. "Psora," is a chronic disease in the same way, though sometimes its manifestations are intensely acute. Another difference between an acute and a chronic miasm is that the acute naturally ends in complete recovery or in death; whereas a "chronic" miasm continues to act in varying or alternating ways throughout life unless it is cured by proper treatment.

Having discovered the existence of a chronically operating poison in the essential character of certain diseases, it was necessary for Hahnemann to find remedies which had corresponding chronic action in order to obtain complete similarity. These he found in the remedies named by him anti-sycotic, anti-syphilitic, and chiefly, anti-psoric. Since Hahnemann's day much has been done in tracing out the life-history of morbid diatheses, and there is no necessity to limit the number of chronic diseases to the three he described. It is open to original minds to find other miasms and their similars. The use of the nosodes in homœopathy, and the use of "vaccines" and "serums" in allopathic imitations of homœopathy are instances of possible developments on these lines.

But no matter what may be the plane on which the points of similarity are sought and obtained, the individual symptoms of each case must in the last resort determine the choice of the remedy. It is not a matter of giving an "antipsoric" for a case of psora; if the case is indeed a psoric case, though some good may be done with a medicine whose disease-making action is not of the psoric order, the case will not be cured. The division of remedies into antipsoric and non-antipsoric is a convenience for narrowing down the choice, as the "chronicity" is the most important feature to be matched; but the choice of the particular medicine of the group is determined by the individual symptoms of each case. Hahnemann's doctrine of chronic diseases is from first to last one of *practical* import.

8. THE GENIUS EPIDEMICUS.

The doctrine of *genius epidemicus* is another practical aid in prescribing. Just as one proving gives only a partial idea of a drug, so one case of an epidemic disease gives only a partial idea of the disease. It is perfectly legitimate homœopathy to take a number of cases and having found the drug disease which corresponds most closely to the disease in all its developments, to give that drug in a routine fashion to all cases which do not manifestly call for some other drug. The use of *Baptisia* in this way in the influenza epidemics has saved me a great deal of brain-work and has cut short, often in a few hours, many an attack of the disease. That does not mean that I have given no other remedy; on the contrary, I have had to use in some case or other almost every remedy in the materia medica; but the knowledge of the doctrine of the *genius epidemicus* has saved a vast amount of trouble, nevertheless.

9. THE HOMŒOPATHIC MATERIA MEDICA.

The last court of appeal, when the choice of a remedy is not clear, is the Homœopathic Materia Medica. In the homœopathic materia medica, as I have already shewn, the symptoms belonging to each remedy are arranged in a certain order, namely, under the headings of the different anatomical sections in which they have occurred, so that the practitioner can find at once any symptom which has occurred in any particular part of the body. All the Eye symptoms, for example, are given in the section "Eyes"; all the Stomach symptoms in section "Stomach," etc. There are some who regret that Hahnemann did not keep his provers' day-books and publish them instead of this classified list of symptoms (which is known in homœopathy as *The Schema*). This regret would be justified if the symptoms were not available in their individual capacity and did not admit of re-combination to an infinite extent. But a definite symptom is available for its value, just as a definite coin is, independently of the particular mint from which it may have been issued. It is this which renders homœopathy the flexible and adaptable instrument that it is; and it is this which makes the *Symptom Register* the essential of the homœopathic materia medica.

Furthermore, the symptoms are not only available in their individual capacity, they will bear reducing to their elements and still be available, just as the symptoms of a patient will bear the same reducing. For instance: a patient complains that he was seized with violent pains in the back immediately on stepping out of a bath. The bath here was evidently the determining condition. But the bath is not the *essential* of the symptom, the essential is the *wetting*. On referring to a repertory, it is under the heading, "Aggravation by wetting," that the corresponding remedy will be found and probably not under *bath*. In this case *Rhus* was the remedy. Conversely, take the example of *Aloe*, which has this symptom: "Just before getting into bed, sudden explosion and clashing in l. ear, as from breaking of glass; the clash of the glass was heard at the bottom of the head, and extended thence towards r. ear." If that symptom were met with in a patient, or any symptom closely resembling it, *Aloe* alone would cure; but the symptom may be generalised and utilised (and I have so utilised it) for sensations of explosions in the head, or a noise as of something breaking. Should a symptom like this occur when the remaining symptoms seem to indicate *Aloe* equally with other remedies, its presence would determine the choice.

10. Symptom Repertories.

This brings me to speak of Symptom Repertories, and among them Bœnninghausen's *Pocket Book*, as I have already said, holds a place of very great importance. Bœnninghausen realised and demonstrated the legitimacy and the utility of paraphrasing and generalising symptoms and their Conditions, and his lists of Conditions of Aggravation and Amelioration, of Sensations, of Desires and Aversions are invaluable.

It frequently happens in practice that a symptom is wanted with some peculiar Condition of aggravation or amelioration. Several medicines are found having the symptom, but not one with the Condition. On referring to Bœnninghausen, one of them is found in the list of remedies having that particular Condition, though it had not been noted in connection with the symptom in question; but that does not destroy its appropriateness. Bœnninghausen showed that when a medicine manifested any symptom occurring under any peculiar Condition, that Condition might, and probably would, indicate the medicine when the same Condition appeared qualifying any other symptom. At any rate it would determine the choice of one of several remedies, all of which had the symptom but only one the Condition.

It is the same with peculiar sensations: the sensation may have been experienced in one part of the body in the prover, but that does not destroy the remedy's appropriateness should the identical sensation appear in a different part in the patient. Hence the utility of Bœnninghausen's list of *Sensations*.

The Totality of Symptoms insisted on by Hahnemann as the basis of correspondence does not refer only to their numerical sum, but to their relative importance. It is not every sensation of a patient that constitutes a symptom from the prescribing point of view. In every case the practitioner has to ask himself what the points are on which he intends to base his prescription. It has been said that if three leading characters of a case are found under a given remedy, there is a "three-legged stool" on which a prescription may be based with every chance of success.

There are some classes of symptoms which are more important than others to be matched, and it may be useful to indicate some. Without attaching much significance to the order, I should name these as of especial importance: (1) Mental concomitants with bodily diseases. (2) Very peculiar symptoms and very peculiar combinations of symptoms. (3) Precise localities. (4) Course and direction of pains and sensations. (5) Alternating symptoms. (6) Conditions of Time: Periodicity and the occurrence of symptoms at particular times of the day or night, or phases of the moon or year. (7) Conditions of Temperature, sensitiveness to heat and cold, and aggravation or amelioration by change of temperature, and at the various seasons.

The use of repertories is in itself an art which the homœopathist must diligently cultivate. I cannot say that I find any one entirely satisfactory. The plan of the *Cipher Repertory* (excluding the cipher) is to my thinking the best; but this is not complete, and many of the completed portions are long out of date. Gentry's *Repertory* is the easiest to use, and I should be sorry to be without it. Kent's great *Repertory* is the fullest and most satisfactory. Among other repertories, Lippe's, that of Curie's *Jahr*, and Winterburn's *Pocket Repertory* may be named. The *Index* to Allen's *Encyclopædia* is indispensable to those who possess that work. There is also a *Repertory* to Hering's *Guiding Symptoms*.

11. Various Materia Medicas.

Among materia medicas, all who can should possess Allen's *Encyclopædia* and Hering's *Guiding Symptoms*. The former contains all the symptoms of the *Materia Medica Pura* and of the *Chronic Diseases* of Hahnemann. Dudgeon's translation of the former is the best in the English language. Among works *about* the materia medica, Farrington's *Clinical Materia Medica* and Dunham's *Lectures on Materia* and Kent's *Lectures* are admirable works. Dudgeon's translation of the *Organon* should be in every library. The want of a full materia medica, giving a full Schema and an explanatory introduction had been long apparent to me, and I endeavoured to supply the want by my *Dictionary of Practical Materia Medica*. A thorough knowledge of the materia medica is only to be gained by *persistently using it ;* by persevering search for the most similar remedy for every case which arises, whenever the remedy is not at first obvious to the prescriber. The search will not always be crowned with success, but let not the practitioner be disheartened by this; the search itself is of use to him as it will have helped to make him familiar with his instruments, the materia medica and the repertories.

The knowledge of remedies in homœopathy is like the knowledge of words in speaking a foreign language. The beginner in homœopathic practice should, in the first instance, make himself absolute master of some dozen of the most widely useful remedies, with all their characteristics and peculiarities, of the conditions under which their symptoms appear and cease, and of their special times of occurrence, if they have any. The following is a list I recommend, the medicines being named in the order of what I regard as their importance:—*Sulphur, Lycopodium, Calcarea, Arsenicum, Thuja, Aconitum, Nux vomica, Pulsatilla, Silica, Hepar, China, Belladonna, Bryonia.* An accurate knowledge of the symptomatology of these drugs will enable the practitioner to deal successfully with the majority of cases he meets. But it will also do more than this for him; it will give him a solid basis on which to build up a knowledge of the rest of the materia medica.

PART II.—CASE-TAKING.*

1. A Suggested Form.

The first step towards making a good prescription is a well-taken case. The homœopathist takes his cases with much more care than do others; for he has a double diagnosis to make—the diagnosis of the disease and the diagnosis of the remedy. The directions given by Hahnemann himself in the *Organon* should be carefully studied, and the spirit of them followed. The patient should be allowed to tell his own story, stating just what he *feels*, and the particular symptoms he is most anxious to be rid of.

---

* The greater portion of this section originally formed part of an Introductory Address delivered to students at the London Homœopathic Hospital. This explains the direct personal note in it which I have not thought necessary to alter here.—J. H. C.

I once had a compliment paid to me by a patient in Hahnemann ward when I was a resident physician in the hospital. It was paid indirectly and was all the more valuable for that. It was contained in a remark made to another patient and overheard by one of the nurses. The speaker was telling his neighbour why he approved of my methods. It was not because I had cured him, for he had not been in hospital long enough for that; it was because, as he put it, "*He lets you have your say.*"

This, I take it, is the foundation on which a true picture of a case has to be constructed in the doctor's mind—the patient's own uninterrupted story of that which he experiences. It is very far from being the whole of the picture, for if the doctor cannot see much more than the patient can tell him, he is not much of a doctor. But the patient's story provides not only the foundation, but also the outline which the imagination of the physician must fill in. It is on this power of correctly filling in the lines and the colours of a case that success in the art of the physician largely depends. When the patient has finished his story then comes the physician's turn. By his questions he elicits the particulars of the patient's past history, his family history, and the cause of his trouble if ascertainable, and he completes the picture by such items as he is able to obtain by physical examination.

Having elicited the evidence, subjective, objective and inferential, the next question is—how is he to preserve the record? In this matter, every practitioner is a law to himself. Some have copious and accurate memories and are able to hold the picture complete in all its details in their own minds. I am not one of these. For me it is a necessity to get all the chief points on written record, so that, without burdening my memory, I can quickly restore the mental picture at any future time, by a reference to my notes.

In my own practice I have found of great service in taking cases detached printed forms such as I here append. The headings of the Hahnemannian Schema are spaced out, and under each I put the symptoms as told me by the patient, or as ascertained in examination. As the Schema form is the only form in which a comprehensive knowledge of a remedy can be retained in the memory, so it is most useful to get the facts and symptoms of a patient's case likewise into Schema form for purposes of comparison. The points of resemblance at once occur to the practitioner who has his knowledge in orderly shape. For it is of vital importance to have our knowledge in proper form; otherwise the unorganised part of it only hampers us in the use of the little we have made our own. And we cannot rightly claim to possess any knowledge that we have not incorporated with our mental organism.

For recording the subsequent progress of a case I have blank papers of the same size as the printed forms. I have them made of the thinnest notepaper, so that they occupy very little space in my pocket-book. Any stationer will supply both the printed forms and the blank papers.

It is simply for convenience of reference that I use this form to enter the symptoms in. I do not elicit them in that shape—I take them in their natural order as they come. The schema is the index of the case, but the body of the case is the picture in your own imagination. For the continuation of the case blank slips are used into which the initial slip fits, and these can be added to indefinitely. In my desk are drawers which hold these slips, and these are arranged in alphabetical order. The four following pages indicate the form I mean.

For cases taken at the bedside I adopt the same plan. At first I used to memorise and write the cases up later at home.

Complaint and History

Generalities

Mind

Head

Eyes

Ears

Nose

Face

Mouth

Throat

Appetite, Eating

Stomach

Abdomen

Bowels

Kidneys, Urine

Generative

Respiratory

Chest

Heart

Neck, Back

Extremities

Skin

Fever

Sleep

Temperature

Time

Motion, Touch, etc.

45

But I found that too troublesome and too great a strain on my memory. I always like to save myself trouble, as most of my friends know, and by dotting down the items at the bedside in the records which I carry in my pocket case I save both trouble and time. Thus far the mechanical part of the process.

Having got your case taken and entered, what are you going to do with it? "Cure it," you say. Certainly; but there is something more to be done before you can get to work on that. The case must be digested in your own mind. If you can put a satisfactory label on it, by all means do so. But that is not sufficient in itself.

Every new case we take on is a new world we enter; and for the time being we must identify ourselves with it, if we are to alter it for the better.

2. "TOTALITY OF THE SYMPTOMS" AND THE INVISIBLE NATURE OF DISEASE.

Among the technicalities of Homœopathy is the phrase "Totality of the symptoms." There is nothing mysterious or sacred about the phrase, but Hahnemann rightly said that this "totality,"—that is, the sum total of the sensations and observable changes in the organism—constitutes the concrete problem in every case with which we have to deal, no matter what name the academicals may give to it.

Disease, we must never forget, is, in Hahnemann's conception, an INVISIBLE thing. It is a derangement of the INVISIBLE VITAL FORCE. To use a modern simile, the symptoms constitute a moving picture like the figures on the screen of a cinema. The visible and tangible part of the human body is the screen; the appearances and sensations of the diseased vital force are the "symptoms" and are analogous to the moving figures; but the operators producing the appearances are hidden from the audience. All the same, it is by looking on the screen that you can read the story of the changes in the invisible life-force in a way you could not do by going behind the screen. "Hence the totality of the symptoms" constitutes the disease *as our senses apprehend it.* The academic name we give to it is a secondary matter. As Hahnemann once said to a patient who asked him what his disease was, and what he was going to give him,—"The name of your disease is no concern of mine, and the name of the medicine I give is no concern of yours." The totality of the signs, pains and sensations is for practical purposes the concrete problem, and the less we trouble about the film and the light, the more clearly shall we be able to follow the story and discern our actual task.

3. "Treating Symptoms." Hahnemann's Case.

Among the many absurd objections which Hahnemann had to meet and which his followers still have to meet is that Homœopathy "only treats symptoms and if it gets rid of them it leaves the disease untouched." The very opposite is the truth. Homœopathy is compelled to extinguish the internal, morbid action before it can cause the external symptoms to vanish. The Allopathic method is to get rid of the symptoms even at the cost of producing other and worse symptoms. The outward and visible signs and symptoms are the guides to the internal and invisible causes—that is all.

There are a number of ways in which the totality may be dealt with when once we have got it. The way Hahnemann favoured was to write out the symptoms in a string, affix to each the remedies which are credited in the *Materia Medica* and repertories with having produced it, and then, having selected the one which corresponds to the greatest number of symptoms, giving it to the patient.

Hahnemann published very few of his own cases, because, as he explained, he did not wish to give his pupils an excuse for treating cases by the names of the complaints, such as *Nux* for indigestion, *Bryonia* for rheumatism, and so on. Each case was to be treated on its own merits, whatever its name.

I cannot do better than quote one of Hahnemann's own cases reported by himself, and this I will do in a few moments. It will show the double-action process which takes place in the homœopath's mind when taking a case.

Whilst what I have termed the film of the disease cinema symptom-complex by being unrolled before the doctor's mind's eye when taking a case, this picture automatically unrolls other picture-films stored up in the doctor's mental theatre. These are the records of the medicinal diseases set forth in our materia medicas. Every person who pretends to practise homœopathy must have his mental world stored with plenty of these. There is nothing but hard work and constant observation which will effect this, and best of all personal experiences. That was how Hahnemann learned his. It is essential to get into our minds the striking and clear-cut characteristics of a number of remedies indelibly engraved on our memories. As examples, I may mention the admirable series of "Drug Pictures" drawn by Dr. Margaret Tyler and published in our journals, the drug pictures of Dr. Hughes' *Pharmacodynamics*, of Kent's *Lectures*, and the introductory parts of the articles in my *Materia Medica*. With a mind well-furnished with an extensive gallery of this kind, the reeling off of a patient's symptom-film will inevitably and without any effort, call up the materia medica pictures which correspond to them, and for the most part the proper remedy will be picked out almost automatically. If the mental picture-gallery is too scanty, or if the details of the picture are not sufficiently clear, there is the Repertory and the printed *Materia Medica* for reference, and these must always be accessible in case of need.

Hahnemann's picture gallery was bitten in, as I have explained, with his own experiences. He had "proved" or tested most of the instruments which he used on his own person, and he took doses for this purpose which were by no means small or highly diluted.

Now I will give you his case which will be found recorded on p. 91 of my *Homœopathy Explained*.

"Sch——, a washerwoman, somewhere about forty years old, had been more than three weeks unable to earn her bread when she consulted me on September 1, 1815.

"1. On any movement, especially at every step, and worse on making a false step, she has a shock in the pit of the stomach, that comes, as she avers, every time from the left side.

"2. When she lies she feels quite well; then she has no pain anywhere, neither in the side nor at the pit of the stomach.

"3. She cannot sleep after 3 a.m.

"4. She relishes her food, but when she has eaten a little she feels sick.

"5. Then water collects in her mouth and runs out of it like water-brash.

"6. She has frequent empty eructations after every meal.

"7. Her temper is passionate, disposed to anger. When the pain is severe she is covered with perspiration. The catamenia was quite regular a fortnight since.

"In other respects her health is good."

This is the case, and whether you choose to call it "indigestion," "gastralgia," "biliousness," or by any other name you are not advanced one bit on the path of cure. But what happened in Hahnemann's mind on the unrolling of this film? It immediately started the unrolling of several corresponding materia medica films. And this is how Hahnemann tells the story of them:—

"Now as regards Symptom 1, *Belladonna, China* and *Rhus toxicodendron* cause shooting in the pit of the stomach on making a false step, but none of them *only on movement*, as is the case here. *Pulsatilla* certainly causes shooting in the pit of the stomach on making a false step, but only as a rare alternating action, and has neither the same digestive derangements as occur here at 4, compared with 5 and 6, nor the same state of the disposition.

"*Bryonia* alone has among its chief alternating actions, as the whole list of its symptoms demonstrates, pain *from movement*, and especially shooting pains, as also stitches beneath the sternum (in the pit of the stomach) on raising the arm, and on making a false step it causes shooting in other parts.

"The negative symptom 2 met with here answers especially to *Bryonia;* few medicines (with the exception, perhaps, of *Nux vomica* and *Rhus toxicodendron* in their alternating action—neither of which, however, is suitable for the other symptoms) show a complete relief to pains during rest and when lying; *Bryonia* does, however, in an especial manner.

"Symptom 3 is met with in several medicines, and also in *Bryonia*.

"Symptom 4 is certainly as far as regards sickness after eating, met with in several other medicines (*Ignatia, Nux vomica, Mercurius, Ferrum, Belladonna, Pulsatilla, Cantharis*), but neither so constantly and commonly, nor with relish for food, as in *Bryonia*.

"As regards symptom 5, several medicines certainly cause a flow of water like water-brash, just as well as *Bryonia;* the others, however, do not produce symptoms similar to the remaining ones. Hence *Bryonia* is to be preferred to them in this particular.

"Empty eructations (of wind only) after eating (symptom 6) is found in few medicines, and in none so constantly, so commonly and to such a degree, as in *Bryonia*.

"To 7, one of the chief symptoms in diseases (see *Organon*, sec. 213) is the 'state of the disposition,' and as *Bryonia* causes this symptom also in an exactly similar manner, *Bryonia* is for all these reasons to be preferred in this case to all other medicines as the homœopathic remedy."

So much for the selection of the remedy. Here we see an admirable display of Hahnemann's mind at work. As he elicited the symptoms one by one, the "films" of all the medicines he names began to unroll themselves in his mind, and the *Bryonia* film fitted much more closely to the case than any of the others. Though much space is required to tell the story, the action in Hahnemann's mind was almost instantaneous.

Now let us have the dosage of the remedy given and the sequel. Hahnemann says:—

"Now as this woman was very robust, and the force of the disease must consequently have been very considerable to prevent her, on account of the pain, doing any work; and as her vital powers, as stated, were not impaired, I gave her one of the strongest homœopathic doses, a full drop of the undiluted juice of *Bryonia* root to be taken immediately, and bade her come to me again in forty-eight hours. I told my friend E., who was present, that within that time the woman would assuredly be quite cured; but he, being but half converted to homœopathy, expressed his doubts about it. Five days afterwards he came again to learn the result, but the woman did not return then and, in fact, never came back again. I could only allay the impatience of my friend by telling him her name and that of the village where she lived, about a mile-and-a-half off, and advising him to seek her out and ascertain for himself how she was. This he did and her answer was: 'What was the use of my going back? The very next day I was quite well, as I am still. I am extremely obliged to the doctor, but the like of us have no time to leave off our work; and for three weeks previously my illness prevented me earning anything.' "

Here most assuredly the academic name of the disease was nothing to the prescriber, and the name of the medicine nothing to the patient. But Hahnemann found the substance into which Nature had packed the vibrations corresponding to the vibrations of the disease, and the former vanquished the latter. The undiluted juice of the root was given, and that must be something stronger than the mother tincture, as it does not appear to have had any alcohol mixed with it. But a cm. potency could not have acted more effectually.

As I have said above, Hahnemann's "medicine-films" had to a large extent been created by his own experiments on himself. It looks a very simple matter for anybody to swallow a drachm of the ϕ (or mother tincture) of *Bryonia* and to experience a great many pains and aches in consequence. Truly this is quite easy. But to observe all these sensations accurately, depict them clearly in all their true characteristics and arrange them so that they may be available for use by all succeeding generations—to conceive of the possibility of doing this, and to execute the work, demanded genius of the very highest order, a supreme artist as well as a master in all that goes to make up medical science. That the world of general medicine does not yet know Hahnemann is by no means wonderful. He is still far and away beyond their range and reach.

In this case we have an illustration of the classical method of practising homœopathy. It contains the essence of all homœopathic medication. But Hahnemann himself discovered a way of shortening the labour. He observed that certain symptoms and certain combinations of symptoms, were of much greater value than others from a prescribing point of view. If these cropped up in any case and had their correspondence in symptoms occurring in the provings of remedies, the remedy was easily found. This suggestion was developed by Drs. Henry N. Guernsey and Adolph Lippe in America, and by David Wilson, Thomas Skinner and others in England, to an extent that has proved very valuable.

So that when we come to digest a case, as I term it, in our own minds, we are always on the look-out for the most peculiar, and, it may be, most absurd symptoms which often contain the entire solution of the mystery we are trying to solve. If a patient says to me "There is one thing I hardly like to tell you, doctor," I don't rest till I get that very "thing" out of him—or her. A patient who consulted me recently had a quite amazing collection of symptoms, but it was not until she confided to me that her greatest trouble was the thoughts that came into her mind unbidden of a blasphemous order, that I was able to find the solution for the chief of her troubles in *Anacardium*.

A symptom of this kind would be nothing more than an absurdity to an allopath, but to the homœopath it is the greatest value and means to the patient all the difference between suffering and relief, and even between life and death.

Thus it will be seen that the taking of the case is not by any means a purely mechanical affair, or a mere matter of counting symptoms, although the mechanical method is not to be discarded or neglected.

4. INDICATIONS FROM HEREDITY AND HISTORY.

Again, in the process of "digesting" our case, there is the question of heredity, and of the possible presence of "chronic miasms," as Hahnemann termed them, the number of which have been added to since his day.

In my work these play a very important part in case-taking, especially in chronic cases. I always "fish" for them, and generally find one or more than one. If a case has "never been the same" since an attack of influenza," whatever else I may give the *Tuberculin of Koch* is certain to have a run. If there is consumption or pulmonary trouble in the history, *Bacillinum* is generally given in one or more potencies. If cancer is thrown up in the history, *Carcinosin*, or one of the numerous other nosodes of cancer may be called for to clear up the symptoms. And perhaps more frequently than any the "Tree of Life"—*Thuja occidentalis*. I have written somewhere that the old axiom, "when in doubt give *Sulphur*," has given place for me to "When in doubt give *Thuja*." *Thuja* is, of course, a sycotic and corresponds to the wart-producing constitution.

Among the questions all patients who come to me have to answer is "How many times have you been vaccinated? When last? and did it take?" *Thuja* is the leading agent to clear the way for other remedies when there is any active vaccinal taint present, and nowadays the taint is pretty nearly universal.

Thuja is also the chief antidote to the effects of Tea, which we all drink. So, in all chronic cases, "When in doubt give *Thuja*," if the more mechanical symptom-matching has not thrown up a clear indication for something else.

Here I cannot do better than cite a case which illustrates this point in case-taking, and though it comes from a lay source—if a Church dignitary can be called a layman—it is none the worse for that. The rôle of Physician and Padre were united not many centuries ago, and when Man has recovered his lost knowledge of Himself, it is probable that they will be united again. Here at any rate is the experience, and I give it because it is better than anything which I have handy of my own.

My very good friend, Canon Roland Upcher, Rector of Stradbroke in Norfolk, sent the article containing it in the form of a letter to THE HOMŒOPATHIC WORLD and it was headed "Consumption and Vaccination." Here it is:—

"*Re* Dr. Fergie Wood's remarks, *Homœopathic World*, August 1924, about *the probable existence and action of Consumption and Vaccinosis miasmata in the human system to be reckoned with in dealing with disease:* This I have proved as fact, on several occasions, and I wish to record one remarkable case, which came under my notice and cure. A woman fifty years of age, was taken into a certain hospital in a former parish of mine—suffering from great pain in the lower abdomen with vomiting, she was unable to keep any food down.

"Two eminent surgeons from a certain county town met the three local practitioners in consultation.

"They unanimously diagnosed the case as undoubtedly cancer of the stomach. The X-ray was not used.

"But as it was in so difficult a position it was judged too dangerous to operate upon; and the poor woman was sent home to die. However, not without a second consultation at her home.

"*Result*—the first diagnosis was confirmed.

"The woman was in such a desperate condition, that she could only lie in bed and groan. She neither could take any food nor retain nor pass anything.

"Under these circumstances, I determined to see whether Homœopathy could do any good.

"First Question: 'Have you any history of consumption in your family?'

"*Answer*: 'Yes! My brother and sister both died of consumption.'

"Second Question: 'Have you ever been re-vaccinated?'

"*Answer*: 'Yes; about five years ago, and I have never been well since.'

"Third Question: 'Did you ever have a bad fall, or blow in your stomach?'

"*Answer*: 'Not lately.'

" 'But did you EVER have a bad fall?'

"*Answer*: 'Yes; when I was about seventeen or eighteen, I fell off a swing on to my stomach.'

"Now follows the treatment according to Homœopathy.

"In the first place I had to knock down two stone walls before the indicated remedy could get through to the local mischief.

"The first wall was that of Consumption. Received 5 globules of *Bacillinum* 30 in single dose. Called three days afterwards, found the woman gone out, had walked a mile and a half down to the town.

"Next day she was greatly excited, so I called again.

" 'Well, Mrs. F., are you mad? What have you been doing, going out walking to town?'

"*Answer:* 'Well, sir, I felt, and still feel, so much better; I can eat and drink and keep it down, and I have less pain.'

"*Wall No.* 1 *knocked down.*

"Next came the Vaccinal wall and she received two doses, one drop of *Thuja* φ, twenty-four hours apart.

"Called at the end of the week. The woman met me at the door with 'Please, sir, a discharge has set in!'

" 'Good gracious! Where from?'

" 'Please, sir, from the womb!'

"This discharge continued for a week and the tumour in the abdomen, with *outside* swelling nearly as big as a football, slowly subsided.

"But as the woman appeared so weak and prostrate with the discharge, I got frightened and judged it well to antidote the *Thuja*, so administered *Pulsatilla* 30, one dose.

"Next day the discharge ceased and the tumour immediately began to swell up again.

"Question? Is wall No. 2 knocked down?

"Cannot tell, but anyhow the woman is a '*Daisy*': so I will try the Homœopathic rule and give her some 'Daisy.' Anyhow, it is God's remedy for bruises. (Why? Because the more the Daisy is cut, trampled on and bruised the better it grows.)

"She accordingly received three drops of *Bellis Perennis* φ, and

I left her with the remark, 'I think you will find that will do your "belly" good!'

"Unable to visit again for a week. When I had to go into the woman's neighbourhood to take a Confirmation class, called, found the woman washing clothes in back kitchen.

" 'Well, how are you, Mrs. F.?'

" 'Quite well, thank you, sir!'

" '*Quite well*? ! ! How's that?'

" 'Well, sir, three days after you gave me that last dose, I had a great bearing down as if I was going to have a baby and THAT thing all came away, 4lb. of it, and I and my husband buried it in our garden!'

"*Reflection.* The two stone walls, having been knocked down by *Bac.* and *Thuja*, *Bellis* was able to get through and do its work.—Q.E.D.

"This happened fifteen years ago and the woman is still alive and flourishing."

Here again, as Hahnemann put it, the *name* of the disease was no concern of the prescriber, and the name of the medicine was no concern of the patient. But the former got the true picture of the invisible disorder of the vital force in his imagination, whether the academicals had given it the right name or not. And his knowledge of the powers of drugs to bring about a like disorder enabled him to counter the morbid vibrations in the order of their origin. The consumptive tendency the patient brought into the world with her. The vaccinal taint was super-imposed on that, and re-imposed still later. The traumatism came after the first vaccination and before the second.

In a complicated case of this kind the most urgent and active of the miasms or causes is generally the first to be tackled.

Then, in addition to the miasms, or chronic disease poisons, there is the highly important question of Causation. This may prove the leading indication and if recent, the only one. Accidents and shocks, physical mental and emotional, are highly important points to be considered in remedy selecting. The remedy which meets these may clear up the entire case, or it may clear away the traumatic element and leave the course open for remedies that are more directly indicated by the symptoms.

Let us take an example from *Arnica*. One day I accidentally ran a piece of wire into my thumb, resulting in very acute pain, as was natural. I had a small vial of *Arnica* ϕ at hand, and removing the cork, placed the injured point over the mouth of the vial and inverted the bottle so that the tincture came into immediate contact with it. The pain vanished, seeming to travel up the arm and away, and there was an end to the trouble.

In a case of traumatism it is very important to get the remedy in action without delay. I have known *Arnica* given *instantly* in the case of falls when nothing was broken or dislocated, remove all trouble almost as completely as in the case of the punctured wound.

5. THE VALUE OF THE NAMES OF DISEASES.

In regard to the question of "Names of Diseases," let me say this by way of qualifying some previous remarks. The fixing of the correct nosological label on each case is both important and useful when it can be done. If it were not so, books like *The Prescriber* would be unnecessary. But, when this is not possible, Hahnemann's method enables the homœopath to steer a safe course through the uncharted sea, whilst the allopath is left completely befogged.

I have been speaking so far of cases of disease which are running a more or less chronic course. In acute cases, case-taking is a somewhat different matter. That is to say the physician must take his points and digest them rapidly, and here the value of the nosological label comes in. The correct name of the disorder goes a long way towards pointing out the corresponding remedy. At any rate it reduces the selection to a group from among which the simile or the simillimum is most likely to be found.

In the case of epidemics there will generally be found one or two remedies which cover the bulk of the cases, and when these are found much of the wear and tear of remedy selection will be saved by the correct nosological name. In other cases, when the "totality" is obtained there will generally stand out certain symptoms which have got to be matched if the simile is to be obtained. Because it is not every sensation of a patient which can be dignified with the name of "symptom" from the prescribing point of view. Generalities are of very little use. Particulars are necessary, and every pain complained of must submit to cross-examination. "Where?" "When?" and "How?" are questions to be answered. The exact *locality* of a pain or sensation is the first point to note. The *time* of its occurrence is the next. Then come the conditions under which it either appears, or grows worse or better. And, in addition, the pains or sensations which occur concomitantly with it. When you have got these particulars about a sensation or pain, you have a real symptom that has character and distinction about it, which makes it possible to match with something equally distinctive in the repertory and materia medica.

This piece of advice let me give you: Never make a prescription without noting down something to indicate *why* you gave that particular remedy. Then, when you see the patient next, you will have something to tell you whether your shot has gone home, or whether you have scored a miss. The mere report of a general expression of "better" or "no better" is not sufficient for this. Generalities are all very well for the allopath, but the homœopath is the servant of Nature, and truth to minute particulars is exacted of all her servants.

A final bit of practical advice is this. In searching the Materia Medica for a remedy in a case it frequently happens that we come across an indication for a remedy suitable for another case we have under treatment. When this happens, at once put down the name of the remedy on the record of the second case and it will be ready when the patient next appears. If it is not entered at the time of finding the chances are that it will be forgotten when it is wanted. The study of the Materia Medica is thus often doubly and even trebly fruitful.

Part III.—PLAN OF *THE PRESCRIBER*, AND HOW TO USE IT.

1. The Plan.

The plan of the work is simple. The names of the diseases are given in alphabetical order: and where a disease has more than one, each name is given with a reference to the one under which the treatment is described. This will generally be found to be the name by which it is most commonly known. Under each heading the names of the medicine or medicines most useful in the particular disease are given. When more medicines than one are named, there will be found prefixed to each the symptoms which would lead the prescriber to choose that in preference to the rest. Where no such differentiating symptoms can be given, the medicines are named in the order of their general applicability, and numbered; it is intended that the prescriber shall use them in that order, if there are no other symptoms in the case pointing to one more than the other.

Where a number of symptoms are given as belonging to one medicine, these will be found separated either by commas or semicolons. All those only separated by commas belong to a single group, and these must all be present in order to indicate the medicine. For example; under **Sciatica** will be found, "Pains made worse by sitting, relieved somewhat by walking, entirely by lying down, *Am. mur.:*" this means that *Ammonium muriaticum* is indicated when the pain of sciatica is marked by all these characters. If in any case the pain were noted as being "relieved somewhat by walking," without the other two, the medicine would probably not be appropriate. Again, under the same heading we have: "Purely neuralgic; accompanying paralysis; in old and debilitated subjects, *Ars.:*" this means that *Arsenic* is likely to benefit all cases that are of a purely neuralgic kind, as opposed to inflammatory or rheumatic; also sciatica in patients suffering from paralysis, also sciatica in old and debilitated patients. Each characteristic is sufficient in itself to indicate the medicine, and this the semicolons are intended to show; should two of the characteristics, or all three, be found in the same patient, the medicine would be still more strongly indicated. But it must be understood that all the medicines given under any heading have a distinct specific relation to the part or the affection under consideration; and whilst I have sought to give the distinguishing traits of each drug, that the best medicine may be chosen first, still all the medicines are more or less homœopathic, and if one fails, the one which seems next in appropriateness should be tried. But it must always be borne in mind that the whole of the symptoms of any patient must be taken into consideration, and not the most urgent only. The drug which corresponds best to the totality of a patient's symptoms will be the most certain to cure.

Under certain headings, such as **Tongue, Taste, Smell,** etc., I have given some characteristic conditions, which, however, do not in themselves constitute disease. They occur as symptoms in various diseases, and as the result of the action of certain drugs, and are often useful in determining the choice of a medicine, if that medicine is in relation to the case as a whole. For example, if a prescriber is in doubt which of two medicines to give in a case of dyspepsia, a reference to the heading **Tongue** may show which of these medicines is capable of producing a condition of tongue most like that present and determine the choice.

2. Rules for Prescribing.

Having found the medicine which corresponds to the case, there remains the questions of attenuation, dose, and frequency of repetition. In these matters dogmatism is out of place, and every man's experience is his best guide. But some guidance is needed before experience is available, and this I have tried to give. In the matter of attenuation, my own experience leads me to believe that all attenuations, from the mother-tincture upwards, are curative, provided the choice of the medicine is correct. When the similarity is very close between drug symptoms and patient's symptoms, the attenuation cannot be too high to cure, and the higher it is the more permanent the cure is likely to be. But the question of attenuation is secondary to that of the selection of the drug.

mother tincture

It is taken for granted that the reader possesses at least an elementary acquaintance with homœopathic pharmacy. It will be sufficient to state here that the sign ϕ following the name of a medicine stands for the strongest preparation of the drug (the sign θ is also used in the same sense by some writers) *dilution* and the numbers 1, 2, 3, etc., or 1x, 2x, 3x, etc., for the different attenuations. The figures 1, 2, 3, etc., refer to the centesimal *100 th* attenuations; the proportion being in "1," one part of the strongest preparation of the substance to 99 of the attenuating medium, and in "2," one part of "1" to 99 parts of the attenuating medium, and so on. The figures 1x, 2x, etc., refer to the decimal scale of attenuation; "1x" meaning one part of the strongest preparation to 9 parts of the attenuating medium, 2x one part of 1x to 9 parts of the attenuating medium, and so on.

1. *The Attenuation.*—After the name of each medicine there will be found the number of the attenuation recommended. When several attenuations are believed to be equally efficacious, the numbers of the lowest and the highest are given, and a bar is placed between them. For example, "*Acon.* 1—3" would mean *Acon.* 1, 3x, 2, or 3, and the prescriber may select any one of those as he thinks fit. When the choice lies between two only, the two numbers are joined by an "or": as "*Cham.* 1 or 6." When no sign or figure follows the name of a medicine the pure substance is meant: e.g., "*Kali i.* gr. ii." means two grains of the iodide of potassium itself.

2. *The Dose.*—In all cases where no mention of dose is made, one drop of the tincture, or one pilule or tablet is intended. The choice between tinctures and pilules is one of convenience chiefly. When tinctures are preferred, one or two drops to a tea-spoonful or a dessert-spoonful of water is the proper dose, or,

if given in powder, one or two drops to a sufficient quantity of sugar of milk. Distilled water, or water that has been boiled, is preferable to tap-water. When triturations are intended, this is always indicated by the number of grains for a dose following the number of the attenuation. For example, "*Silic.* 3, gr. iii." means three grains of the third trituration of *Silica*. Triturations may be given dry on the tongue, or suspended in water, as preferred by the patient.

3. *The Repetition of the Dose.*—For the sake of simplicity and uniformity, the times of the repetition of the dose are given in terms of hours and minutes. After the name of a medicine with its attenuation, "1h." means that the medicine is to be given every hour; "2h." every two hours; "6h." every six hours, or four times a day; "8h." every eight hours, or three times a day; "10m." every ten minutes.

In acute cases HAHNEMANN directs that the medicine should be given at short intervals, in chronic cases at longer. The rule laid down was to give one dose in a chronic case, and wait until its effects were exhausted. This may be done in some cases; in others it is well to repeat the dose at short intervals until a decided effect is produced, and then wait until the action is exhausted before again repeating it. If the same symptoms return the same remedy must be repeated; if they are changed, a different remedy must be sought.

In the latest edition of the *Organon*, the sixth, Hahnemann taught that the cure of chronic cases could be expedited by repetition of the remedy, but before each dose the bottle containing the mixture should receive ten forcible succussions. In this way the potency is raised with each dose, and the remedy can be repeated without fear of troublesome aggravations. The practice of prescribing medicine mixed already by the chemist is thus preferable to that of ordering quantities of the tincture to be mixed at home.

The practice of giving a single dose and allowing time for it to evolve its action is an excellent one when it is possible to carry it out and observe the effects. Dr. R. T. Cooper treated many cases of chronic disease with great effect by administering unit doses of ϕ tinctures, allowing them to act for two or three weeks without repetition. Dr. Cooper directed that the dose should be taken on an empty stomach—at least two hours after a meal, no food to be taken for at least one hour after the dose.

4. *The Time of Day.*—The best time for giving medicine (when the repetition of the dose is not too frequent to allow of choice) is from an hour to half-an-hour before food. In ordering a medicine every six hours (four times a day) the first dose may be given on rising, the second an hour before lunch, the third an hour before dinner, and the last at bedtime. An exception must be made in the case of the lower attenuations of *Arsenic* and *Iron*. These should be given immediately after food.

5. *Alternation.*—Remedies may sometimes be alternated with advantage, but this should not be adopted as a routine method. If two medicines seem almost equally indicated it is best to decide upon one of them, and give that. When the prescriber has seen whether it answers his expectations or not, he will be able to decide on the propriety of giving the other. To give both at the same time destroys the value of the observation, and tends to weaken the prescriber's powers of diagnosing the remedy.

6. *Sleep.*—Except in dangerous acute cases patients should not be awakened from sleep to receive their medicine. When it is necessary to give the dose during sleep, it is often possible to do it without arousing the patient.

3. EXAMPLES OF PRESCRIPTIONS.

1. *Acon.* 3, 4h. This may be ordered from a homœopathic chemist in this way:—

℞ Acon. 3, gtt. lxii.
Aquæ puræ ℥vi.
Misce. Signetur, ʒii., quartis horis.

(Take of *Acon.* 3, seventy-two drops. Of pure water six ounces. Mix. Direct:—A dessertspoonful every four hours.)
or if ordered in the tincture form:—

℞ *Tinct. Acon.* 3, ʒii.
Signetur, gtt. iii. ex aqua ʒii., quartis horis.

(Take of *Acon.* 3 two drachms. Direct.:—Three drops in a dessertspoonful every four hours.)

If a mixture is desired free from alcohol it may be ordered thus:—

℞ *Acon.* 3 (or 30), glob. x.
Aquæ puræ ℥vi. Solve.
Signetur: ʒii., quartis horis.

(Take of *Acon.* 3 (or 30) ten globules, of pure water six ounces. Dissolve. Direct.:—A dessertspoonful every four hours.)

If it is proposed to give the dose in powder form it may be ordered in this way: Take of Tincture of Aconite three drops, of Sugar of Milk a sufficient quantity. Make a powder; send of such twenty-four (or whatever number is desired.) One powder on the tongue every four hours.

If pilules (or tablets or discs) are intended to be given, the prescription would be as follows:—

Take of pilules (or tablets or discs) of Aconite 3, two drachms. One pilule (or tablet or disc) to be taken every four hours.

2. *Silic*. 3x, gr. iv. 6h.

This may be expanded as follows:—

Take of trituration of Silica 3x four grains; make a powder; send of such twenty-four. One powder to be taken four times a day. Or—

Take a trituration of Silica 3x two drachms, or a quarter of an ounce. As much as would lie on a six-penny piece to be taken four times a day. (Small horn scoops are sold by the chemists made to hold one, two, or three grains each. In prescribing triturations it is often convenient to order one of these, and direct, "a scoopful to be taken," etc.). But it is more practical to order of the chemist as many powders as are likely to be required.

Bacill. 200, gl. iv. once a week.

This may be ordered as follows:—

Take of *Bacillinum* 200 four globules; of Sugar of Milk two grains. Make a powder. Send as many as required. One to be taken dry on the tongue once a week. Plain powders of Sach. Lact. may be ordered in the interval if the patient cannot be made to understand the prolonged action of single doses. Or if other medicines are called for by special symptoms, they may be given between the doses without interfering with the constitutional action of the remedy.

In giving remedies for chronic conditions it is a good plan to prescribe the doses at bed-time or on rising and at bed-time. The patient has then no need to be thinking of getting the doses in during the day. In giving doses at intervals of several days it is convenient to prescribe a series of numbered powders, directing them to be taken at bedtime or at bedtime and on rising as the case may be. I find it useful to make the prescription in this way—

$$\text{R } \textit{Thuja } \frac{30}{1,\ 8,\ 15,\ 22} \text{ gl. vi.}$$

mitte xxiv., Sig. One to be taken at bedtime, in numerical order. This means that of the 24 powders, numbers 1, 8, 15 and 22 have each six globules of the remedy. The rest of the powders are not *directly* medicated, but that does not mean that they are not medicated at all. According to my observation they are medicated by contact in varying degrees and their variation is rather helpful than otherwise in developing the curative action of the remedy.

Part IV.—LIST OF REMEDIES

Abbreviations and Signs.

Abbreviations		*Names of Medicines*
Abies n.	.	Abies nigra.
Absinth.	.	Absinthium.
Acet. ac.	.	Aceticum acidum glaciale.
Aco. or Acon.	.	Aconitum napellus.
Act. rac.	.	Actæa racemosa.
Adrenalin.	.	Extract of supra-renal capsules.
Æsc. hip.	.	Æsculus hippocastanum.
Æthiops ant.	.	Æthiops antimonialis.
Æth. c.	.	Æthusa cynapium.
Agar.	.	Agaricus muscarius.
Agn. cast.	.	Agnus castus.
Ail.	.	Ailanthus.
All. c.	.	Allium cepa.
All. sat.	.	Allium sativum.
Aln	.	Alnus
Aloe	.	Aloe.
Alm.	.	Alumen.
Alumia	.	Alumina.
Amb.	.	Ambra.
Amm. bro.	.	Ammonium bromidum.
Amm. c.	.	Ammonium carbonicum.
Amm. mur.	.	Ammonium muriaticum.
Amyl nit.	.	Amyl nitrosum.
Anac.	.	Anacardium orientale.
Angust.	.	Angustura vera.
Anhal.	.	Anhalonium lewinii.

Abbreviations			*Names of Medicines*
Anthrac.	.	.	Anthracinum.
Ant. c.	.	.	Antimonium crudum.
Ant. tar.	.	.	Antimonium tartaricum.
Apis	.	.	Apis mellifica.
Apocy.	.	.	Apocynum cannabinum.
Apom.	.	.	Apomorphia.
Aral. rac.	.	.	Aralia racemosa.
Arb. a.	.	.	Arbutus andrachne.
Arct. l.	.	.	Arctium lappa.
Arg. m.	.	.	Argentum metallicum.
Arg. mur.	.	.	Argentum muriaticum.
Arg. n.	.	.	Argentum nitricum.
Arn.	.	.	Arnica montana.
Ars.	.	.	Arsenicum album.
Ars. i.	.	.	Arsenicum iodatum.
Ars. sul. rub.	.	.	Arsenicum sulphuratum rubrum.
Artem.	.	.	Artemisia.
Arum t.	.	.	Arum triphyllum.
Asa.	.	.	Asafœtida.
Ascl.	.	.	Asclepias tuberosa.
Astacus	.	.	Astacus fluviatilis.
Ast. r.	.	.	Asterias rubens.
Atr..	.	.	Atropinum.
Atrop. s.	.	.	Atropinum sulphuratum.
Aur.	.	.	Aurum metallicum.
Aur. bro.	.	.	Aurum bromatum.
Aur. iod.	.	.	Aurum iodatum.
Aur. mur.	.	.	Aurum muriaticum.
Aur. m. n.	.	.	Aurum muriaticum natronatum.
Aviare	.	.	Nosode of fowl-phthisis.

Abbreviations		*Names of Medicines*
Avena s. .	.	. Avena sativa.
Bacill. .	.	. Bacillinum.
Bac. test. .	.	. Bacillinum testium.
Bad. .	.	. Badiaga.
Balsam of Peru .		. Balsamum Peruvanium.
Bap. .	.	. Baptisia.
Baryt. c. .	.	. Baryta carbonica.
Baryt. iod. .	.	. Baryta iodata.
Bell. .	.	. Belladonna.
Bellis. .	.	. Bellis perennis.
Benz. ac. .	.	. Benzoicum acidum.
Benzoin .	.	. Benzoin odoriferum.
Berb. .	.	. Berberis vulgaris.
Berb. aq. .	.	. Berberis aquifolium.
Bism. .	.	. Bismuthum.
Blatt. .	.	. Blatta orientalis.
Borac. ac..	.	. Boracicum acidum.
Bor.	.	. Borax.
Bov.	.	. Bovista.
Brom.	.	. Bromium.
Bry.	.	. Bryonia alba.
Bufo	.	. Bufo rana.
Bufo sah..	.	. Bufo sahytiensis.
Cact.	.	. Cactus grandiflorus.
Cadm. s. .	.	. Cadmium sulphuratum.
Calad.	.	. Caladium.
Calc. ac. .	.	. Calcarea acetica.
Calc. ars..	.	. Calcarea arsenicosa.

Abbreviations			*Names of Medicines*
Calc. c.	.	.	Calcarea carbonica.
Calc. caus.	.	.	Calcarea caustica.
Calc. chlor.	.	.	Calcarea chlorata.
Calc. fluor.	.	.	Calcarea fluorata.
Calc. iod.	.	.	Calcarea iodata.
Calc. lact.	.	.	Calcarea lactica.
Calc. m.	.	.	Calcarea muriatica.
Calc. ov. t.	.	.	Calcarea ovi testæ.
Calc. phos.	.	.	Calcarea phosphorica.
Calc. pic.	.	.	Calcarea picrata.
Calc. s.	.	.	Calcarea sulphurica.
Calend.	.	.	Calendula.
Calot. g.	.	.	Calotropis gigantia.
Camph.	.	.	Camphora.
Cann. Ind.	.	.	Cannabis Indica.
Cann. sat.	.	.	Cannabis sativa.
Canth.	.	.	Cantharis.
Caps.	.	.	Capsicum.
Carb. a.	.	.	Carbo animalis.
Carb. v.	.	.	Carbo vegetabilis.
Carb. ac.	.	.	Carbolicum acidum.
Carbon tetrachloride	.		Carbon tetrachloride.
Carb. sul.	.	.	Carboneum sulphuratum.
Carcin.	.	.	Carcinosinum.
Carcin. adeno stom.	.		Carcinoma adeno (stomach).
Card. m.	.	.	Carduus marianus.
Carl.	.	.	Carlsbad.
Carron oil	.		Carron oil.
Caul.	.	.	Caulophyllum.
Caust.	.	.	Causticum.

Abbreviations			*Names of Medicines*
Cean.	.	.	Ceanothus.
Cedr.	.	.	Cedron.
Cham.	.	.	Chamomilla.
Chel.	.	.	Chelidonium majus.
Chen. anth.	.	.	Chenopodium anthelminticum.
Chim.	.	.	Chimaphila umbellata.
China.	.	.	Cinchona officinalis.
Chin. ars..	.	.	Chininum arsenicosum.
Chin. sul..	.	.	Chininum sulphuricum (Quinæ sulphas).
Chloral.	.	.	Chloralum hydratum.
Cholest.	.	.	Cholesterinum.
Cr. k. s.	.	.	Chromium kali sulphuratum.
Cic. v.	.	.	Cicuta virosa.
Cimicif. r.	.	.	Cimicifuga racemosa (*see* Act. rac.).
Cina	.	.	Cina.
Cinchona rub.	.	.	Cinchona rubra.
Cinerar. marit.	.	.	Cineraria maritima.
Cinnab.	.	.	Cinnabaris.
Cistus.	.	.	Cistus Canadensis.
Cit. ac.	.	.	Citricum acidum.
Clem.	.	.	Clematis erecta.
Coca	.	.	Erythroxylon coca.
Cocc.	.	.	Cocculus Indicus.
Coc. cact..	.	.	Coccus cacti.
Cod.	.	.	Codeinum.
Coff.	.	.	Coffea cruda.
Colch.	.	.	Colchicum.
Collin.	.	.	Collinsonia.
Coloc.	.	.	Colocynthis.
Como.	.	.	Comocladia.

Abbreviations			*Names of Medicines*
Con.	.	.	Conium.
Conch.	.	.	Conchiolinum.
Cop.	.	.	Copaiba.
Coquel.	.	.	Coqueluchin.
Coral. r.	.	.	Corallium rubrum.
Cratæg.	.	.	Cratægus oxyacantha.
Croc.	.	.	Crocus sativus.
Crotal. h. .	.	.	Crotalus horridus.
Crot. t.	.	.	Croton tiglium.
Cundur.	.	.	Cundurango.
Cupr.	.	.	Cuprum metallicum.
Cupr. acet.	.	.	Cuprum aceticum.
Cupr. ars.	.	.	Cuprum arsenicosum.
Cycl.	.	.	Cyclamen.
Dign.	.	.	Digitalinum.
Dig.	.	.	Digitalis.
Dinitroben.	.	.	Dinitrobenzolum.
Diosc.	.	.	Dioscorea villosa.
Diphth.	.	.	Diphtherinum.
Dolichos	.	.	Dolichos pruriens.
Dros.	.	.	Drosera rotundifolia.
Dulc.	.	.	Solanum dulcamara.
Durum	.	.	Durum.
Ecchin.	.	.	Ecchinacea angustifolia.
Elap.	.	.	Elaps corallinus.
Epihyst.	.	.	Epihysterinum.
Epithel.	.	.	Epitheliominum.
Eucal.	.	.	Eucalyptus globulus.

Abbreviations			*Names of Medicines*
Eup. perf.	.	.	Eupatorium perfoliatum.
Eup. purp.	.	.	Eupatorium purpureum.
Euphor. cor.	.	.	Euphorbia corallata.
Euphorb. het.	.	.	Euphorbia heterodoxa.
Euphorb.	.	.	Euphorbium.
Euph.	.	.	Euphrasia.
Ferr.	.	.	Ferrum.
Ferr. ac.	.	.	Ferrum aceticum.
Ferr. magn.	.	.	Ferrum magneticum.
Ferr. mur.	.	.	Ferrum muriaticum.
Ferr. iod.	.	.	Ferrum iodatum.
Ferr. phos.	.	.	Ferrum phosphoricum.
Ferr. picr.	.	.	Ferrum picricum.
Ferr. redact.	.	.	Ferrum redactum.
Ferr. pyrophos.	.	.	Ferrum pyrophosphoricum.
Ficus r.	.	.	Ficus religiosa.
Fil. mas.	.	.	Filix mas.
Fluor. ac.	.	.	Fluoricum acidum.
Frag. vesc.	.	.	Fragaria vesca.
Frax. Am.	.	.	Fraxinus Americanus.
Gal. ap.	.	.	Galium aperine.
Gamb.	.	.	Gambogia.
Gels.	.	.	Gelsemium.
Gent. l.	.	.	Gentiana lutea.
Ginseng	.	.	Ginseng.
Glon.	.	.	Glonoinum.
Gnaph.	.	.	Gnaphalium.
Granat.	.	.	Punica Granatum.

Abbreviations			*Names of Medicines*
Graph.	.	.	Graphites.
Grat.	.	.	Gratiola.
Grind.	.	.	Grindelia squarrosa.
Guaco	.	.	Guaco.
Guaiac.	.	.	Guaiacum.
Gunp.	.	.	Gunpowder.
Gymno.	.	.	Gymnocladus.
Ham.	.	.	Hamamelis.
Hecl.	.	.	Hecla.
Hed. hel.	.	.	Hedera helix.
Hell. n.	.	.	Helleborus niger.
Helod.	.	.	Heloderma.
Helon. d.	.	.	Helonius dioica.
Hep.	.	.	Hepar sulphuris.
Hippoz.	.	.	Hippozæninum.
Hydras.	.	.	Hydrastis cenadensis.
Hydrastia mur.	.	.	Hydrastia muriatica.
Hydrastinin. mur.		.	Hydrastininum muriaticum.
Hydro.	.	.	Hydrocotyle asiatica.
Hydrocy. ac.	.	.	Hydrocyanicum acidum.
Hydrob.	.	.	Hydrophobinum.
Hyo.	.	.	Hyoscyamus niger.
Hyper.	.	.	Hypericum perfoliatum.
Iberis	.	.	Iberis.
Ign.	.	.	Ignatia.
Ind.	.	.	Indigo.
Infl.	.	.	Influenzinum.
Iod.	.	.	Iodum.

Abbreviations			*Names of Medicines*
Iodof.	.	.	Iodoformum.
Ipec.	.	.	Ipecacuanha.
Iris t.	.	.	Iris tenax.
Iris v.	.	.	Iris versicolor.
Jab..	.	.	Jaborandi.
Jac. c.	.	.	Jacaranda caroba.
Jatr.	.	.	Jatropha curcas.
Jug. c.	.	.	Juglans cinerea.
Jug. r.	.	.	Juglans regia.
Kali bich.	.	.	Kali bichromicum.
Kali brom.	.	.	Kali bromatum.
Kali c.	.	.	Kali carbonicum.
Kali chlor.	.	.	Kali chloricum.
Kali cy.	.	.	Kali cyanatum.
Kali i.	.	.	Kali iodatum.
Kali m.	.	.	Kali muriaticum.
Kali n.	.	.	Kali nitricum or Nitrum.
Kalm.	.	.	Kalmia latifolia.
Kreas.	.	.	Kreasotum.
Lac can.	.	.	Lac caninum.
Lach.	.	.	Lachesis.
Lact. v.	.	.	Lactuca virosa.
Lathyrus s.	.	.	Lathyrus sativus.
Lavender oil	.		Oil of lavender.
Led.	.	.	Ledum palustre.
Lept.	.	.	Leptandra.
Liat.	.	.	Liatris spicata.

Abbreviations			*Names of Medicines*
Lil. t.	.	.	Lilium tigrinum.
Lith. c.	.	.	Lithium carbonicum.
Lobel.	.	.	Lobelia inflata.
Luet.	.	.	Lueticum (Syphilinum).
Lyc.	.	.	Lycopodium clavatum.
Lyss.	.	.	Lyssin (Hydrophobinum).
Macrotin..	.	.	Macrotinum.
Magnes aus.	.	.	Magnes australis (South Pole of Magnet).
Mag. c.	.	.	Magnesia carbonica.
Mag. m.	.	.	Magnesia muriatica.
Mag. phos.	.	.	Magnesia phosphorica.
Maland.	.	.	Malandrinum.
Mang.	.	.	Manganum.
Medo.	.	.	Medorrhinum.
Meli.	.	.	Melilotus alba.
Menin.	.	.	Meningococcinum.
Menth. pip.	.	.	Mentha piperita.
Merc. bin.	.	.	Mercurius biniodatus.
Merc. c.	.	.	Mercurius corrosivus.
Merc. cy.	.	.	Mercurius cyanatus.
Merc. d.	.	.	Mercurius dulcis.
Merc. i. fl.	.	.	Mercurius iodatus flavus.
Merc. s.	.	.	Mercurius solubilis Hahnemanni.
Merc. sul. r.	.	.	Mercurius sulphuratus ruber (*see* Cinnabaris).
Merc. v.	.	.	Mercurius vivus.
Mez.	.	.	Daphne mezereum.
Mill.	.	.	Millefolium.
Morbil.	.	.	Morbillinum.

Abbreviations		*Names of Medicines*
Morgan (Bach) .	.	Morgan Bach.
Morph. .	.	Morphia.
Mosch. .	.	Moschus.
Mur. ac. .	.	Muriaticum acidum.
Mur. p. .	.	Murex purpurea.
Naja .	.	Naja tripudians.
Naphthal. .	.	Naphthalinum.
Nat. ars. .	.	Natrum arsenicicum.
Nat. cacod. .	.	Natrum cacodilicum.
Nat. c. .	.	Natrum carbonicum.
Nat. hypochl. .	.	Natrum hypochlorosum (Liquor sodæ chlorinatæ).
Nat. m. .	.	Natrum muriaticum.
Nat. sal. .	.	Natrum salicylicum.
Nat. sel. .	.	Natrum selenicum.
Nat. phos. .	.	Natrum phosphoricum.
Nat. s. .	.	Natrum sulphuricum.
Nit. ac. .	.	Nitricum acidum.
Nit. mur. ac. .	.	Nitro-muriaticum acidum.
Nit. s. d. .	.	Nitri spiritus dulcis.
Nitrum .	.	Nitrum (*see* Kali nit.).
Nuph. .	.	Nuphar lutea.
Nux j. .	.	Nux juglans (*see* Juglans Regia).
Nux m. .	.	Nux moschata.
Nux v. .	.	Nux vomica.
Oc. can. .	.	Ocimum canum.
Œnanth. .	.	Œnanthe crocata.
Olean. .	.	Oleander.

Abbreviations			*Names of Medicines*
Ol. an.	.	.	Oleum animale.
Ol. jec. as.	.	.	Oleum jecoris aselli.
Op. .	.	.	Opium.
Orig.	.	.	Origanum.
Ornith. u.	.	.	Ornithogalum umbellatum.
Osm.	.	.	Osmium.
Oxal. ac. .	.	.	Oxalicum acidum.
Pæon.	.	.	Pæonia.
Pall.	.	.	Palladium.
Pareir. b. .	.	.	Pareira brava.
Parot.	.	.	Parotidinum.
Pest.	.	.	Pestinum (or Plaguinum).
Petr.	.	.	Petroleum.
Petrosel.	.	.	Petroselinum.
Phaseol.	.	.	Phaseolus nana.
Phell.	.	.	Phellandrium.
Phos.	.	.	Phosphorus.
Phos. ac. .	.	.	Phosphoricum acidum.
Physos.	.	.	Physostigma.
Phyt.	.	.	Phytolacca.
Pic. ac.	.	.	Picricum acidum.
Pit. w. g. .	.	.	Pituitary whole gland.
Plant.	.	.	Plantago major.
Plat.	.	.	Platina.
Plumb.	.	.	Plumbum.
Plumb. ac.	.	.	Plumbum aceticum.
Pod.	.	.	Podophyllum peltatum.
Pru. s.	.	.	Prunus spinosa.
Psor.	.	.	Psorinum.

Abbreviations			*Names of Medicines*
Pumpkin seed	.	.	Pumpkin seed (Cucurbita pepo).
Puls.	.	.	Pulsatilla nigricans.
Pyr.	.	.	Pyrogen (also called Sepsin).
Querc.	.	.	Quercus.
Quinæ arsenias.	.	.	*See* Chinin ars.
Quinæ sulphas.	.	.	*See* Chinin. sulph.
Rad. b.	.	.	Radium bromidum.
Ran. b.	.	.	Ranunculus bulbosus.
Ran. s.	.	.	Ranunculus sceleratus.
Ratan.	.	.	Ratanhia.
Rhe.	.	.	Rheum.
Rho.	.	.	Rhododendron.
Rhus t.	.	.	Rhus toxicodendron.
Rhus v.	.	.	Rhus venenata.
Rob.	.	.	Robinia.
Rum. c.	.	.	Rumex crispus.
Rut.	.	.	Ruta.
Saba.	.	.	Sabadilla.
Sabal. serr.	.	.	Sabal serrulata (Saw Palmetto).
Sabin.	.	.	Sabina.
Samb.	.	.	Sambucus nigra.
Sang.	.	.	Sanguinaria Canadensis.
Sanguis.	.	.	Sanguisuga officinalis.
Sant.	.	.	Santonine.
Sarsa.	.	.	Sarsaparilla.
Scarlat.	.	.	Scarlatininum.
Scil.	.	.	Scilla maritima.

Abbreviations			*Names of Medicines*
Scill. acet.	.	.	Acetum scillæ.
Scirrh.	.	.	Scirrhinum.
Sec.	.	.	Secale cornutum.
Sel. .	.	.	Selenium.
Senec.	.	.	Senecio aureus.
Seneg.	.	.	Senega.
Senna	.	.	Senna.
Sep.	.	.	Sepia.
Septicæmin.	.	.	Septicæminum.
Sil. .	.	.	Silica.
Solan. acet.	.	.	Solania acetica.
Sol. t. œ. .	.	.	Solanum tuberosum œgrotans.
Solidago v. a.	.	.	Solidago virgo aurea.
Spig.	.	.	Spigelia.
Spon.	.	.	Spongia.
Stan.	.	.	Stannum.
Staph.	.	.	Delphinium staphisagria.
Staphylo. .	.	.	Staphylococcinum.
Stell. med.	.	.	Stellaria media.
Stict.	.	.	Sticta pulmonaria.
Still.	.	.	Stillingia sylvatica.
Stram.	.	.	Stramonium.
Stroph.	.	.	Strophanthus hispidus
Strych.	.	.	Strychnia.
Strych. liq.	.	.	Liquor strychniæ.
Strych. nit.	.	.	Strychninum nitricum.
Sul. ac.	.	.	Sulphuricum acidum.
Sulphuros. ac.	.	.	Sulphurosum acidum.
Sul. .	.	.	Sulphur.
Symp.	.	.	Symphytum.

Abbreviations			*Names of Medicines.*
Syz.	.	.	Syzygium.
Tab.	.	.	Tabacum.
Tamus.	.	.	Tamus.
Tara.	.	.	Taraxacum.
Tarent.	.	.	Tarentula Hispanica.
Tarent. Cub.	.	.	Tarentula Cubensis.
Tell.	.	.	Tellurium.
Tereb.	.	.	Terebinthina.
Teucr.	.	.	Teucrium marum verum.
Thlasp. b. p.	.	.	Thlaspi bursa pastoris.
Thio.	.	.	Thiosinaminum.
Thyr.	.	.	Thyroidin (Extract of Thyroid glands).
Til..	.	.	Tilia Europœa.
Thuj.	.	.	Thuja Occidentalis.
Trombid..	.	.	Trombidium.
Tuberc. k.	.	.	Tuberculinum Kochii.
Typhoidin.	.	.	Typhoidinum.
Uran. n. .	.	.	Uranium nitricum.
Urt. ur.	.	.	Urtica urens.
Ustil.	.	.	Ustilago maydis.
Uva. u.	.	.	Uva ursi.
Vaccin.	.	.	Vaccininum.
Vacc. myrtil.	.	.	Vaccininum myrtillus.
Valer.	.	.	Valeriana.
Vanad.	.	.	Vanadium.
Variol.	.	.	Variolinum.
Verat.	.	.	Veratrum album.

Abbreviations				*Names of Medicines.*
Verat. v.	.	.	.	Veratrum viride.
Verb.	.	.	.	Verbascum thapsus.
Vetterin (ointment)		.		Vetterin.
Vib. op.	.	.	.	Viburnum opulus.
Vinc. m.	.	.	.	Vinca minor.
Viol.	.	.	.	Viola odorata.
Viol. t.	.	.	.	Viola tricolor.
Xanth.	.	.	.	Xanthoxylum.
Zinc. met.		.	.	Zincum metallicum.
Zinc. m.	.	.	.	Zincum muriaticum.
Zinc. phos.		.	.	Zincum phosphoricum.
Zinc. pic.	.		.	Zincum picricum.
Zinc. s.	.	.	.	Zincum sulphuricum.
Zinc. valer.		.	.	Zincum valerianicum.

N.B. This LIST OF REMEDIES contains all the main remedies specified throughout *The Prescriber*. Occasional reference is made to little known and seldom used remedies, for which the reader should consult Dr Clarke's extensive *A Dictionary of Practical Materia Medica*.

Explanation of Signs Used.

m. = minute
h. = hour
r. = on rising
h.s.s. = at bed-time
gl. = globule
gtt. = drop
gr. = grain
ʒi. = one drachm, or one teaspoonful
ʒii. = two drachms, or one dessert-spoonful
ʒss. or ʒiv. = half an ounce, or one table-spoonful
Ʒi. = one ounce, or two table-spoonfuls
Oi. = one pint
< = worse, or aggravation
> = better, or amelioration

THE PRESCRIBER

Abdomen, DISTENDED.—In fat scrofulous children, *Calc. c.* 6, 6h. Intercurrently, *Bacil.* 30, once a week. In thin, rickety children, *Silic.* 6, 6h. Intercurrently, *Bacil.* 30, once a week. When due to worms, *Cina* 3, 6h. If due to flatulence with or without constipation, *Lyc.* 6, 6h. If from flatulence, with great pain, the bowels being open or loose, *Diocor.* 12, 6h. Hysterical distension, (1) *Ign.* 12, 2h. (2) *Asaf.* 12, 2h. As if a living animal were there, *Thuj.* 12, 2h.

DROPSICAL. *See* **Ascites** and **Dropsy.**

Abortion. *See* **Miscarriage.**

Abscess, or Suppuration.

THREATENING.—Redness, pain and throbbing, without much swelling, *Bell.* 12, 1h. Much swelling with or without redness, burning, throbbing, stinging pain, *Apis* 3x, 1h. After *Bell.* or *Apis*, if either of these is insufficient to check the inflammatory action, *Merc. sol.* 6, 2h. Tissues bluish, intense burning pains, (1) *Tarent cub.* 6, 2h. (2) *Ars.* 3, 2h. Abscess near the rectum, (1) *Calc. s.* gr. vi. 3h. (2) *Silic.* 6, 3h. (Instead of poultices bathe with hot *Calendula* lotion every 2 or 3 hours.)

FORMED.—When matter has actually formed, to assist the process and bring it to a favourable termination, *Hepar s.* 6, 3h. When suppuration has taken place and is slow to evacuate, *Silic*. 6, 3h. Locally, fomentations with hot *Calendula* lotion (*Calend. φ* a teaspoonful to half a pint of hot water) two or three times a day. Pains of acute gathering can be relieved by applying compresses of lime water (*Liq. calci*. B. P.) and changing frequently. (I never allow poulticing, and I find the marks remaining after opening under this treatment are far less conspicuous than those which follow premature lancing.)

DISCHARGING.—When an abscess has been opened or has opened spontaneously, *Calc. s*. 6x, gr. v. 4h. If the discharge is thin and watery, *Silic*. 6, 4h.; if yellow, purulent discharge, "pus with a vent" *Calc. sulph* 6x or 6. 3 or 4 times daily, locally, a compress of *Calendula φ* (one teaspoonful to half a pint of water), to be kept applied, and changed frequently. As soon as the bulk of the discharge has come away *Calendula* ointment should be substituted for the wet dressing.

CHRONIC SUPPURATION.—(1) *Silic*. 6, 6h.; locally, *Calendula* lotion as above. (2) *Gunp*. 3x, gr. vi. 6h. With hectic fever; debility from great loss of fluids, *Chi*. 3, 2h. With great debility, low fever, red tongue, thirst, restlessness, anxiety, *Ars*. 12, 2h. Fistulous openings, *Ac. fluor*. 6, gtt. iii. 6h. Symptoms of blood-poisoning, (1) *Gunp*. 3x, gr. vi. 4h. (2) *Arn*. 3, 4h. (3) *Pyrogen* 30, 4h.

Accidents. *See* **Brain,** CONCUSSION OF; **Bruise, Sprain, Wounds.**

Acidity.—*Acid. Sulph*. 3, 4h. With gastralgia and eructations of wind, *Arg. nit*. 6, 4h. After food; everything taken (especially fat, oils, and sugar) "rises acid"; the kind of dyspepsia that precedes tubercle, *Calc. c*. 6, 4h. Regurgitation of food tasting acid, an hour after eating; sinking sensation at epigastrium, *Sulph.* 6, 4h. With distended feeling after the least food, constipation, thick urine with red deposit, *Lyc.* 6, 4h. Constant eructations and vomiting of intensely sour fluid, principally at night, *Robinia* 3, 4h. With much stomach flatulence, *Carbo v.* 6, 4h.

See also Dyspepsia.

Acne.—Simple and recent in young persons, *Carb. v.* 6, 6h.; if plethoric, *Bell.* 3, 4h.; if pale, *Puls.* 3, 4h. More chronic, (1) *Kali brom.* 3x—30, 4h. (2) *Rad. bro.* 30, once a week. (3) *Arct. l.* 3x, 4th. From cold drinks, *Bellis* 3x, 4h. [*Sulphur* 6, 8h. may be given intercurrently with any of the other medicines; and it is often useful to apply at the same time a lotion of *Sulph. φ* (a teaspoonful to the ounce) with a camel-hair brush to the spots.] Thuja 30. 3 doses in one day, then wait, is often a most useful remedy. Berberis Aquifolium φ mins 10 in a little water 3 times daily after meals. This may be given in conjunction with the homœopathically indicated remedy.

Acne Rosacea.—(1) *Carbo an.* 6, 6h. (2) Especially when connected with uterine derangement, *Hydrocotyle* 3x, 6h. From spirit-drinking, *Nux v.* 3, 4h. With much redness and active irritation, (1) *Rad. bro.* 30, once a week. (2) *Rhus t.* 3, 6h. With blueness and tendency to chilblains, *Agar.* 3, 4h. Severe and inveterate cases, (1) *Ars. iod.* 3x, gr. ii. night and morning, after food. (2) *Sulph. iod.* 3, gr. viii. night and morning.

See also Face.

Acromegaly.—(1) *Thyroidin*, one or two tablets of the crude preparation three times a day. (2) *Conch.* 3, gr. v. 8h. (3) *Hecl.* 5, gtt. v. 8h.

Actinomycosis.—(1) *Nit. ac.* 3x, gtt. v. 8h. (2) *Hippoz.* 5, gtt. v. 8h.

Addison's Disease.—(1) *Adrenalin* 2x—30, 4h. (2) *Nat. m.* 6, 4h. (3) If these fail to do good in three or four weeks, *Arg. n.* 3x, 4h. (4) *Silica* 30, 8h. I should also suggest *Bacil.* 30—200, gl. v. once a week.

Adenoids.—In pale, fat children, cold clammy feet, head perspiring at night, *Calc. c.* 30, 8h. In children with consumptive family history, *Bac.* 100, gl. v. once a week. Much clear mucous discharge, *Agraph. n.* 3x, 8h. Thin children, large, pale tonsils, *Calc. ph.* 3x, gr. iv.—30, 8h. Children who are always hungry, irritable skins, averse to be washed, *Sul.* 30, 8h. Psoric subjects, offensive catarrh, *Pso.* 30, 8h. Mentally weak, *Baryt. iod.* 3x—30, 8h. Dark-eyed, dark-haired children, *Iod.* 3x—30, 8h.

After-Pains. *See* **Labour.**

Agalactea. *See* **Lactation.**

Ague. *See* **Intermittent Fever.**

Ague-cake. *See* **Spleen.**

Alcohol Habit.—A single dose of *Sulph.* 30 or 200 every two or three weeks, in conjunction with any other treatment. To relieve the craving for alcohol in persons who wish to give up the habit, *Cinchona rubra* φ, gtt. xxx. in a wineglassful of water three times a day. If the *Cinchona* does not appear to have the desired affect, or if its effect should decrease, *Sulph.* 3, three times a day. Whirling vertigo, foul breath, gnawing at stomach pit, *Querc.* 1, gtt. x. 8h. Nervous collapse, sinking sensations and craving, *Avena* φ, gtt. v.—x. 8h. After these *Stroph.* φ, gtt. i.—v. 8h. When the craving comes on, it may sometimes be allayed by eating a few raisins. An orange eaten before breakfast lessens the craving.

Alcoholism.—ACUTE. *See* **Delirium Tremens.**

CHRONIC.—Total abstinence. Morning vomiting, tremulousness, *Nux. v.* 3, 4h. Irritability and nervous depression, (1) *Avena s.* φ, gtt. v. 8h. (2) *Zinc.* 6, 4h. Chronic vomiting, with white tongue, *Ant. tart.* 6, 4h. *See also* **Liver:** CIRRHOSIS. *Sulph.* 30 or 200. *see* above. Old drunkards, *Quercus* φ—3x, 4h.

Alopecia. *See* **Hair.**

Amaurosis.—Recent; sudden blindness from cold bathing in hot weather, *Aco.* 3, 2h. Sudden blindness, *Gels.* 3, 2h. With appearances of bright objects, *Bell.* 3, 4h. Night-blindness (or moon-blindness), *Bell.* 3, 4h. From abuse of alcohol or tobacco, (1) great general sensitiveness and irritability; sensitive to light; morning sickness, *Nux v.* 3, 2h.; (2) after *Nux;* sees different colours; letters look red when reading, *Phos.* 3, 2h.; (3) sees badly by candlelight; sight becomes dim when reading; photophobia, *Hep. s.* 6, 8h. From other causes, *Tabac.* 3, 4h. With conditions of nervous exhaustion and irritability, *Phos.* 3, 4h. With paralytic conditions, *Plumb. acet.* 6, 6h. *See* **Eyes:** SIGHT.

Amblyopia (Weak Sight: Commencing Amaurosis).—As a result of exhausting disease, *Chi.* 3, 4h. From sexual excess, *Ac. Phos.* 1x, 4h. From abuse of alcohol or tobacco, (1) *Nux v.* 3; (2) *Phos.* 3. *See under* **Amaurosis.** From over-use of the eyes, *Ruta grav.* 3, 4h. From over-use of the eyes, with coloured vision, *Sant.* 3x, 6h.

Amenorrhœa. *See* Menstruation.

Anæmia.—From exhausting diseases, discharges, or hæmorrhages, *Chi.* 3, 4h. Simple iron deficiency anæmias, there are many excellent iron preparations on the market these days. *Ferrum* 6. once daily for 1 week, followed by *Ferrum* 12 for 1 week followed by *Ferrum* 30 for 1 week will produce a rapid rise in hæmoglobin. (If iron does good at all, it does it rapidly, and it should be stopped as soon as the improvement ceases. If there is no improvement at first, it should never be continued.) With constipation; palpitation on lying down; earthly complexion, *Nat. mur.* 6, 6h. Constipation very obstinate, *Plumb. acet.* 3, gr. ii. 8h. With much sickness, inability to retain any food, *Petrol.* 3, 4h. Especially in splenic anæmias, *Rub. t. φ*, gtt. x. 8h. In patients who have been heavily dosed with tonics, *Puls.* 3x, gtt. v. 8h. Anæmia, resulting from accidental stoppage of the menses, *Puls.* 3, 4h. Anæmia with excessive menstrual loss, the period coming on before its normal time, *Calc. c.* 6, 4h. With marked indisposition to bodily or mental exertion, and great increase of urates and phosphates in the urine, *Picr. ac.* 3, gr. ii. 8h. In pale, flabby children, with tendency to enlarged tonsils, *Calc. phos.* 3, gr. v. 8h. Chlorosis (green sickness), with mental depression, irritability, debility, and increase of phosphates in urine, *Helonias φ—3*, 4h. Anæmia in infants, thin and puny, with tendency to rickets, *Silica* 6, 8h. Anæmia with vomiting, acute epigastric pain and tenderness, palpitation and fainting, *Arg. n.* 6, 1h.

Anæmia, Acute Pernicious. Vitamin B_{12} Wasting, thirst, anxiety, restlessness, cachectic conditions, (1) *Ars.* 3, 4h.;

(2) *Carcin.* 30—200 once a week. In goitrous subjects; nervous weakness; palpitation, chilly, *Thyr.* 3x, gr. v. 8h. Tuberculous subjects; rapid loss of energy, puffy about eyes, (1) *Phos.* 30, 8h. (2) *Bacil.* 30—200, once a week. Anæmia depending on gastric or intestinal ulcer, or other known cause, *see* **Stomach,** ULCERATION OF, etc.

Anasarca. *See* **Dropsy.**

Aneurism.—(Where possible, complete rest in the horizontal position should be enjoyed.) Failing specific indications, begin in general with *Baryt. c.* 3x, gr. v. 8h. If that fails, *Lycopod.* 6, 4h.; special indications being: constipation with flatulence and loaded urine. If both fail, *Kali iod.*, gr. i. or gr. x. 8h.; special indications—great emaciation, cachectic, or syphilitic subjects. Burning pressive pain or stitches in chest (right side), *Carb. an.* 30, 4h. When accompanied by symptoms of heart weakness, (1) *Cratæg. φ*, gtt. v. 8h.; (2) *Ars. i.* 3x, gr. ii. thrice daily, after food. *See under* **Heart.**

Anger, VIOLENT FITS OF.—*Nux v.* 3, 2h. Anger with violence alternating with fits of repentance, *Croc.* 3, 2h. Suppressed anger; or uncontrollable outbreaks, *Staphis.* 3—30, 2h.

EFFECTS OF.—Febrile disturbance, *Acon.* 3, 2h. Bilious fever, *Cham.* 6, 2h. Hysteria, *Ign.* 3, 2h. Colic, *Colocynthis* 6 every hour until relieved.

Angina Pectoris.—PAROXYSM.—Palpitation, anxiety, small pulse; associated with epilepsy, *Ac. hydrocy.* 3x, ¼h. Violent beating as if heart would burst chest open, laboured breathing, pains radiating in all directions, down left arm with weakness of it, *Glon.* 3, ¼h. Pressure and oppression; darting, shooting, stabbing, or lacerating pain, faintness and dyspnœa; pain down left arm; effects of tobacco or alcohol, *Spig.* 3, ¼h. Nervous irritation depression, pains at the heart, and tremulous irritability of the heart, *Naja* 6, ¼h. Pain as if the heart were gripped with an iron hand, constriction of the chest, *Cact.* 3, 1h. Pain at the heart with rheumatic symptoms, *Act. r.* 3, 1h. Angina with asthmatic symptoms and cramps, *Cupr. met.* 6, ¼h. Oppression of breathing, with great restlessness; tobacco angina; dragging-down sensation, *Lil. t.* 30, 8h. Pain at heart in morning, on bending forward in bed; or before, and during urination, *Lith. carb.* 6, 8h. If other measures fail to relieve the pain, inhalations of *Nitrite of Amyl* may be given 3 drops on cotton wool. In the absence of specific indications, *Naja* 30, a dose every half hour for 2—3 doses, will speedily relieve, if it is going to be useful.

THE DISEASE.—In the intervals between the attacks, the medicines, as indicated above, should be given three or four times a day. If there is organic disease and weakening of the heart muscle, *Ars. iod.* 3x, gr. ii. night and morning immediately after food. [When the digestion is disordered, the most scrupulous attention must be paid to the dieting. Very often medicines given with a view to meeting the digestive symptoms will relieve the heart as well. When there is excessive flatulence, *Carbo v.* 6, half an hour before food, is most useful.]

Anidrosis.—Dry, white, leathery skin, *Æth. c.* 3, 4h. Skin of whole body becomes dry and cracked, *Nat. c.* 6, 4h. Skin dry and wrinkled, *Phos.* 6, 4h. Skin dry, absolute lack of perspiration, *Plumb.* 30, 4h. Skin dried up, rough, like hogskin, *Kali. i* 30, 4h.

Ankles, SWOLLEN.—Simple, *Apis* 3x, 4h. From debility, *see* **Debility**. From rheumatism, *see* **Rheumatism**. From varicose veins, *Hamam.* 3, 4h.; *see* **Varicose Veins**. Rest.

WEAK.—Almost all cases, *Calc. phos.* 3, gr. v. 8h. For pale children, *Calc. carb.* 6, 8h. Thin, rickety children, *Silic.* 6, 8h.

Ankylostoma Duodenale.—*See under* **Worms**.

Antrum of Highmore.—Catarrh of; discharge semi-purulent, offensive; opening communicating with the mouth, *Phos.* 2, 3h. Pulsating pain, swelling; tumour of, *Mag. c.* 6, 2h.—8h. Swelling, with tearing towards eye, *Merc. c.* 6, 2h. Burrowing, tearing pain, *Chel.* 1, 2h. Bones affected, *Hecla* 6, 8h.

Anus, BLEEDING FROM.—Difficult stool, with some blood; painful bleeding piles; bleeding after wine or whisky, *Alumen* 6, 4h. Severe bleeding whilst urinating; hard, knotty stools, followed by bleeding; clots of blood; dripping of blood during evacuation of the bowels, *Alumina* 6, 4h. Thin, watery, non-coagulating blood, *Sanguis.* 5, 4h. *See also* **Hæmorrhoids**.

FISSURE.—Sharp, cutting, sticking pain during stool and after; constipation, stool in hard masses, *Nit. ac.* 6, 6h. Pain, smarting and sore, stool in small lumps and covered with mucus, *Graph.* 6, 6h. Burning soreness in anus, stool large, hard, dry, knotty, much pain in the back, *Æscul. hip.* 3, 6h. Burning in anus more after than before or during stool, stitches like stabs with penknife, stool loose or constipated, *Ratanhia.* 3, 6h.

ITCHING.—With itching of pudendum, *Ambra* 6, 8h. From ascarides, *Teucr.* 1x, gtt. iii. 8h. With worm fever, *Cin.* 3, 8h. Violent itching, and crawling in anus and rectum,

Ignat. 3, 8h. While walking in open air, and after stool, *Ac. nit.* 6, 6h. Pricking as with pins; itching burning in anus, *Alumina* 6, 6h. Burning itching, smarting at night, *Ant. crud.* 6, 8h. (Locally, and ointment made of *Verbasc.* φ ʒi. to ung. Cetac. or Vaseline ʒi. is useful.)

PROLAPSE.—In children, *Ferrum phos.* 6x, gr. v. 8h. With diarrhœa, bleeding and tenesmus, *Aloe* 3, 8h. From moderate exertion at stool, *Ign.* 3, 8h. After every stool or sudden motion, as sneezing; with diarrhœa, especially in the morning, *Pod.* 6, 8h. With diarrhœa, green or yellow, with burning pain; or with hard insufficient stool and violent urging, *Gambog.* 3, 8h. Prolapse whilst urinating, *Mur. ac.* 6, 4h. Alternate protrusion and retraction during stool, *Sol. t. æ.* 6, 8h. Prolapse on slightest attempt at stool, *Ruta* 1, 8h.

Anxiety, Care, Grief, Worry, EFFECTS OF.—(1) *Ign.* 3, 2h.; (2) *Mag. c.* 200, 4h.

Aphasia.—*Chen. anth.* 30, 4h. In paralysis with imbecility, *Anac.* 30, 4h. Amnesic aphasia with depression, *Kali bro.* 30, 4h. Loss of speech from loss of hearing. *Lyc.* 30, 4h. Has to exert himself a long time before he can utter a word, *Stram.* 30, 4h. Loss of memory with incoherent talk, *Gels.* 30, 4h.

Aphonia. *See* Voice.

Aphthæ or Thrush.—Simple, in children or adults, *Borax*, 3x (gr. ii. or gtt. i.), 2h. The mouth to be washed every two or three hours with a lotion of *Borax*, one grain to the ounce. In children with vomiting of milk, *Ant. tart.* 6, 2h.; locally, solution of *Potas. permang.* one grain to the ounce—or Condy's fluid (purple) five drops to the teacupful—every two or three hours. Heat in mouth, < by cold water, *Caps.* 6, 2h. With herpetic eruption on lips, *Nat. m.* 6, 2h. With salivation and tenderness of salivary glands, *Kali chloric.* (chlorate of potash), 3, 2h.; wash of chlorate of potash, one grain to the pint. With salivation and slimy diarrhœa, *Merc. cor.* 6, 2h.; with Condy's fluid wash. Marasmic cases; ulcerous cases; profound prostration and low fever, with or without diarrhœa, *Ars.* 3, 2h.; Condy's wash.

Apoplexy, THREATENED.—Giddiness, headache, fullness in the head in plethoric subjects, *Nux v.* 3, 3h.; avoidance of all stimulating drink or food, and all excitement. Numbness and tingling, with arterial excitement, *Acon.* 3, 2h. Rush of blood to head, *Ast. r.* 12, 1h.

EARLY SYMPTOMS.—Full, throbbing head with flushed face, *Bell.* 3, 2h. Hot fomentations to the head.

FIT OF.—Quick, full pulse, *Acon.* 12, every quarter of an hour. Great redness of the face, and signs of active congestion of the head, *Bell.* 12, every quarter of an hour. In cases of less active congestion and fever, where there have been errors of diet, *Nux v.* 3, every quarter of an hour. Dusky-red face, coma stertor, *Opium* 3, every quarter of an hour. Absence of signs of active congestion. *Arn.* 3, every quarter of an hour. *Ferr. phos.* 6x, in water, a teaspoonful every hour until sensibility is recovered.

AFTER-EFFECTS.—When sensibility is recovered, *Arn.* 3, 1h. *Kali m.* 6x, four times daily, is a very useful remedy, and may be used in alternation with *Arn.* 3. It is advisable to continue its use for several weeks. Resulting paralysis, *see* **Paralysis.**

Appendicitis.—Fearful pain in ileo–cæcal region, great tenderness to pressure on one spot; deathly sensation in stomach-pit, *Ir. t.* 2x—30, 2h. (*Iris tenax* is the most specific of all appendicitis remedies and may be regarded as a routine prescription to begin with.) Cutting or tearing pain right side of abdomen, distension, sensitiveness, irritability, *Lach.* 6, 2h. (*Gunp.* 3x may be alternated with *Lach.* 6, every 2h. in threatened attacks, *Pyrogen* 6 or 30 should also be considered. Relapsing appendicitis. Latent pyrogenic process, patient continually relapsing after apparent similimum. 30th potency 3 times daily for 3 days or 6th potency twice daily for a week then once a day for a week. Pain and tenderness in region of appendix, fever, headache, *Bell.* 3, 1h. (Paint the part with *Belladonna* liniment and apply hot fomentations over this.) Bruised pain in appendix region; symptoms < at night *Merc. c.* 6, 2h. Burning pain, swelling in cæcal region, anguish, restlessness, prostration, fever, thirst, *Arsen.* 3, 2h. Low, typhoid fever restlessness, tearing pain, *Rhus t.* 3, 2h. Quarrelsome delirium, pain and soreness across abdomen, full, bounding pulse. *Verat. v.* 3, 2h. Application of liniment of *Veratrum viride* φ (one part to thirty of water).

Appetite, DISORDERS OF.—Usually symptomatic of depraved bodily conditions, and best remedied by measures directed to those conditions.

DEPRAVED.—For salt things, *Calc. c.* 6, 6h. For cold raw food, *Sil.* 6, 6h. For vinegar, *Sep.* 6, 6h. For beer, *Puls.* 6, 2h. For sour, highly flavoured pungent things, *Hep.* 6, 6h. For sour, refreshing things, *Carb. a.* 6, 6h. Longing for unknown things, *Chi.* 3, 6h. For dry food, *Alumina* 6, 6h.

LOST.—Want of appetite, which returns while eating, *Chi.* 3, 6h. Aversion to meat, *Calc. c.* 6, 6h. Bitter taste; tongue coated yellow at back, *Nux v.* 3, 6h. Complete loss of appetite for food, drink and tobacco, without disgust or bad taste for these things, *Ign.* 3, 6h. Loss of appetite for everything, *Rhus t.* 3, 6h. Fullness after a few mouthfuls, as if too much had been eaten, *Pru. s.* 3, 6h. Simple loss of appetite, or after acute illness, *Gent. lut.* φ—3x, gtt. v. ½h. before meals.

INCREASED.—Canine hunger, *Iod.* 3x, 6h. Feels faint if he does not eat every three or four hours, *Iod.* 3x, 6h. Gnawing hunger, *Iod.* 3x, 6h. Sensation of emptiness with debility, *Ign.* 3, 6h. Sinking feeling, *Act. r.* 3, 6h. Canine hunger without appetite, *Rhus t.* 3, 6h.

Arteries, DISEASES OF.—Suspected atheroma, (1) *Phos.* 3, 6h. (2) *Vanad.* 6, 6h. *See* **Aneurism.**

Arthralgia. *See* **Joints.**

Arthritis. *See* **Joints.**

Ascarides. *See* **Worms.**

Ascites.—Whenever the ascites is the principal trouble, if the symptoms indicate no other remedy, *Apocy.* φ, gtt. i. 3h. (Some patients are very sensitive to *Apocy.*, so its action should be carefully watched at first.) *See also* **Dropsy.** Treat the patients according to the conditions on which the ascites depends.

Asthenopia. *See* **Eyes:** SIGHT.

Asthma.—PAROXYSM.—Recent and uncomplicated, *Hydrocy. ac.* 3x, 15m. Pure spasmodic asthma, spasm very prominent

all over body, vomiting after the attack, *Cupr. met.* 6, 15m.
Attack occurring early in morning: frequently induced by
disorders of stomach, *Nux vom.* 3, 15m. In hydrogenoid
subjects; with morning diarrhœa, *Nat. sul.* 3, gr. iv. 4h.
Occurring periodically at midnight or 2 a.m., *Ars.* 3, 15m.
Occurring from 3 to 5 a.m., *Kali c.* 6, 15m. Pulse full,
anxiousness, restlessness, fear, *Acon.* 3, 15m. Useful in many
cases, especially in stout people and when there is a malarial
element, *Blatt.* 2x—3x, 2h. in the attack, 6—30, 6h. in
interval. Convulsive breathing, nausea or vomiting, cold
sweat on the face, *Verat. v.* 3, 15m. Nausea and great
depression of heart, *Lobel.* 3, gtt. i. 15m. Old asthmatics,
Senega 1, 4h. Where the asthma is not pure, but associated
with catarrh and cough, if the mucus is scanty, *Ipec.* 3, 15m.
If the mucus is profuse, *Ant. t.* 6, 15m. When there is a
history of former attacks of bronchitis and pneumonia, *Ars.
i.* 3x, gr. ii. or gtt. ii. after meals. If these fail, *Stramonium*
cigarettes may be smoked as a palliative. If possible, however, this should be avoided as the use of them is a distinct
hindrance to the *cure* of the condition.

INTERVALS.—Spasmodic variety; vomiting after attack, *Cupr.
m.* 6, 6h. Attacks occurring early in morning, stomach
disorders, *Nux v.* 3, 6h. Where there is, in addition to the
attacks, general debility, loss of flesh, tendency to night
sweats, bowels loose or regular, tongue clean or red, relief
by heat, attacks worse in cold, damp weather, *Ars.* 3, 6h.
Chronic asthma; sudden suppression of chronic eruptions;
psoriasis; gout; tendency to skin eruptions; patient subject
to fainting spells; sinking sensation in the forenoon; flushes
of heat, *Sulph.* 3, 6h. Malarial or sycotic cases; in **damp**

localities, near lakes or rivers; < early morning, *Nat. sul.* 3, gr. viii. 4h. (Asthma is usually constitutional, and each case must be treated according to the constitutional symptoms of the patient.) In most cases a course of *Bacil.* 30—200 once a week will be of marked advantage.

Atheroma. *See* Arteries.

Athetosis.—After a severe or instrumental labour the child should receive *Arn.* 30, gtt. i. ½h. If spasmodic symptoms set in, (1) *Cicut. v.* 3, ½h.—2h. Later, if spasms, rigidity, and increased reflexes are present, (1) *Lath. s.* 3x, 2h.; (2) *Liq. Strychniæ* 3x, gtt. ii. t.d. Galvanism: positive pole on spine, negative on muscles involved.

Atrophy.—*Iod.* 3x, 6h. With fever, *Ars.* 3, 6h. Chilliness, earthy complexion, constipation; wasting from above downwards, *Nat. m.* 6, 6h. Wasting of muscles and paralysis, *Plumb. acet.* 6, 6h. Neck emaciated; skin in folds, *Sarsa.* 6, 4h. General marasmus; legs most wasted; from below upwards, *Abrot.* 30, 4h.

Axilla.—Pain in (right), extending down arm, *Jug. c.* 1, 4h. Irritation; eruption; abscess in, *Jug. reg.* 1, 4h. Eruption with inflamed glands, *Elaps.* 30, 4h. Inflamed glands, *Baryt. c.* 6, 4h. Abscess in, *Hep.* 6, 2h. Perspiration: excessive, *Kali carb.* 12, 4h.; offensive, *Nit. ac.* 1, 4h.; like garlic, *Lyc.* 6, 4h.

Back.—ACHING.—From over-exertion, *Arn.* 3, 3h. *Bellis.* 3, 3h. From uterine affections, *Act. r.* 3, 3h. In pregnant women, with sense of weakness in the back, *Kali carb.* 6, 6h. Intense, neuralgic backache, *Variol.* 200 8h. With oxalates in urine,

Oxal. ac. 6, 4h. With scanty urine, *Terebinth.* 3, 2h. With piles, *Æscul. h.* 3, 6h. *See also* **Lumbago** *and* **Menstruation**, PAINFUL.

WEAKNESS OF.—In rickety subjects, *Silic.* 6, 8h. In hysterical subjects, *Ign.* 3, 6h. After exhausting disease, (1) *Chi.* 3, 6h.; (2) *Calc. phos.* 3, gr. v. 8h. With sexual weakness and from sexual excess, *Phos.* 3, 4h.

Baker's Itch. *See* **Lichen.**

Barber's Itch. *See* **Beard.**

Balanitis.—(1) *Merc. sol.* 6, 8h. (2) *Jac. car.* 6, 8h. Cleanse thoroughly every four hours, and bathe with a lotion of *Calendula* (ten drops to the ounce).

Baldness. *See* **Hair.**

Beard.—PUSTULAR ERUPTIONS.—*Hepar s.* 6, 8h. Ointment of *dilute acid Nitrate of Mercury* may be applied at bedtime. Sycosis (ringworm of the beard), (1) *Bacil.* 100, gtt. v. once or twice a week; (2) *Calc. c.* 30, 6h. (3) *Rad. bro.* 30, once a week. *Acid. sulphuros. dil.* may be applied at bedtime.

Bed-sores.—PREVENTION.—Bathe with whisky the parts that are exposed to pressure. Put the patient on a water-bed. Glycerine or glycerine cream, is one of the best preventives of bed sores. When sores have formed, apply *Hypericum Oil* (made by extracting *Hypericum* in hot olive or linseed oil). This is a most valuable remedy, and is obtainable from homœopathic pharmacies. The prevention and management of bed-sores is a matter of nursing chiefly. The medical treatment must be directed to the general condition. If the bed-sores themselves become the most important feature of the case, *see* under **Ulcers** and **Gangrene.**

Belching. *See* Eructations.

Beri-Beri or Endemic Neuritis.—Numbness, pain, œdema, anæmia, (1) *Ars.* 3—6, 2h.; (2) *Rhus t.* 3x—30, 2h. Paralysis, wasting, rheumatic stiffness, *Phos.* 3—30, 2h. Paralysis of lower extremities, *Gels.* 3, 2h. With rigidity, *Lath.* 3x, 8h. Swelling of whole body, short breath, fever with sweat, *Sep.* 6, 8h. The patient must have abundance of nourishing food and fresh air.

Bilious Attack.—When the attack has come on, with vomiting of bile or acid, violent headache, diarrhœa, *Iris v.* 3, ½h. With constipation, light stools, sharp pain in liver, tongue like wash-leather, frontal headache, depression, *Bry.* 3, ½h. Complete suppression of bile, white stools, yellow skin, *China* 3, 2h. Pains in the eyes and over them, blackish, fœtid, liquid stools, *Leptand.* 3, ½h. Morning diarrhœa, green or yellow stools, *Podoph.* 6, 1h. After over-indulgence in alcohol, or over-eating, in spare, sedentary persons, constipation, depression, *Nux v.* 3, ½h. After fat or rich food, *Puls.* 3, ½h. Sharp pains in the liver, pains in the loins and constipation, *Berb.* 6, 1h. (Bilious attacks are generally the expression of a morbid constitutional state, usually the psora of Hahnemann. This must be treated constitutionally. *See* Biliousness.)

See also Diarrhœa, Dyspepsia, and Vomiting.

Bilious Fever. *See* Remittent Fever.

Biliousness.—Patients who are subject to periodical attacks of biliousness should take regular exercise, avoid alcoholic drinks of all kinds, eat sparingly of meat, and avoid rich or fat food. The removal of the tendency may be assisted by the following medicines, which must be given according to the symptoms of the patient over a length of time:—In bloodless subjects, with pale or flushed face, and throbbing head, *Fer. metal.* 6, 4h. In persons of costive habit, subject to one-sided headache, *Kali c.* 6, 8h. In dark, sallow, spare persons of sedentary life, subject to constipation, *Nux v.* 3, 8h. Persons who suffer from acidity, sinking at pit of stomach in forenoon, fainty spells, constipation and piles, *Sulph.* 6, 8h. In gouty subjects, with loaded urine, *Nat. sulph.* 6x, gr. v. 8h. When there is abdominal flatulence, constipation, and scanty urine, *Lyc.* 6, 8h. Discomfort in the region of the liver, constipation, the stools being composed of very minute lumps, packed together like sheeps', *Magnes. mur.* 6, 8h. *Chel.* φ 5—10 drops in a little water 3 times daily after meals is an extremely valuable adjunct to treatment. *Chionanthus* φ similarly, either of these two remedies can be taken in addition to other treatment. *See also* Anæmia, Liver, Constipation, Diarrhœa, etc.

Bites. *See* Stings and Hydrophobia.

Black-eye.—*Arn.* 3, ½h. If skin unbroken, *Arn.* 1x, ten drops to the ounce of water, to be applied as a lotion. If the skin is broken, a lotion of *Hamamelis* φ, five drops to the ounce, to be applied instead. From a blow, *Led.* 200, 2h. With pain in eyeball, *Symphyt.* 30, 1h.

Bladder, IRRITABLE.—Frequent desire to pass water, which is natural or increased in quantity and slightly burning, *Apis* 3x, 2h.; constant desire, only a few drops voided, *Canth.* 3, 2h. Burning, cutting, or sticking pain in urethra (especially the female urethra) during and after urinating; frequent desire, *Berb.* φ, gtt. ii. ½h.—4h. Burning in region of

kidneys, bladder, and ureter, strangury, *Tereb.* 3, ½h.—4h.
Irritation of the neck of the bladder and urethra in women,
Copaib. 3x, 4h. Incontinence of urine, chiefly during the
day, *Ferr. phos.* 6x, gr. v. 6h. Irritable bladder in gouty or
alcoholic subjects; irritability of bladder and rectum, with
urging, at the same time, with little or no result, *Nux v.* 3,
4h. Involuntary passage of urine in sleep, *Senega* 3, 6h. In
sleep during the daytime, or during the night, *Bell.* 1, 6h.
Involuntary passage of urine on coughing or sneezing,
Caust. 1—6, 6h. *See under* Urine.

PARALYSIS OF.—(1) *Op.* 1, 2h. (2) *Canth.* 3, 2h. When there
is a continuous sensation as if imperfectly relieved of its
contents, *Secale* 1, 4h. *See also* Strangury; and Urine,
RETAINED.

ACUTE INFLAMMATION OF.—*Canth.* 3, 2h. If caused by chill in
damp weather, *Dulc.* 3, 2h. Symptomatic of kidney affection
or calculus, with much secretion of mucus, *Pareira* φ, gtt.
x. 4h.

CHRONIC INFLAMMATION OR CATARRH OF.—*Canth.* 3, 6h. With
incontinence of urine in bed at night, *Puls.* 3x, 6h. Water
smelling like horse's, (1) *Benz. ac.* 3x, 6h. (2) *Nit. ac.* 5,
4h. If these fail, *Chimaphila* φ, gtt. v. 6h.

Blepharitis. *See* Eyes: EYELIDS.

Blepharospasm.—Involuntary twitching of eyelids, *Codeia* 3,
6h. If continued, with spasmodic affection of muscles of
eyeballs, *Agar.* 1, 4h. With dazzling of sight, *Puls.* 3, 4h.
With ciliary spasm, patient unable to read without pain and
frontal headache, aggravated by light, *Physostig.* 3x, 6h.

Blindness. *See* **Amaurosis; Amblyopia;** and **Eyes:** Sight.

Blood-poisoning.—[This is a general term and includes affections of the blood resulting from bad smells, poisoning with foods that have gone bad, impure drinks, excluding specific poisons and infection from specific diseases.] Acute cases with low fever, delirium, thinks his limbs are separated from his body, *Baptis.* 1x, 2h. Depressed, dull headache, aching in back, weakness of limbs, chills run up back; from dissection wounds, *Echin.* φ, gtt. iii. 2—4h. When skin affections, boils or abscesses result, *Gunp.* 3x, gr. vi. (or iii. 2-gr. tablets) 4h. (This remedy has a very wide range of usefulness in these cases.) Fever of typhoid type, putrefaction of fluids and tendency to suppuration, *Pyro.* 5, gtt. v. 4h. From poisoned wounds, infection spreading along lymphatic, *Lach.* 6, 2h. Chronic blood-poisoning with fever, thirst for cold drinks, restlessness, anxiety, red tongue, *Ars.* 3, 4h.

Blood-spitting. *See* **Hæmoptysis.**

Blood-vomiting. *See* **Hæmatemesis.**

Bloody Flux. *See* **Dysentery.**

Blushing.—Too Easily.—In general, *Amyl. nit.* 30, 8h. When eating, *Carb. a.* 6, 8h. After eating, *Carlsbad* 30, 8h. From bashfulness, *Ambr.* 6, 6h.

Boils.—As a routine remedy when no special indications for others presents, *Gunp.* 3x, gr. vi. (or 3 tablets) 3h. Preventive, when there is tendency to them, *Arn.* 3, 8h. When just beginning to form. *Bell.* 3, 2h. When further advanced, *Silic.* 3, gr. v. 6h.; a lotion of *Calc. mur.* 1x (a drachm to three ounces), may be kept constantly applied from the beginning. When matter has formed, *Hep. s.* 6, 4h. Boils after fevers, *Phyt.* 1, 4h. When crops of boils are constantly appearing, *Sulph.* 3, 6h., given for a length of time, will probably check the tendency. Succession of boils, *Anthrac.* 30—200, 6h. With low fever, *Echin.* φ, gtt. v. 4h.

Bone.—BRUISED.—*Ruta* 1, 2h.; *Ruta* φ (ten drops to the ounce) for a lotion.

PERIOSTITIS.—Simple, *Mezer.* 3, 3h. Syphilitic, *Aur. mur.* 3x, gtt. ii. 2h. Rheumatic, *Merc. sol.* 6, 4h. Scrofulous, *Silic.* 6, 4h. Of forehead and face, *Phytolac.* 3, 2h. With increased formation of bone, *Phos.* 3, 3h. Of long bones, *Angust.* 3, gr. v. 6h.

NECROSIS.—*Phos.* 3, 3h. After *Phos.*, *Silic.* 6, 4h., if necessary.

CARIES.—*Bacil.* 30—200, gl. iv. once a week. In children if thin and puny, *Silic.* 6, 8h. In fat children, *Calc. c.* 6, 8h. In syphilitic subjects, *Ac. fluor.* 3, 6h. In scrofulous subjects, *Silic.* 6, 8h. In tuberculous subjects, *Phos.* 3, 8h. Of long bones, *Angust.* 3, gr. v.—6, 6h.

NODES.—With burning and boring pain in the bones, and redness and swelling, *Aur. mur.* 3x, gtt. ii. 6h. Especially on bones of head, *Kali bich.* 3x, gr. ii. 4h. Soft, on forehead, *Nux v.* 3, 2h. With nightly pains in the bones, *Mezer.* 3, 6h. If these fail, *Stilling.* 1x, 6h. *See also* **Rheumatism: Syphilitic.**

EXOSTOSES.—Syphilitic, *Merc. cor.* 3, 6h. Of the head, *Kali bich.* 3x, 6h. Painful, *Helca.* 6, 6h. On the jaws, *Plumb. acet.* 3 gr. v. 8h. Near epiphyses, *Conch.* 3, gr. v. t.d. *Calc. Fluor* 6 or 30. 6 may be given twice daily or 30 once or twice per week, discontinue when improvement is shown. Repeat when improvement ceases.

PAINS IN.—Nightly, in syphilitic patients, *Mezer.* 3, 6h. If very chronic, *Aur. mur.* 3x, gtt. ii. 6h. Lightning pains, *Fluor. ac.* 3, 6h. As if bruised, *Ruta* 3, 6h. On the approach of stormy weather, *Rhod.* 3, 6h. In influenza, or malaria, *Eupat. perf.* 3, 3h.

Borborygmi.—*Rumex crisp.* 6, 4h. Preceding a loose stool; sound as if a bottle were being emptied, *Jatropha* 3, 4h. With constipation and abdominal distention, *Lyc.* 6, 4h. With worm symptoms, *Cina* 3, 4h.

Bowels. *See* **Abdomen, Anus, Colic, Constipation, Diarrhœa,** and **Peritonitis.**

Brain.—CONCUSSION OF.—(1) *Arn.* 30, gtt. ii. ½h, for a few doses, then every hour, discontinue when reaction comes on and consciousness returns, *Cicuta* and *Hypericum* may have to be considered, if convulsions follow. *Nat. Sulph.* for mental states consequent upon head injury.

CONGESTION OF.— Flushed face, bright eyes, dilated pupils, active delirium, *Bell.* 3, 1h. Non-inflammatory, arising from exposure to intense cold, from sea-sickness, or suppressed menses, *Bry.* 3, 1h. Cerebral stasis, *Bellis per.* 3, 3h. Brain affections of infants with great drowsiness, *Nux mosch.* 30, 2h. Retrocession of eruptions; difficult dentition, *Cupr. acet.* 3, ½—1h. Determination of blood to the head; congestion after great losses of blood, *Ferr. pyrophos.* 1x, gr. ii. 6h. Vertigo, sensation of band round temples, inability to concentrate thought, *Gels.* 3, 3h. Tight sensation from sunstroke, *Cact.* 3, ¼h. Violent throbbing, congestion from exposure to sun or heat from suppression of menses, or in pregnancy, *Glon.* 3, 2h. Oppression, drowsiness, constipation, *Op.* 3, 1h. With predisposition to apoplexy, *Nux v.* 3, 2h. Chronic cases heat at vertex, faint feeling, feet cold or else burning, *Sul.* 3, 6h. *See also* Sunstroke.

DROPSY OF. *See* Hydrocephalus.

SOFTENING.—The symptoms of this disease vary so very much that each case must be treated by itself; but two medicines will be found very generally of service—*Phos.* 3, and *Baryt. c.* 6. If no other medicine is indicated, they may be given, each four times a day, on alternate weeks. *Vanad.* 6, 6h., may also be considered. In over-worked subjects, *Bellis p.* 3, 6h.

Brain-fag.—Nervous prostration, *Phos. ac.* 1x, gtt. ii. 6h. Great indifference; lack of will-power to undertake anything *Pic. ac.* 3, 6h. Weak memory, dull intellect, (1) *Zinc.* 6, 6h.; (2) *Zinc. pic.* 3, gr. viii. 8h. From loss of sleep, *Zinc. acet.* 1x, gtt. x. 4h. Distracted and incapable of mental exertion from much mental work of different kinds in rapid succession, *Æthus. cynap.* 3, 6h. Loss of memory "funk" before an examination, *Anacard.* 3, 3h. Pale subjects with tendency to large tonsils; brain weakness after much worry, or after illness, *Calc. phos.* 3, gr. ii. 8h. Chronic headache, nervousness, and loss of memory from overwork; sufferings < by cold and > by warmth, *Silic.* 6, 8h.

Brain Fever. *See* Mania and Typhus Fever.

Breast.—ABSCESS OF.—Threatening; as soon as the first symptoms of pain or hardness come on, *Bry.* 3, 1h. This will often abort the process. If *Bry.* fails to check it in forty-eight hours, give *Phytolac.* 1, 2h., and apply a lotion of

Phytolac. φ (gtt. x—℥vi.). Less hardness than *Bry.* red streaks radiating from a central point to the circumference, *Bell.* 3, 1h. Should suppuration occur, give *Hepar* 6, 3h. Foment with hot *Calendula* lotion (ten drops to the ounce) every two hours, and if necessary make an incision as soon as pointing occurs. After incising leave off poultices, support the breast well, and bathe it twice a day with hot *Calendula* lotion (ten drops to the ounce) and dress with *Calendula* ointment giving *Silic.* 6, 3h. Sinuses left after breast abscess, *Silic.* 6, 3h. Retracted nipples, *Sarsap.* 6, 8h. For breast troubles during weaning, *see* Lactation.

CONTUSION OF.—(1) *Bellis* 3x, 2h. (2) *Conium* 3, 2h.

PAIN IN.—Sharp, piercing pain in right breast just below nipple; difficult to take a deep inspiration; extending to the stomach; to the shoulder, making it difficult to raise the arm; before menses, *Sang.* 3, 2h. Painful *empty* feeling in breasts in nursing women, intolerable when child nurses, > by pressure, *Bor.* 30, 4h. Breasts painful before menses: if the menses are scanty, *Con.* 3, 2h.; if menses are copious and early, *Calc. c.* 30, 4h., for a week before the period is expected.

PAIN BELOW LEFT BREAST (INFRA-MAMMARY PAIN).—In unmarried females, *Act. rac.* 1, 2h. With scanty menses, *Puls.* 3, 6h. Rheumatic, *Ranunc. b.* 1, 3h. With leucorrhœa, *Cean.* 1, 6h.

Breast Pang. *See* Angina Pectoris.

Breath. FETID.—(1) *Arn.* 3, 3h. (2) *Merc. sol.* 6, 3h. (3) When mercurial, *Nit. ac.* 6, 3h. Putrid, *Aur. met.* 30, 8h. Bad odour from mouth after dinner; sour-smelling breath, *Nux v.* 3, 3h. Odour of onions, *Petrol.* 3, 4h. Stercoraceous, *Querc.* 3x, 4h. Like carrion, *Pyro.* 6, 4h.

Breathing. *See* **Croup, Asthma, Heart,** etc.

Bright's Disease. *See* **Kidneys.**

Bronchial Glands.—Disease of.—*Bacil.* 30—200, gl. iv., once a week. (*See under* **Glandular Swellings,** Chronic.) When there is distressing spasmodic cough, *Calc. c.* 6, 2h. If the cough is accompanied by flushing of the face, and comes on when lying down at night, *Bell.* 3, 1h.

Bronchiectasis.—Treatment must be according to the catarrhal symptoms, as indicated below under **Bronchitis.** If sputa very offensive, inhalations of *Kreasote* (gtt. xxx. in an inhaler, thrice daily) may be given in addition to other treatment.

Bronchitis.—In the earliest stage, chills, fever, oppression, dry, tickling cough, *Acon.* 3, 1h. Fever established, dry, hacking cough, or with a little mucus, hoarseness, soreness along trachea; pains between shoulders, sharp pains in chest; tongue white, constipation, *Bry.* 3, 1h. Short dry cough from tickling in larynx; dry spasmodic cough with vomiting; stitches in chest; headache, redness and heat of face; bronchitis after ether anæsthesia, *Bell.* 1—30, 1h. Cough looser, tendency to perspiration, *Merc. sol.* 6, 3h. Cough spasmodic, great dyspnœa, little expectoration, dry sounds in chest in day, moist at night, symptoms worst at night; with gastro-intestinal disturbance and persistent nausea, *Ipec.* 3, 1h. Oppression of chest, great depression, cough and hoarseness, much expectoration, clear or white; tongue white, creamy, disgust for food, inclination to vomit; capillary bronchitis in children, *Ant. tart.* 6, 2h. Acute or chronic bronchitis, where the mucus is tough and stringy and difficult to raise, *Kali bich.* 3x, 2h. Cough spasmodic, waking the patient up in the night, very little expectoration, *Ars.* 3, 2h. Bronchitis with fever and night sweat, purulent expectoration; phthisical symptoms; great weakness, *Ars. iod.* 3x, gr. iii. thrice daily immediately after food. Broncho-pneumonia, *Phos.* 3, 2h. Spasmodic cough, dry or with copious expectoration, oppression of the chest, with stitches or burning; often accompanied with nasal catarrh, *Sang.* 3, 1h. Somewhat chronic bronchitis, profuse yellow expectoration, hoarseness, sensation of a clot of mucus, or internal swelling when swallowing, *Hep. s.* 6, 2h. In delicate blonde subjects, lax fibre, abundant expectoration; cough < on lying down; compels the patient to sit up in bed; < in warm room, *Puls.* 3, 2h. Chronic cases, after subsidence of acute symptoms, tendency to headache, liver sluggish, asthmatic, constipation; < when warm in bed at night, *Sulph.* 3, 4h. Acute or chronic cases, much oppression at chest; cough worst night and morning; dry except after night's rest; short or spasmodic general health affected, *Nit. ac.* 6, 2h. In old persons with blue nails and cold extremities, hoarse, profuse expectoration without power to raise it, *Carb. veg.* 6, 2h. Long-standing bronchitis in old people, physical powers depressed, expectoration difficult to raise from want of power, *Amm. carb.* 3x, 1h. In old people, cough irritating and shaking, *Senega* 3, 2h. Where there is irritability of the bladder, the cough causing expulsion of urine, *Caust.* 6, 3h. Spasmodic cough with difficult expulsion of phlegm, and feeling of soreness all down trachea and under sternum; < in cold air, *Rumex crisp.* 6, 2h. Cough coming on on lying down, *Hyoscy.* 3, 2h. Short, dry cough from tickle under middle of sternum, coming on when lying down at night, *Conium* 3, 2h. (These two medicines may be given at night, whilst others are given by day, should the general symptoms indicate other medicines, and the night cough call for one of these.) Bronchitis of Influenza, suspiciously like Tuberculosis, *Aviare* 30, 4h. After effects, *Kali iod.* 30, 4h. *See also* **Cough.**

CROUPOUS BRONCHITIS.—*Kali bichrom.* 3x, 2h.

Brow Ague.—Recent, *Chin. sulph.* 3x, 3h. Chronic *Ars.* 3, 3h Of clock-like periodicity, *Cedr.* 3, 3h. *See also* **Headache.**

Bruises.—Of the soft parts, *Arn.* 3—30 1h. A lotion of *Arn.* φ or 1x (five drops to the ounce), or *Arnica oil* should be applied to the part if the skin is unbroken. If the skin is broken, a lotion of *Hamam.* φ (ten drops to the ounce). Bruises of the bones, *Ruta*, 3, or any potency up to 30, depending on severity of injury, 2h.; and *Ruta* φ (ten drops to the ounce) for a lotion. Of the female breast, *Bellis.* 3x, 2h. After *Bellis*, *Con.* 3, 2h. Of parts rich in nerves (especially fingers, toes, and matrix of nails); injuries to the spinal cord and resulting paralysis, *Hypericum* 3, 3h.; a liniment consisting of equal parts of *Hyperic.* φ, spirit of wine, and distilled water, to be rubbed with the hand on the injured part (if the spine) three times a day: or to be kept applied on lint or soft linen (if it is in the extremities, and the injury is recent).

Bubo.—Whether simple or syphilitic, *Merc. sol.* 6, 2h. If the patient is already under the influence of mercury, *Nit. ac.* 6, 2h. Should these fail to check the disease after three days' trial, (1) *Badiag.* 6, 4h.; (2) *Carb. an.* 6, 4h. (Under this treatment it will frequently disperse; and so long as there is any chance of this, poultices should be avoided.

They may be resorted to with advantage when suppuration and discharge are inevitable.) When discharge has taken place, the same medicine may be continued, and a lotion of *Calend.* φ (ʒi.—ʒi.) applied frequently. Should the wound become phagedænic, iodoform powder should be dusted freely on the wound after frequent cleansing with warm water irrigation: internally, *Kali. iod.* gr. v. 6h.

Bunion.—The true bunion from pressure, *Silic.* 6, 8h. Use as a lotion, and apply as a compress at night, *Kali iod.* gr. x—ʒi. of water. Rheumatic enlargement of the bursa, *Rhod.* 3, 3h. (If inflamed, a liniment of equal parts of *Verat. v.* φ, of spirit of wine, and distilled water may be applied.) In gouty subjects, *Benz. ac.* 3x, 8h. *Rhus-tox* 6—12. twice daily. *Urtica urens* φ 5 drops in a wineglass of hot water, 3 times daily. (An ointment of *Benz. ac.* 1x, ʒi., to Cetacean ointment, ʒi., may be applied.)

Burns and Scalds.—If slight without vesication, *Urtica urens* φ (one part to four of water) to be applied as a lotion and the rags kept wet with it, without being removed. Or, in burns of first degree, a lotion of *Hamamelis* φ, gtt. x.—ʒi. may be used in the same way. Nelsons Burn Ointment is a most useful and soothing application to small burns. If there is vesication, *Canth.* φ (one part to ten of water) to be applied in the same way, and *Canth.* 3, 1h., given internally. If the burn is extensive, it should be covered with lint soaked in Carron oil (equal parts of *linseed oil* and *lime water*), and *Canth.* 3, 1h., given internally. Or a one per cent. solution of *Pic. ac.* may be applied on lint. If the burns are deep, destroying the skin, *Kali bichr.* 3x, 2h.; Carron oil dressing. Suppuration after burns, *Hep.* 6, 4h.

After effects of burns or scalds, *Caust.* 30, 8h. Anything more than a superficial burn, should receive skilled medical attention.

Bursitis. *See* **Housemaid's Knee.**

Cæcum, INFLAMMATION OF. *See* **Appendicitis.**

INFLAMMATION OF PERITONEUM AROUND. *See* **Peritonitis and Perityphilitis.**

Calculus.—BILIARY (GALL-STONES, PASSAGE OF).—*Calc. c.* 30, 15m. Should this fail to relieve within three hours, *Berb* φ, 15m. Pains radiating from gall-bladder; > by moving about, or bending backward, *Diosc.* φ or 30, ½h. When pain is felt in left lobe of liver, *Card. mar.* φ, gtt. x. 4h. Those subject to gall-stones should not go too long (not more than six hours during the day) without food. Pure olive oil may be taken freely by those subject to biliary obstruction. For prevention of their formation, *China.* 6, 8h., for four weeks, and then at increasing intervals, "Poland Water" is the best drinking water in these cases. In cases of gall-stones *Chel.* φ, 5 drops in a little water three times daily after meals for several weeks or longer will promote free flow of bile and together with *China* 6, night and morning for 14 days then morning only for 14 days will help a high percentage of cases.

RENAL, PASSAGE OF.—Agonising pain, twists about, screams and groans; red urine with brick-dust sediment, *Oc. can.* 30, 15m. Writhing with crampy pains, must move about, *Diosc.* φ—30, 15m. Violent sticking pains in bladder, extending from kidneys into urethra, with urging to urinate, *Berberis* 6, 15m. Should this fail, *Pareira brava* φ, ʒss. in a wineglassfull of warm distilled water every half-hour.

PREVENTION.—Gravelly urine, pain in back and loins, *Berb.* φ, 6h. Tendency to store uric acid in the tissues; gouty subjects, *Urt. ur.* φ, gtt. v. 8h. Drink distilled water.

VESICAL, TENDENCY TO. *See* Gravel.

OF THE LUNG.—Coughing up of calcareous nodules, *Calc. c.* 6, 4h.

Callosities.—*Ant. c.* 6, r. and h.s.s. Or, *Rad. b.* 30, unit doses.

Cancer.—DIATHESIS.—Worn, jaded look, yellow or sallow complexion, "hide-bound" state of skin, low spirits, loss of appetite, chronic constipation, *Hydrast.* 1, 8h. Tendency to fatness, sluggish circulation, lazy disposition, tendency to glandular enlargements, *Phyt.* 1, 8h. Thin, wiry, anxious patients, of cachectic appearance, poor appetite, inactive digestion, with tendency to diarrhœa and various skin affections, with burning pains, *Ars. iod.* 3x, gtt. ii. or gr. ii. thrice daily (immediately after food). In all cases of chronic illness having a cancerous heredity or the constitutional symptoms of the diathesis a course of treatment with *Carcin.* 30—200 once a week will be likely to benefit.

EPITHELIOMA OF TONGUE AND OTHER PARTS.—In doubtful cases, *Thuja* 3x, 6h.; locally, *Thuja* φ to be painted on with camel's-hair brush night and morning. Decided cases, *Hydrast.* 1, 6h.; locally, a mixture of equal parts of *Hydrast* φ and glycerine to be painted on night and morning. If after five or six weeks of this treatment there is no improvement in cancer of the tongue, *Kali cyanat.* 3x, gr. ii. night and morning. Of lip (1) *Lyc.* 6—30, 8h. (2) *Sepia* 3, gr. ii. 8h. (3) *Cann. sat.* φ, gtt. ii. in powder once a fortnight. Epithelioma of lip or elsewhere, *Ars. i.* 3x, gr. ii. thrice daily, after food; locally, a solution of *Arsen.* 3x (ten drops to the ounce) to be painted on night and morning. Occasional doses of the cancer nosodes, *Carcin.* 30—200 or *Epithel.* 30—200 will be advantageous. When in accessible parts exposure to *Radium* rays is very successful in many of these cases.

OF BREAST.—*In all cases let all pressure or friction be avoided and the breast kept cool.*

IN DOUBTFUL CASES.—Where there is a painful nodule on the breast, of which it is impossible to decide the nature, *Bry.* 1, 8h. A painless, stationary enlargement, *Calc. iod.* 3x, gtt. iv. 8h. If there is debility and decided increase, *Ars. i.* 3x, gr. ii. thrice daily, after food. Where there is cancerous heredity: indrawn or divided nipples, *Carc.* 30—100, once a week.

UNDOUBTED CASES.—In all cases the nosode *Scirrh.* 30—200, or *Carcin.* 30—200 in weekly doses should be given either alone or in addition to any of the following:—(1) *Hydrast.* 1x, 6h. *Hydrast.* lotion (ʒi to ʒiii.) may be applied locally. (2) If the disease advances in spite of this, after one or two months of trial, *Ars.* 3x—3, 6h. (3) Especially indicared if there are cracks at the commissures of the lips, *Cundurango* 1x, 6h. Should these fail, the following may be given according to indications:—Torpid constitution, melancholy, irritable, menses scanty or suppressed and painful when the affection has resulted from a blow, *Coni.* 1, 3h. Irritable, nervous, fanciful patients; tumour not very sensitive to pressure, great pain in the arm, with rigidity and loss of power, *Cicuta v.* 3x, 3h. Stitching pains shooting out of the nipples, *Ol. an.* 30, 8h. Induration resulting from a blow;

patient liable to acne and boils, *Bellis. per. φ*, gtt. iii. 8h.
If the whole breast is hard, bluish-red, and covered with
protuberances, *Kreas.* 3, 3h. Hard, painful lumps in breast,
Aster. rubens. 12, 8h. Sycotic patients, *Thuj.* 30, 8h. Paget's
disease, *Lobel erin. φ*, gtt. ii., unit doses every ten days.

OPEN CANCERS.—THREATENED ULCERATION.—Thin, anxious
patients, puckering of the skin over the tumour, *Ars. i.* 3x,
gr. ii. (or *Nat. cacodyl.—see above*), thrice daily, after food.
Cachetic, melancholic patients, tendency to constipation,
skin hardening over the tumour, *Hydrast.* 1x, 4h.; locally,
an ointment of *Hydrast. φ*, a drachm to the ounce of vaseline.
Blood-poisoning fever symptoms, *Echin. φ*, gtt. v. 4h.

ACTUAL ULCERATION.—Fœtid discharge (1) *Bufo* 30, 4h. (2)
Bapt. 1x, 3h.; a lotion of *Bapt. φ* (five drops to the ounce
of water) to be injected into the wound every few hours. If
the ulceration is angry, irritable, and increasing, *Hydrast.*
1x, 3h. being given internally, *Hydrast.* ointment (a drachm
to the ounce of vaseline) to be painted on with a camel-hair
brush, after syringing with a lotion of *Hydrast. φ* ten drops,
strong *carbolic acid* five drops, water one ounce. Should
this fail to relieve, *Galium apar. φ*, 6h.; locally, an application of equal parts of *Galium ap. φ* and glycerine. Where
there is bleeding, *Sang. c.* 1x, 2h.; locally a lotion of *Ham.
φ* (ten drops to the ounce). A useful ointment in open
cancers is *Ruta* ointment, made by extracting the whole
fresh plant in vaseline. The ordinary *Boracic acid* ointment
is also useful in many cases.

OF THE UTERUS.—The same indications as for cancer of the
breast, with much hæmorrhage, *Epihyst.* 30—200, once a
week. *Ruta φ*, gtt. ii. in powder once a fortnight. As local

measures when needed, washing or syringing with lotion of *Hydrastis* and *Carbolic acid* (as above), and application of plugs of lint charged with *Hydrastis* ointment. If there is much bleeding, *Hamamelis* may be substituted for *Hydrastis*, both in lotion and ointment, and in the same proportion. The use of antiseptic dressings that can be burned will be found of great advantage.

OF BONE.—(1) *Phos.* 6—30, 6h. (2) *Symph.* φ—30, 4h., with application of *Symph.* φ, or poultices of the herb. (3) *Aur. iod.* 3x, 6h.

FUNGUS HÆMATODES (BLEEDING CANCER).—(1) *Phos.* 30, 6h. (2) *Thuja* 30, 6h.; application of dry lint, and pressure by a bandage.

AFTER REMOVAL of cancer of the breast a prolonged course of constitutional treatment is essential. Weekly doses of *Carc.* 30—200 or *Scirrh.* 30—200, and remedies indicated by the constitutional state, chiefly *Nat. cacod.* gr. ¼, bis die after food, *Iod.* 3x, 6h., and *Kali i.* gr. v. 8h.

FOR the PAINS of cancer, *Euphorb.* 6—30, 2h. Burning pains, *Euphorb. het.* 6—30, 2h.; if other remedies fail, *Opium* φ, gtt. ⅓, 1—3h.

Cancrum Oris.—*Merc. cor.* 3, 1h.; application of glycerole of *Muriatic acid* (*Ac hydrochlor. dil.*, B. P., gtt. v., *Glycerine* ℨss.) every two hours. Should *Merc. cor.* fail, *Ars.* 3, 2h.

Carbuncle.—In general, *Anthrac.* 30, 2—4h. (This will often abort the case, and if it does not do that will conduct most cases to a favourable result.) When there is low fever

as from blood-poisoning, *Echin.* φ, gtt. v. 2—4h. Heat, redness, throbbing, swelling, *Bell.* 3, 2h. When there is considerable thickening, *Hepar s.* 6, 2h. Application of lotion
of *Liquor. Calc. chlor.* (1x, a drachm to the ounce). Much
œdema and swelling of tissues around, *Apis* 3x, 1h., and
Calc. chlor. lotion. Dark blue appearance, *Arn.* 3, 1h.;
lotion of *Arnica* φ (5 drops to the ounce). Dark blue appearance, coldness of the extremities, low vitality, *Carb.* v. 6, 1h.;
with burning, stinging pain, *Tarent. cub.* 30, 2h. General
prostration and symptoms of blood-poisoning, *Lach.* 6, 1h.
Dry tongue, thirst, typhoid condition, *Ars.* 3, 1h. Indolent
carbuncle; also after it has begun to discharge, *Sil.* 6, 8h.;
dress with boracic acid ointment (powdered *Boracic acid*,
one drachm to an ounce of vaseline or prepared lard) or
Calendula ointment. *Gunp.* 3x, gr. vi. 2—4h., given alone
or in alternation with one of the other remedies will clear
up many cases.

Caries. *See* **Bone.**

Catalepsy.—*Can. ind.* 3—30, 3h. If after a fair trial lasting
over some weeks this fails, *Cicuta vir.* 3, 3h. Coming on at
monthly period, *Mosch.* 30, 8h. With opisthotonus, *Angust.*
6, 1h. With opisthotonus; with emotional disturbance, *Ign.*
3—30, 1h. After fright: (1) *Acon.* 3, 4h.; (2) *Gels.* 30, 4h.;
(3) *Op.* 30, 4h. From jealousy, (1) *Hyo.* 30, 4h.; (2) *Lach.*
30, 4h. From joy, *Coff.* 30, 4h.

Cataract.—Soft, *Colch.* 1, 4h. From injury, *Con.* 3, 4h. Capsular opacity, *Euphras.* 3x, 4h.; lotion of *Euphras.* φ (ten drops
to the ounce) three times a day. Hard, cataract in the early
stage, concentric opaque laminæ, *Calc. c.* 6, 4h. Afterwards,

if necessary, *Phos.* 3, 4h. Later stages, *Silic.* 6, 4h. *Calc. fluor* 30—200. One dose per week for 4 weeks followed by *Sulph.* 30—200 one dose per week for 2 weeks followed by *Calc. flour.* again for 4 weeks then *Sulph.* again for 2 weeks —repeat etc. etc. Many cataracts will recede under this treatment. *Calc. iod.* 30—200 is also useful. For diabetic cataract, *see* treatment for **Diabetes.**

Catarrh, NASAL.—GENERAL TENDENCY TO.—*Merc. sol.* 6, 8h. In pale, fair, strumous subjects, *Calc. c.* 6, 8h. In patients subject to irritation of the skin, *Sulph.* 6, 8h. In chilly subjects with unhealthy complexion and constipation, *Na. mur.* 6, 8h.

ACUTE NASAL. *See* **Cold.**

CHRONIC NASAL.—In weakly, debilitated subjects, *Ars. i.* 3x, gr. ii. 8h. Where there is constipation and tendency to skin eruptions about the orifice, or behind the ears, *Graph.* 6, 8h. Fluent, intermittent; with much sneezing; chilliness; constipation, *Nat. m.* 3—6, 8h. Depression, offensive discharge, bones of nose sore, syphilitic or mercurialised subjects, *Aur. mur.* 3x, gtt. ii. 8h. Constant dropping of mucus from back of nose into throat, affection of Eustachian tube, *Hydrast.* 3, 4h. Yellow or white stringy discharge, or thick plugs, *Kali bichrom.* 3x, gtt. ii. 4h. Stinging and tickling in nose, with irritative swelling, with or without free discharge, *Sang.* 3, 4h. Swelling of nose and redness; obstinate catarrh; caries of bones, *Hippoz.* 6, 6h. *See* **Ozæna.**

CHRONIC CATARRH OF LARYNX, TRACHEA, AND BRONCHI.— Copious white expectoration, rattling in chest; white tongue, **nausea,** dyspnœa; vital depression, *Ant. tart.* 6, 6h. Broad, flabby tongue, clear mucus, *Merc. sol.* 6, 6h. In chilly subjects; enlarged spleen; constipation, *Nat. m.* 6, 6h.

CHRONIC CATARRH OF ALIMENTARY TRACT.—Strumous subjects, *Calc. c.* 6, 8h. Patients with tendency to eruptions, *Sulph.* 6, 8h. Blonde, impressionable subjects, *Puls.* 3, 8h. White, loaded, foul tongue, nausea, thirst, much mucous expectoration from the throat, *Ant. crud.* 6, 8h.

CATARRH of almost any mucous surface; yellow or white; tough and stringy, *Hydrast. c.* 1—3, 4h.

Catarrhal Pneumonia. *See* **Pneumonia.**

Catheterism.—A dose of *Acon.* 1 or 3 given shortly before passing a catheter will prevent pain if there is any difficulty. *See* **Traumatic Fever.**

Cellulitis (INFLAMMATION OF CONNECTIVE TISSUE: FIRST STAGE OF ABSCESS.)—*Silic.* 6, 4h. *See also* Abscess.

Cerebro-Spinal Meningitis. *See* **Meningitis.**

Chafing. *See* **Excoriation.**

Chancre.—HARD.—*Merc. sol.* 6, 8h.; application to the sore of water-dressings only. *See* **Syphilis.**

SOFT.—*Merc. sol.* 6, 8h.; to be constantly kept cleansed. Should the sore become PHAGEDÆNIC whilst taking *Merc.*, give *Nit. ac.* 1, 2h.; application of *Iodoform powder*, and repeated irrigation. If no *Merc.* has been given before phagedæna appears, *Merc. cor.* 3, 2h., and *Iodoform* externally. *See* **Bubo.**

Change of Life, SUFFERING FROM.—Nervousness, numbness in various parts, "sinking" sensation, flushings, constipation, sensation of ball in the throat, *Ign.* 3, 6h. Restlessness, sleeplessness, "sinking," unhappy state of mind, *Act. r.* 3, 4h. Flushings, symptoms worse on waking from sleep, external pressure (even of clothing) intolerable, melancholic, irritable, *Lach.* 6, 6h. Flushing < evening and when exercising, perspirations, *Sul. ac.* 5, 4h. Rush of blood to head and heat of face; nose-bleed, *Graph.* 30, 4h. Flushes and sudden perspiration, *Jab.* 6, 2—4h. Leucorrhœa, sacral pain, persons of dark complexion and fine delicate skin, *Sep.* 6, 6h. Loss of appetite, "biliousness," taste of bile in mouth on waking, flushings, *Kali. c.* 6, 6h. Great irritability and nervousness, depression of spirits, sensation of ball in the throat, sleeplessness, *Valer.* 3, 6h. Skilful constitutional prescribing is of unquestionable value.

Chapped Hands. *See* **Hands.**

Charbon. *See* **Malignant Pustule.**

Cheloid.—(1) *Silic.* 3, gr. v. 8h.; (2) *Fluor. ac.* 6, 8h.; (3) *Graphit.* 3, gt. v.—30, 8h.; (4) *Nit. ac.* 12, 8h. (5) *Carcinosin* 30 or 200. 3 doses in one day at 6 hourly intervals in addition to the low potency remedy *viz. silic.* 3; *Fluor. ac.* 6; *Graph.* 3; etc.

Chest, PAINS IN.—From taking cold, *Acon.* 3, 2h. From overexertion *Arn.* 1, 2h. Sharp, cutting pains catching the breath, worse by motion or touch, *Bry.* 3, 2h. Pressure with stitches, breathing, motion and contact all painful, left side especially affected, *Ran. b.* 3, 2h. Stitches beneath the right ribs, *Chel.* 1x, 2h. Pain under left breast, with amenorrhœa, *Puls.* 3, 2h. Rheumatic pains in the chest, *Act. r.* 3, 2h. Sharp pain through lower part of left side of chest, *Oxal. ac.* 3, 2h.

STERNUM.—Pressure external and internal, *Ruta* 3, 2h. Oppression, and pressure beneath, *Samb.* 3, 2h. Pain internally behind sternum; spasmodic pressure behind middle of, *Chel.* 1x, 3h. Pressure in lower part; painful to touch, *Ran. b.* 3, 2h. Cutting under sternum when coughing; pressing pain beneath sternum when coughing, with a feeling of warmth and rattling, *Kali. nit.* 3, 4h. Aching in sternum and oppression of breath; cutting in middle of chest; shooting pains beneath; stitches, *Sul.* 3, 4h. Violent continual gnawing behind lowest part, external painfulness, *Ran. s.* 3, 2h. Burning soreness behind xiphoid cartilage, *Ran. s.* 3, 2h. Burning sensation under sternum, *Sang.* 3, 2h. Suffocative post-sternal pain occurring on walking, *Jug. cin.* 3, 2h.

DROPSY OF. *See* Hydrothorax and Pleurisy.

TIGHTNESS, OPPRESSION, ETC. *See* Lungs, Heart, Pleurisy, Breathing, and Cough.

Chicken-pox.—For initial fever, *Acon.* 3, 2h. When the vesicles form, *Ant. tart.* 6, 2h. When the fever is over, *Merc. sol.* 6, 4h. If there is much itching, application of *Camphorated oil* (*Camphora*, ʒi., *Ol. oliv.* ʒiv.) to the pocks with a camel-hair-brush.

Chilblains.—TENDENCY TO.—Blonde girls with delayed menstruation; more painful when hot, *Puls.* 3, 8h. Strumous subjects, *Calc. c.* 6, 8h. Patients with irritable skins, *Sulph.* 3, 8h. In nervous subjects with tendency to enlarged thyroid; chilly, stout persons, *Thyr.* 3, gr. v. 8h.

SIMPLE CHILBLAINS.—More painful when cold, *Agar.* 1, 3h.; *Tamus* φ, applied with brush, night and morning. If in girls with delayed and scanty menses, *Puls.* 3, 6h.; *Tamus* φ externally. From defective circulation, *Calc. mur.* 3x, gr. viii, 8h. Locally *Tamus* ointment, at very first sign of chilblains, rubbed in night and morning is most useful.

INFLAMED.—Dusky red, much burning, *Rhus t.* 3, 6h. Application of *Rhus* ointment (*Rhus t.* φ, ʒi., Vaseline ʒi.). Dark, purplish, *Verat. v.* 3, 3h.; application of lotion of *Verat. v.* (*Ver. v.* φ, ʒii., Spirit of Wine, ʒii., Aq. ad. ʒi.).

BROKEN.—*Petrol.* 3, gtt, i. 3h. *Calend.* ointment (ʒi.—Vaseline ʒi.) to be kept applied. Suppurating, *Hep. s.* 5, 6h.

Chilliness. *See* **Shivering.**

Chlorosis. *See* **Anæmia** and **Menstruation.**

Cholera Asiatica.—PREVENTION.—Wear next the skin a plate of copper (6 in. by 4, for a man of large size; 5 in. by 3 for a small man, and for a woman; 4 in. by 2 for children). Let it be fastened round the waist by straps attached to longitudinal slits cut in the ends of the plate, which should be oval. Let the plate rest on the front of the abdominal wall and let it be made slightly concave, so as to adapt itself to the shape of the body. The plate should be worn day and night. It may be cleansed from time to time by rubbing with vinegar. When Cholera is epidemic, *Tincture of Camphor* should be taken once or twice a day, in doses of two or three drops on sugar. Can cause nausea if taken in water.

In addition to this, if the person to be protected is much exposed to the disease, one or two drops of *Cuprum aceticum* 3x should be given in a little water night and morning.

PRELIMINARY SYMPTOMS.—In cholera times, whenever diarrhœa occurs, give Rubini's *Tincture of Camphor*, three drops on a lump of sugar, every fifteen minutes to every hour, according to the urgency of the symptoms, until the diarrhœa is completely removed.

Should an attack come on without premonitory diarrhœa, sudden coldness and lividity seizing the patient, give Rubini's *Camphor*, three drops every ten minutes. This may be given if there is diarrhœa at the same time, provided it is not excessive.

The patient should now be kept at rest, and as warm as possible, hot flannels being applied to the abdomen, and hot bottles to the feet. No solid food whatever should be given; water may be taken *ad libitum;* and small pieces of ice may be given to suck. Milk is the best food, if it is tolerated. Movement is to be avoided. It is better to treat patients at their own homes if at all possible, as the very fact of moving a patient into hospital may make the difference between death and recovery.

If under *Camphor* reaction does not come on, but, on the contrary, the patient becomes worse, vomiting and purging setting in with violent pains in the body, cold sweat on forehead, give *Veratrum album* 1, gtt. ii. 10m. If the patient complains much of cramps with the vomiting and purging, *Cuprum acet.* 3x. gtt. ii. 10m. If the collapse deepens in spite of treatment, and the patient is in danger more from general depression than the discharges, *Arsenicum alb.* 3x. gtt. i. every ten minutes. When the collapse is most profound, respiration slow, deep, gasping, the patient appearing dead in the intervals; collapse supervening on cessation of discharge, *Hydrocy. acid.* 1, gtt. ii. 10m. Rice-water stools, painless, *Ricin.* 1, gtt. ii. 1h. With tympanites, *Colch.* 3x. gtt. ii. ½—1h.

Cholera Infantum.—Watery diarrhœa, crying, complaining, biting fists, sleepless, *Acon.* 3, ½h. Anxiety, crying, intolerance of milk, regurgitation of food an hour after taking, tendency to convulsions, *Æthus. cyn.* 3, ½h.

Cholerine—English Cholera—Cholera Nostras.—Bilious vomiting and bilious stools, *Dios. v.* 3, ½h. Violent cramps, *Cupr. arsen.* 6, ¼h. Blueness, cramps, vomiting, watery diarrhœa, *Verat. alb.* 3, ½h. Explosive stools, *Elater.* 1, 2h.

Chondritis. *See* **Perichondritis;** *also* **Bones.**

Chordee.—This is generally an accompaniment of gonorrhœa, and will yield to the treatment prescribed for that disease. If it should occur independently, or refuse to yield to the ordinary treatment, give *Kali brom.* gr. iii. at bedtime, to be repeated in an hour if necessary. *See* **Gonorrhœa.**

Chorea.—Twitching, jerking, restless; in children with bluish faces and fingers; subject to chilblains; the most commonly indicated remedy *Agaric.* 3, 3h. If this fails to cause improvement within two weeks, *Ver. v.* 3, 3h.; and application, to the spine, with the hand, night and morning, of a lotion consisting of equal parts of *Verat. v. φ*, Spirit of Wine, and water. When of emotional origin, or when accompanied by emotional symptoms, *Ign.* 3, 3h. When due to fright, and when the patient is frightened at animals and imaginary things, *Stram.* 3, 3h. When fear of the original fright remains, give *Opium* 200, 3 doses at four hourly intervals in one day. Await results. Where there are symptoms of rheumatism, restlessness at night, *Act. r.* 3, 2h. If there is general debility, *Arsen.* 3, 6h. In scrofulous children, *Calc. phos.* 3, gr. v. 8h. Inveterate cases, *Cupr. acet.* 3, 8h. [In all cases the patient should be well fed; cod-liver oil should be given to children when it is tolerated.]

Chronic Diseases.—In the treatment of cases of chronic disease homœopathy has very great advantages over the old school, but in my experience there are few homœopaths who take full advantage of it. It is necessary, in the first place, for the practitioner to understand the conditions of success, and in the next place it is necessary for the practitioner to make the patient understand. The first condition is —TIME. A constitution cannot be radically changed for the better in a week or a month, and it is seldom accomplished in a year. Hahnemann demanded at least two years for the cure of a chronic case. It is well when such a case comes for treatment for the first time to refuse to undertake it unless the patient will promise all the time required. Or a patient may be told that his immediate condition may be ameliorated, but he must not consider himself cured, and must not be surprised by a return of the symptoms at some future time. The young homœopath will be saved much disappointment if he understands this. A case comes to him, and the first prescription answers admirably. The patient thinks he is cured, and if the doctor does not understand the real nature of the case, he is apt to think so too. If he is aware of the chronically operating cause, he is prepared for the backward swing of the pendulum, and knows how to meet it. Another point to be remembered is that cases of this kind do not need to be seen frequently (except for intermediate acute phases). As a rule, once a month is quite often enough. If they are seen too frequently, there is not time to properly apprehend the evolution of the medicinal action, and the practitioner is in danger of changing it too frequently and spoiling his case. The true nature of chronic disease was first pointed out by Hahnemann, and his elucidation is most helpful in practice. The term "chronic disease" in his sense has a different meaning from the same term in ordinary medical writings, and though both schools would apply the term to the same case in many instances, it is necessary to clearly understand the difference in the signification. In ordinary medical language a case of acute rheumatism which fails to clear up properly, but goes lingering on for months or throughout the rest of life, is said to have become "chronic"; or a case may never have had an acute stage, and having a slow, non-febrile course, it is also "chronic rheumatism." Arthritis deformans is always a "chronic disease" from first to last. These, in the language of ordinary medicine, are "chronic diseases." With Hahnemann a chronic disease is a condition of chronic constitutional poisoning analogous to an acute disease due to poisoning with an acute poison. Typhoid is an acute disease due to an acute poison which has an evolution ending in recovery or death. *Syphilis*, on the other hand, is a "chronic disease," due to a chronic poison. *Psora* is another chronic poison having a chronic evolution, and if not cured lasts throughout life, manifesting from time to time in some form or another, in the intervals subsiding into latency. *Sycosis*, or the chronic state of ill-health which manifests itself in the production of fig-warts, completes the trinity of "chronic miasms" as described by Hahnemann. Under the last is sometimes included another, the Cow-pox dyscrasia, or "Vaccinosis," of which the leading vegetable antidote is *Thuja occidentalis*. Most of the "chronic diseases" of ordinary medicine are phases or manifestations of one or other of the chronic poisons or "miasms" of Hahnemann. Hahnemann took a larger view of the history of a patient. He saw in these skin affections, asthma, intestinal catarrh, neuralgias, tumours, or what not, manifesting in the same patient at different times, not so many different diseases, but only so many different manifestations of one continuously acting chronic poison. Thus it happens that the term "chronic disease" as understood by him would apply to many cases of chronic disease as understood by old-school writers; only, with him it would apply not to the particular manifestation then present, but to the entire pathological history of the patient. It was not until Hahnemann recognised the unity underlying diverse disease-manifestations that he was able to treat these cases successfully; and it is the shortsighted view of modern medicine in regarding every manifestation of disease as a separate and independent or local affair that has given surgery its present tremendous vogue.

The treatment of chronic diseases is the test of a homœopath. It cannot be described in detail in a treatise like this. The treatment of the active manifestations of the chronic miasms will be found, indeed, throughout the work under the appropriate headings. As in the case of intermittent fever, in which the best time to give the curative remedy is *after* the paroxysm, so the best time to treat a constitutional state is after an acute manifestation is over.

The chronic miasms act in a direction *from without inward*. This is evident in syphilis and sycosis and in the initial skin affections of psora. But all three may be hereditary, and, in my experience, psora, as at present seen, generally *is* hereditary. But, in any case, as Hahnemann pointed out, in order to cure it, it is necessary to find remedies whose action is *from within outward*. Hence, in the process of a constitutional cure, it frequently happens that an eruption appears on the skin or an old eruption reappears. This is to be regarded as a favourable indication, and by no means is the skin affection to be treated as a local affair.

In diagnosing the constitutional remedy for any patient, the totality of symptoms will always rule, but there are some points which are of more importance than others. I have dealt with this subject in the *Introduction*, but it will be useful here to take by way of illustration the *Sulphur* type, as *Sulphur* is the chief of antipsorics. It is so by reason of its own symptoms corresponding more closely and extensively to psora than those of any other remedy. The typical eruption of *Sulphur* is a crop of itching and itch-like pustular vesicles, the itching being relieved by scratching. The most characteristic organismic symptom is the "sinking," all-gone sensation at the epigastrium, occurring in the forenoon, and more especially at 11 o'clock. When patients say they cannot eat breakfast, but must have something to eat at 11 o'clock *Sulphur* must be thought of. The characteristic mental type of the *Sulph.* patient is somewhat melancholy, with a turn for theological and philosophical speculations. The head is hot and the feet cold. Often we have only to shake hands with a *Sulphur* patient to learn his remedy: the hot sweaty hand of *Sulph.* is very characteristic. The feet may be cold, but more generally they are hot and perspiring. The symptoms are < by washing, < at night, and < by warmth. When patients complain that all their sufferings are worse as soon as they get warm in bed, *Sulph.* is most likely required.

In connections with *Sulph.* it is necessary to study *Calcarea*, as it is in many ways the antithesis of *Sulph.* The *Calc.* patient has irritability of temper, chilliness, cold, perspiring head, cold, clammy hands and feet, the legs feeling as if damp stockings were on. The *Calcarea* patient seeks warmth. *Calcarea* has sinking sensations like *Sulph.*, though not at the same characteristic times. It frequently happens that there is a mixture of the characteristics of these remedies present, and then choice must be made between them. *Lyc.*, *Nat. mur.*, *Silic.*, *Psor.*, all the nosodes and many others must be studied in this connection.

In prescribing for constitutional states it is well to give remedies in the attenuations. I prefer the 30th. The repetition must depend on circumstances. I sometimes give one dose a day or one a week. A placebo may be given in the interval according to circumstances. In treating chronic cases, it is almost essential to success for the practitioner not to reveal the name of the remedy to the patient.

Cicatrix.—For the Removal of.—(1) *Thiosin.* 6, 8h. (2) *Phyt.* 1x, 8h. Inflammation of, *Fluor. ac.* 6, gtt. ii. 8h.

Cheloid.—*Sil.* 3, gr. v. 8h. *Carcinosin* 30 or 200. 3 doses at four hourly intervals in one day, in addition to any other remedy recommended under this heading.

Circulation.—Feeble.—Frequent and regular open-air exercise; sponging with cold or tepid water in which sea-salt has been dissolved, and rapid friction. Great blueness of surface, *Rhus t.* 3, 8h.; Coldness of the hands and feet, unhealthy complexion, *Nat. mur.* 6, 8h. Cold feet, hot head; sinking sensation in forenoon, *Sul.* 30, 8h. Cold hands and feet, legs feel as if damp stockings were on, *Calc. c.* 6—30, 8h. Sensitive to slightest draught of air, *Sil.* 6—30, 8h. *See* **Chilblains, Heart, Liver, Anæmia.**

Cirrhosis. *See* **Liver.**

Clavus Hystericus.—In general, *Kali carb.* 6, ½h. Great impressionability of the senses, nervousness, restlessness, chilliness, agonising at height of attack, and often passing off with copious flow of limpid urine, *Ign.* 3, 1h. In spare, active, dark subjects, *Nux v.* 3, 1h. In blonde persons, especially if occurring on left side of the head, *Puls.* 3, 1h. In the intervals, the same medicine as indicated by the attack may be given thrice daily in the third attenuation, and proper diet and regimen prescribed, if these are not what they should be. In persons who have been much vaccinated, *Thuja* 30 once a week. *See also* **Headache.**

Clergyman's Sore Throat. *See* **Throat.**

Climacteric Sufferings. *See* **Change of Life.**

Coccygodynia (PAIN AT THE EXTREME POINT OF THE SPINE).—Drawing or bruised pain, *Caust.* 6, 8h. Sensation of a heavy load hanging on the end of coccyx, dragging the patient down, *Ant. t.* 6, 4h. Tearing, jerking, *Cicuta v.* 1, 6h. Soreness on pressure, *Silic.* 6, 8h. Pain in, whilst sitting; < by walking or touch, *Kali bichr.* 3x, gr. ii. 6h. Consequences of a fall on coccyx, *Hyper.* 6 or 30, 4h. Coccyx seems elongated, extremely sensitive to pressure, aches all the time, must have cushion, *Xanth.* 1, 4h.

Cold.—Soon after the exposure to cold, whilst the chill is still present, *Camph.* 1x, gtt. ii., on sugar (or *Camph.* φ pilules ii.) every 15 minutes until the chill passes off and glow succeeds. Some time after the exposure to cold, when the actual feeling of chill has to a large extent or entirely passed off, *Acon.* 1, ½h. for six doses; afterwards every two hours. Exposure to wet and cold when overheated, or from iced-drinks, *Bellis p.* 3, 2h. If coryza has already set in, sneezing and running from the nose, *Euphras.* 1x, 2h. Cold fully established, thick, unirritating discharge, *Merc. sol.* 6, 3h. Thin, irritating discharge, *Ars.* 3, 2h. Catarrh, with inflamed swelling of the nose, which is painful; pressure on larynx; hoarseness, *Hep.* 6, 2h. Fluent, watery, acrid coryza; constriction in throat; tickling, dry cough; tight chest, *Sang.* 1, 2h. Tightness at root of nose; tickling cough from inspiring cold air; constant sneezing, acrid coryza, > out of doors; chilly, *All. cep.* 6, 2h. Thin, unirritating discharge, nose red and swollen, *Kali iod.* 1x, 2h. "Stuffy cold," nose blocked, but little discharge, tightness at the chest, *Nux v.* 1—3, 2h. Loss of smell with cold, *Sul.* 1, 4h. Loss of taste with cold, *Puls.* 1, 4h. Loss of taste and smell with cold, *Mag. mur.* 6, 4h.

INFLUENZA COLD.—(1) *Arsen.* 3, 2h. (2) *Nat. mur.* 6, 2h. If the bone pains are very distressing, *Eupat. perfol.* 3, 2h.

TENDENCY TO BACILLINUM—INFLUENZINUM 30 (combined) one dose per month. May be used in conjunction with other treatment. Is purely prophylactic and will not assist acute phase of cold. *Nat. mur.* 6, 8h., continued for one or two months. In women with too frequent and too profuse menstruation, *Calc. c.* 6, in the same way. *See also* **Catarrh, Nasal.**

Coldness.—Coldness of back, *Aco.* 3, 2h. As if cold water running down the back, *Arsen.* 3, 2h. As if a lump of ice in lumbar region, *Agar.* 3, 2h.

Colic.—With Diarrhœa, see **Diarrhœa.** Cutting colic relieved by pressure or bending double; sensation as if the intestines were being squeezed between two stones, diarrhœa, *Coloc.* 3, 20m.—2h. Griping, drawing, bursting, or cutting pains; flatulent spasms, < by pressure, by doubling up, > by standing erect and by moving about, *Dioscor.* 3, 20m.—2h. When a spot is as if gripped with the nails; when the transverse colon is distended like a pad, *Bell.* 1, 20m.—2h. Flatulent colic when the flatus collects in several spots; intolerance of pain, < at night and by warmth, *Cham.* 6, 20m.—1h. Colic from anger, *Staph.* 3, 1h. In young children, the pain > by firm pressure; pain coming on gradually and passing off gradually, *Stan.* 6, 20m.—1h. Flatulent colic in older children, with or without worms, *Cina* 1, 20m.—2h. Flatulent colic accompanying menstruation, *Cocc. i.* 3, 20m.—1h. With obstinate constipation, *Plumb. acet.* 3, gr. ii.—6, 2h. Flatulent colic in spare, dark subjects, with constipation, *Nux v.* 1, ½h. With blueness, cold sweat on forehead, and symptoms of collapse, *Verat. alb.* 1, ½h.

FROM LEAD.—*Opium* 1x, 2h. Should this fail *Alumen* 3, gr. iii—6, 3h.

Colitis.—*See* **Mucous Colitis.**

Collapse.—Cold, blue, cold sweat on forehead, *Verat.* 30, ½h. Head hot, hot sweat, craves air, cold breath, *Carb. v.* 30, ½h. Skin cold, livid, will not be covered, *Camph.* φ, ½h.

Coma must be treated according to the disease of which it is a symptom. *See* **Apoplexy, Sleep, Delirium, Diabetes, Fevers,** etc.

Coma Vigil.—*Hyosc.* 3, ¼h.

Comedo (Retained secretions of sebaceous follicles).—(1) *Baryt. c.* 6, 8h. (2) *Selen,* 6, 8h. (3) *Sulph.* 30 once a week, for three or four weeks, on purely local indications. When there is also inflammation of the follicles, *see* **Acne.**

Concussion. *See* **Brain, Spine, Bruises.**

Condylomata.—*Thuja* 1 or 30, 6h.; *Thuja* φ to be painted on the growths night and morning. About anus, *Euphras.* 1—30, 6h. Figwarts, *Sabin* φ—30, 6h. Syphilitic exuberant, cauliflower-like, easily bleeding, *Nit. ac.* 1 or 30, 6h.; and ointment of the *Acid Nitrate of Mercury* (B. P.) may be applied night and morning. (4) *Medo.* 100, 2 or 3 times a week.

Congestion.—General.—*Verat. v.* 1, 2h. *See* **Brain, Liver, Lungs,** etc.

Conjunctivitis. *See* **Eye,** Inflammation of.

Constipation.—In sedentary people, dark, spare; ineffectual urging; frequent desire, but only very little passes, *Nux v.* 1—30, 8h. After *Nux,* if this is insufficient; in persons who are subject to skin eruptions; who suffer from fainting spells, flushing of heat to the head, or sinking sensation at the pit of the stomach, especially about 11 a.m.; frequent ineffectual urging to stool, insufficient stool, sensation as if something remained behind in rectum, piles which bleed periodically, *Sul.* 3—30, 8h. Torpor of bowels, stool hard, large, dry, *Bry*. 3, 6h. Torpor of bowels; stool small, hard pieces like marbles; dark brown, with drowsiness, *Op*. 3, 6h. Drowsiness, chilliness, flatulence, *Nux mos*. 30, 6h. Very obstinate constipation, dry, lumpy stool; painless, or with severe colic and retraction of abdomen, *Plumb. acet*. 3, gr. ii. —6, 6h. Hard, scanty stool, painful in passing, burning in rectum, passage of blood, *Nit. ac*. 1, 4h. Large, knotty stool, covered with white shreds of mucus, expelled with much effort; associated with delayed menses. *Graph*. 6, 6h. Hard knotty stool, with or without blind piles, much pain in the back; sensation of fullness in rectum after stool; sensation in rectum as if full of small sticks, *Æsc. h*. 1, 6h. Accumulation of fæces in rectum, *China*. 1, 2h. Stool like sheep's dung; pain in region of liver, *Magnes. mur*. 5, 6h. Stool tough, shiny, knotty, like sheep's dung, oily; pressure in rectum as if fæces lodged in it, *Caust*. 5, gtt. ii. 4h. Stool hard, small, dry, crumbling, *Zinc. met*. 6, 4h. Black, pitchy stool, *Zinc. mur*. 3, 4h. Stool retained, sensation as if rough fæces remained in rectum, feeling of constriction at anus arresting it; especially in ill-nourished persons with unhealthy complexion; associated with deficient menses, *Nat. m*. 3, gr. ii.—6, 6h. Slow, insufficient stool; sensation of weight or ball in anus not relieved by stool, *Sep*. 6, 4h. With distention of the abdomen, flatulence passing downwards, water high-coloured, with deposit of lithates, hard, difficult stool, *Lyc*. 6, 6h. Dilated and paralysed rectum; lumpy stools, *Alumina*, 6, 6h. Stools hard as stones; passes much blood; constipation of uterine or rectal cancer, *Alumen*, 30, 6h. No desire for stool; constipation alternating with looseness of the bowels; constipation with dull headache; after abuse of purgatives; with foul tongue; with piles, *Hydrast*.

1, 6h. Stool difficult to pass on account of hardness and size, *Verat. a.* 3, 6h. *Palliatives:* A satisfactory evacuation can often be obtained by *Merc. dulc.* ix. gr. iii. 4h. for a few doses. Persons who have been in the habit of taking purgatives and fear to leave them off, *Sul. φ*, at bedtime. A glass of cold water drunk fasting will often suffice to ensure a good evacuation. Or a glass of cold water may be taken at bedtime; or, if cold water is not tolerated, hot water instead. Or this: a tablespoonful of coarse treacle put into a tumbler of water overnight, and drunk by sips in the morning whilst dressing. In constipation in infants, manna used for sweetening their food is often of great service. *See under* DIET—INFANTS. If other things fail, *Hydrast φ*, gtt. iii. in a wine-glassful of water, taken in the morning fasting, acts as a mild aperient. A sitz-bath every second night (65°—75°F.), for five or ten minutes, the body and limbs being kept thoroughly warm during the time, is often of great assistance where there is torpor of the bowels. A cold water or tepid water compress may be worn across the body at night. Whenever constipation is one of many symptoms of disordered health, the medicines directed to the chief disorder will usually remove the constipation also: *Spigelia* in heart affections, *Iris v.* in migraine, *Gels.* in headaches.

Constitutional Treatment. *See* **Chronic Diseases.**

Consumption, Phthisis Pulmonalis, Tuberculosis Pulmonalis. Whenever available, modern orthodox treatment should be sought.—THREATENED.—Acid dyspepsia, intolerance of milk, in subjects inclined to be fat, *Calc. c.* 6, 6h.; the same in thin subjects, *Calc. iod.* 3x, 6h. Where rapid wasting is

the most prominent symptom, *Iod.* 2x, 6h.; or *Bacillinum**
30, 100, or 200, three or four globules once every one, two,
or three weeks, according to Dr. Burnett's directions (the
value of which I have amply confirmed). This given alone,
or with indicated remedies in the intervals, will prove
marvellously efficacious in all states of "consumptiveness,"
threatened consumption, or illness other than consumption
in patients whose family is consumptive. A convenient way
of dispensing *Bacillinum* is to order four globules to be put
into five grains of *Sacch. Lact.* and made into a powder.

CHRONIC TUBERCULAR, CONSUMPTION FOLLOWING CHRONIC
PNEUMONIA, FORMATION OF CAVITIES IN THE LUNGS.—
Bacillinum 30—200, may be given as directed above in
almost all cases. It will not help all cases, and where no
apparent benefit follows or where there is aggravation of
symptoms it must be discontinued. In general the most
useful medicine is *Ars. iod.* 3x, gr. iv. or gtt. ii., thrice
daily, immediately after food. (This is apt to cause pains in
the abdomen, and even diarrhœa after a time, and then it
should be omitted for a few days. I have generally found this
attenuation the most satisfactory, but I have also used the
30th with great advantage. The lower triturations do not
keep well, but the tincture does, and is very effective. If the
Ars. iod. does no good, and when it ceases to do good, a
selection may be made from the following.) Chronic pneumonic phthisis with tendency to bleeding, *Calc. ars.* 3x, gr.
v. 8h. In strumous subjects with tendency to enlarged
tonsils, *Calc. phos.* 3x—3, gr. v. 8h. Vomiting, *Kreas.* 3, 6h.
Stitching pains in the chest, cough between 2 and 3 a.m.;

* See *Cure of Consumption with its own Virus*, by Dr. J. C. Burnett.

expectoration of small granules; (Hahnemann said cases could hardly be cured without *Kali. c.*), *Kali. c.* 3, gr. v.— 200, 2h. Short cough, with expectoration of coagulated blood, *Nit. ac.* 30, 8h. (follows *Kali. c.* well). Chronic inflammation of small patch of lung with rusty expectoration, *Phos.* 3, 2h. Chronic inflammation of a considerable portion of lung; with night-sweat, constipation, loaded urine, *Lyc.* 6, 2h. Consolidation of lung, rattling of mucus in chest, hoarse cough, < at night, profuse yellow expectoration, *Hep. s.* 6, 2h. Where the cough is worst in the morning, and there are cutting pains about the chest, pain between the shoulders, *Bry.* 3, 2h. Where the cough is spasmodic, causing retching and vomiting of food, *Dros.* 6, 2h.; profuse perspiration, abundant sputa, yellowish or green, of sweet taste, *Stannum* 6, 2h. Where the skin is eruptive; in gouty or rheumatic persons; sinking sensation at 11 a.m., hot fainty spells, *Sul.* 3, 4h. (*Sulphur* should always be well indicated by the symptoms when given in cases of phthisis, and should never be continued beyond the time when these symptoms are well relieved.)

BLEEDING.—In "bleeding consumption" (Phthisis florida), where there is a great deal of bleeding and very little to be made out on examining the chest, *Ferr. acet.* 1x, gtt. ii. 10m. during an attack; as a preventive, 8h. In bleeding, where there is active congestion, dry skin, and fever; blood comes up with an easy hawking or a slight cough, nervousness, restlessness, fear of death, *Acon.* 3, 10m.—1h. according to urgency. Frequent bleedings of small amount, *Phos.* 3, 2h. Dry cough followed by spitting of blood, *Acalyph. ind.* 1x, ½—2h. Florid frothy blood without much cough, *Millefol.*

1x—30, ¼h. Florid frothy blood with cough and tickling behind sternum, *Ferr. acet.* 1x, gtt. ii. 10m.—1h. Dark or clotted blood, *Ham. φ*—3, ¼h. The same with cough and tickling behind sternum, especially if accompanied by nausea, *Ipec.* 3, ¼h. For the prevention of hæmorrhage the best treatment is that directed to the general state as indicated by the general phthisical symptoms.

HECTIC FEVER.—In a general way, *Arsen. iod.* 3x, gr. v. 8h. will keep this within bounds. If the fever is low and approaching typhoid, *Baptis,* 1, 2h. Dry skin, restlessness, irritating cough, *Acon.* 3, 1h.

PERSPIRATIONS.—Like the hectic fever, perspirations are as a rule best controlled by the remedy most indicated by the general condition. When they are so profuse as to constitute the leading symptom, *Jaborandi* 3x, 2h.

ACUTE TUBERCULAR CONSUMPTION (RAPID CONSUMPTION).— In premonitory dyspepsia, *Calc. c.* 6, 6h. In actual disease, *Calc. c.* 6, 2h. The same remedies as in chronic consumption, according to indications.

For particular indications of cough and pain in the side, *see* Cough, Chest, and Pleurisy.

Contusions. *See* Bruises.

Convulsions.—INFANTILE (DURING THE SEIZURE).—Flushed face, prominent throbbing fontanelle, from whatever cause, *Bell.* 3, ¼h. Pale face, sunken fontanelle, excitement without signs of congestion, *Zinc. sulph.* 3, ¼h. (If these characteristics are not prominently marked, the following indications will serve as guides.) During teething, in fretful children,

green watery stools, *Cham.* 6, ¼h. From eating indigestible
fruit, *Nux v.* 3, ¼h. With worm symptoms, *Cina.* 3, ½h.
With gastro-intestinal disorder and great pain, anguish,
intolerance of milk, *Æthusa cyn.* 3, ¼h. In whooping-cough,
Cupr. m. 6, ¼h.

PREVENTION.—The above-named medicines, according to the
indications given, at longer intervals (four times a day).
Diet and regimen must be attended to. In scrofulous and
rickety children the constitutional remedies must be given,
either alone or in alternation with any of the above. *See*
Scrofula and Rickets.

Cornea. *See* Eye.

Corns.—RECENT OR PAINFUL.—(1) *Ferr. picric* 3, 6h. (2) *Rad. br.*
30, once a fortnight. Inflamed or ulcerated, *Nit. acid.* 1, 6h.
A solution of *Salicyl. ac.* 1 in 5 painted on the corn at bed-
time every two or three nights is often very useful, or
Hydrastis ointment (*Hydr.* φ, ʒj, *Vaseline* ʒj).

Corpulence.—In addition to suitable regimen and diet, *Phytolacca Berry* φ Tablets ii. gtt. 8h. If this fails to do good
after a month's trial give (1) *Amm. brom.* 3x, 8h. (2) *Calc.
c.* 3, gr. v.—6, 8g. (3) *Calc. ars.* 3x, gr. ii. 8h. (A tablespoonful of lemon-juice in a little water, sweetened, may
be taken three times a day if it does not disagree.) *Thyroid*
tablets, gr. v. may be given once or twice a day.

Coryza. *See* Cold.

Cough.—*According to* GENERAL CHARACTERISTICS. *Short, dry,
irritative* cough; cough during sleep, *Aco.* 3, 2h. *Spasmodic,*
coming on in the night, waking the patient from sleep,

ending in bringing away a little phlegm, *Ars.* 3, 6h. Cough from tickling, as if from a feather in the throat or dust in the larynx; constant tickle under the middle of the sternum, causing a *hacking cough;* cough during and after eating, *Calc. c.* 6, 2h. Cough from rawness in larynx, < at night in bed before falling asleep; violent *spasmodic* cough with copious expectoration of mucus, *Sul.* 3, 2h. *Spasmodic* cough coming on between 2 and 3 a.m., stitches in the chest, *Kali. c.* 6, 6h. Cough on waking, on moving about in the morning, some expectoration at first (sometimes bloody), afterwards *dry*, < on entering a warm room, sharp pains in chest; cough with pain in head and chest as if they would burst; cough on lying down at night, must sit up, *Bry.* 3, 2h. *Dry hacking* cough from pharyngeal or laryngeal irritation, *Alumina* 6, 6h. *Irritative laryngeal* cough, < in evening and early night, *paroxysmal*, heat and redness of face and sparkling eyes; provoked by tickling in larynx as if dust were at the back of it, compelling a *hard dry* cough; induced by exertion, lying down, or very deep respiration; feeling of soreness in larynx, as if internally hot and sore, this soreness is felt when pressing the larynx externally; oppression and heat in chest, dyspnœa, *Bell.* 3, 2h. *Dry hollow, hoarse* cough in single shocks, or fits of coughing; with worm symptoms, *Cina* 3, 4h. *Dry* cough, but with sensation as if something were in the trachea which might be raised, or comes partly up and then goes back again; provoked by tickling in trachea (below that of *Bell.*), induced by touching trachea or pressing on it, or pressure of clothes, which the patient therefore loosens, or by throwing the head back, also by eating; occurring on awaking from sleep; accompanied by some hoarseness and sore throat,

which shoots up into the ear, and by chronic tonsillitis
with oily white granules, *Lach.* 6, 6h. Cough *dry*, or with
scanty rusty sputa ; night and day; provoked by tickling in
the trachea pretty low down, and by a feeling of rawness
and soreness in trachea and bronchi; induced by a very
deep inspiration; accompanied and characterised by a *hoarse
barking* sound, by rawness of trachea and whole chest, and
by a peculiar and distressing weight across the chest;
hoarseness, *Phos.* 3, 2h. *Dry* cough in evening, provoked by
tickling high in trachea, in long *paroxysms*, induced by
speaking; provoking discharge of urine, voice almost gone;
trachea sore and raw, but not the chest, *Caust.* 6, 4h. *Dry,
short*, and *paroxysmal* cough or constant hack, in evening
and night on going to bed; provoked by tickling in supra-
sternal fossa; induced by pressure in that region and by in-
haling a breath of cool air, by a deep inspiration, and by
any variation in breathing; accompanied by great fatigue
from coughing and by stitches through the left lung,
Rumex crisp. 6, 3h. *Dry* cough with acrid coryza and lachrymation; induced by tickling in larynx, and each cough
seems as if it would split the larynx in two; patient cringes
under the pain, *All. cepa* 6, 2h. *Dry* cough, with dyspnœa,
from tickling high up in the throat; uninterrupted in the
evening; provoked by speaking or stooping, increases more
and more, and then stops [no soreness of larynx or fever
(*Bell.*), not affected by respiration (*Rumex*), not excited by
pressure on trachea (*Lach.*)], *Hep. s.* 6, 4h. *Violent* cough as
if he would *suffocate*, ending in *vomiting*, afterwards a feeling
as of a hard body in the epigastrium; then spitting of blood,
Hep. s. 6, 4h. *Dry laryngotracheal* cough, with *hoarseness*,
induced by attempting to draw a long breath, accompanied

by difficult inspiration, stitches in the lungs, and pain and burning behind the sternum, *Brom.* 12, 2h. *Barking* cough, with hacking and loss of voice, *Spong.* 3, 2h. Pains in larynx with desire to cough; smarting and lancinating pain in trachea; hoarseness; *croupy* cough; cough from tickling in throat, induced by effort to expand chest; increased by movement, *Iod.* 3x, 2h. *Chronic dry laryngeal* cough with stinging and smarting as if a small ulcer in the larynx, generally on one side, *Nit. ac.* 1—12, 2h. *Chronic asthmatic* cough, whether dry or moist; < night and morning; with constipation, *Nit. ac.* 1—12, 2h. *Chronic catarrhal* cough, mucous expectoration, easy and profuse, *Ant. tart.* 6, 3h. *Dry* cough even to vomiting, with anxious sweat at nights; cough with hoarseness, shaking the abdomen; tickling and soreness in trachea and chest; cough with raising of thick, yellow, lumpy, purulent expectoration, in large masses, offensive, *Sil.* 6, 4h. *Catarrhal inflammatory* cough, burning soreness from fauces down sternum, hoarseness, pains about the chest, *Merc. sol.* 6, 3h. Cough with excessive secretion (with much pale urine), *Scilla* 3, 2h. Cough loose by day, with much mucous expectoration, *dry and tickling* on lying down at night, disappears on sitting up in bed, *Puls.* 3, 2h. *Explosive* cough with fetid expectoration and fetid breath, *Caps.* 3, 2h. *Very noisy, dry, hard* cough, in violent short bursts, coming from low down shaking the whole body, *Osmium* 6, 2h. *Violent cough with little or no expectoration,* jarring the head, and straining the abdominal muscles; tickling in trachea, in middle of sternum, provoking cough; cough induced by exertion; after eating; when lying on back; in early morning after midnight; tightness of breath, *Nux v.* 3, 2h. Cough caused by itching in larynx, hoarse, *spasmodic ;* caused by a feeling as if vapour of sulphur were in trachea; < in evening and before midnight; < by cold and when eating or drinking, especially cold things; sputa greenish and tough, or yellow and purulent; Less often watery, offensive, *Carb. v.* 6, 2h. Cough > lying down and at night, *Mang.* 6, 2h. *Irritative shaking* cough of old people, *Seneg.* 3, 2h. *Dry night* cough, *Verbascum* φ, 2h. *Dry night* cough, constant when lying down, > by sitting up, *Hyos.* 3, 2h. *Periodical dry* cough, excited by itching, grating, tickling in throat and behind sternum; *in short bouts,* especially by lying down, laughing or talking; < at night, *Coni.* 3, 2h. Cough *waking the patient* after two hours sleep, *Aral. racem.* 3, 2h. *Suffocative cough* of children, waking them up in the middle of the night, *Samb.* φ, gtt. i. 1h. *Spasmodic choking* cough in nervous subjects, *Ambra* 6, 2h. *Whooping-cough; spasmodic, hysterical* cough, "minute-gun cough," *Corall. r.* 6, 2h. Cough from tickling in the larynx, with vomiting of food, *Dros.* 6, 2h. *Dry, violent laryngeal* cough, especially with constipation, *Nit. ac.* 30, 2h. *Spasmodic* cough with catarrh; with retching, *Ipec.* 3, 2h. *Incessant spasmodic* cough threatening to tear the chest; excited by peculiar tickling in fauces which is brought on by a sense of suffocation in the throat, *Lactuca* 3, 2h. *Incessant dry irritative* cough, excited by drawing the least cold air into the larynx, reading aloud or smoke, *Menth. pip.* 3, 2h. *Spasmodic* cough and *dyspnœa* in lymphatico-nervous constitutions; cough < by day, *Viola od.* 1, 2h. *Stomach* cough; *tormenting dry* cough, and insufferable tickling in throat, robbing the patient of rest; cough in asthmatic subjects, *Lobel.* 3, 2h. *Stomach* cough; < when the stomach is empty, *Bism.* 1, gr. iii. 3h. Spleen cough; a spasmodic cough, which seems to come from the region of the spleen; or cough with pain in spleen, *Scil. acet.* φ, gtt. v. 8h. Cough sympathetic of heart trouble; spasmodic and asthmatic coughs, wheezing and whistling in trachea and bronchi; soreness under sternum; prevalent at all times but < night; dry, harsh, rasping, hoarse, *Pru. virg.* φ, gtt. v. 4h.

COUGH ACCORDING TO CIRCUMSTANCES.—On entering a warm room, *Bry.* 3, 2h. During and after eating, *Calc. c.* 6, 2h. During eating, *Lach.* 6, 2h. After eating, *Nux v.* 3, 2h. Caused by exertion, *Bell.* 3, 2h. Excited by effort, *Ipec.* 3, 2h.

COUGH CAUSING OTHER SYMPTOMS.—Causes headache, *Nat. m.* 6, 2h.; in occiput, *Sul.* 6, 2h; stunning headache, *Æthus.* 3, 2h.; maddening, as if the skull would burst, *Nux v.* 3, 2h.; pain in heart, *Agar.* 1, 2h.; expulsion of urine, (1) *Caust.* 6, 2h.; (2) *Ferr.* 6, 2h.; (3) *Puls.* 3, 2h.; involuntary emission of urine, with tearing pain, *Alumina* 6, 2h. Night cough with involuntary passing of urine, *Colch.* 3x, 2h. Spasmodic dry cough, causing tears to come in eyes, and passing of urine, *Caps.* 3, 2h. Irritating cough, causing taste of blood in mouth, *Amm. c.* 3x, 2h. Cough causing taste of blood in the mouth, *Kali. bi.* 30, 2h. Cough causing taste of blood in mouth; cough arising from pit of stomach by paroxysms, but not in the night, *Nit. ac.* 30, 2h. Cough causing shattering in chest and abdomen; and sensation of a lump in the chest, *Sul.* 3, 2h. Cough causing soreness of chest and throat, *Ant. sul. aur.* 3, gr. v. 4h.

PECULIARITIES OF COUGHS.—Cold expectoration, *Coral.* 6, 4h.; sensation as if air-passages full of smoke, *Brom.* 6, 4h.;

painful sensation as of something lodged in the chest to be coughed up, nothing comes up, and coughing aggravates, *Abies n.* 3x, 2h.

See also **Bronchitis, Throat, Trachea, Whooping-cough.**
In many chest troubles a teaspoonful of pure glycerine taken three times a day has a healing effect.

Cracks in Skin.—HANDS. *See* **Hands,** CHAPPED.

NOSE.—Ulcerated nostrils, with stopped catarrh, *Petr.* 3, 6h.; vaseline locally. Scurf within nose, bleeding when blowing it, painful, disordered smell, *Graph.* 6, 6h.; Crusts about alæ nasi, *Nit. ac.* 6, 6h. vaseline locally.

LIPS.—Cracked and sore, *Graph.* 6, 6h. Cracked in centre, *Nat. mur.* 6, 6h. Painful cracks in corners of mouth, (1) *Petrol.* 3, 6h.; (2) *Cund.* φ, 8h. (Vaseline may be used locally at night in any case.)

Cramp.—IN THE CALVES.—From fatigue, *Arn.* 1, 2h. From no special cause, coming on in the night, *Nux v.* 3, 8h., to be repeated in the night if necessary. Should this fail, *Cupr. met.* 6, 8h. In the soles of the feet, *Colch.* 3, 4h. Cramps in the calves with icy coldness of the legs, *Camph.* 200, 8h. Cramps in calves, soles and toes, *Ferr.* 6, 8h.

Croup. — SPASMODIC — LARYNGISMUS STRIDULUS — MILLAR'S ASTHMA.—Pure spasm, without any cough, hoarseness, or signs of catarrh of the larynx. *Moschus* 3x, inhalations (a few drops of the tincture dropped into a small quantity of water, shaken, and held under the nose); internally, *Cuprum met.* 6, every ten minutes. Application to throat of sponge wrung out of hot water. Waking the patient from sleep,

Lach. 6, 10m. Hoarseness, sawing sound with breathing, *Spo*. 3, 10m. Air enters easily but cannot be expelled, *Chlor*. 1x—30, 15m.

PREVENTIVE TREATMENT.—In strumous subjects *Calc. c.* 6, 8h. Children of convulsive tendency, *Bell*. 3, 8h. Nervous, jerky children, with tendency to chorea, *Agar*. 3, 8h. Where the disease has been brought on by fright, *Ignat*. 3, 8h. Where there is a consumptive history, *Bacil*. 30—200 once a week. [These remedies may be continued for one or two months at a time, and after an interval of a week or two resumed if deemed necessary. Cold sponging and friction in morning, and the administration of cod-liver oil, are useful aids.]

CATARRHAL (Catarrh of the Larynx with Spasm of the Glottis). —Hoarse cough with or without expectoration, suffocative symptoms; dry skin, restlessness, anxiety, fear; from exposure to dry air, *Acon*. 3, gtt. i. every ten minutes. After *Acon*., dry hoarse barking cough, with sawing sound, no loose rattle, worse before midnight, *Spong*. 3, gtt. i. every ten minutes; application to the throat of sponge wrung out of hot water. Suffocating cough in infants, waking them in the middle of the night, accompanied by rough sibilant wheezing, but without true croup, *Samb*. φ—30, gtt. 1, ¼h. Rattling, choking cough, child chokes with every coughing fit; coughs till he chokes: attack comes on or grows worse after midnight, *Hep*. 6, 10m. till relieved. *See* **Laryngitis** and **Cough**. [Bœnninghausen's sequence of remedies for croup consisted of three powders—*Acon*. 200, *Hep*. 200 and *Spo*. 200, given in this order.]

MEMBRANOUS.—Inspiration very difficult, larynx drawn down, child chokes whilst drinking, *Brom*. 3x, 15m. Inhalations of

steam from hot water into which a few drops of *Bromine* 1x
have been dropped: the child's bed should be surrounded by
a tent, and the vapour conducted within. Tough, stringy,
yellowish expectoration, which is brought up with difficulty,
Kali bichrom. 6, ½h. Wheezing, sawing respiration, dry
barking cough, especially in children with dark hair and
eyes; child grasps throat with hand, *Iod.* 3x, 15m. Spasm of
glottis; air enters easily but cannot be expelled, *Chlor.* 1x—
30, 15m. If the child lies with neck stretched out, head bent
back, and gasping, *Ant. t.* 6, ¼h. *Spong.* and *Hepar.* when
the symptoms correspond to those described under last
heading. If the prostration is great, *Ars.* 3, ¼h.

ACCOMPANYING DIPHTHERIA.—The symptoms as described
under the remedies named in the two preceding sections
will decide the remedy to be chosen. The most commonly
indicated is *Iod.* 3x, ½h. Care must be taken not to raise the
child up into the sitting position if there is much prostration.
See **Diphtheria.**

Crusta Lactea. *See* **Impetigo.**

Cuts. *See* **Wounds.**

Cyanosis.—Congenital or idiopathic, (1) *Rhus t.* 3, 6h. (2)
Hydrocy. ac. 12, 8h. When from acquired heart disease, or
when symptomatic of other disorders, the patient must be
treated for the central disease.

Cystitis. *See* **Bladder.**

Dandruff.—Dry scurf, *Ars.* 3, 6h. Moist, *Sepia*, 6, 6h. Thick,
Sulph. 30, 6h. It may be advisable to use a mild sulphur

ointment at the same time. I find an ointment one-fourth the B.P. strength very effective. *See also* **Pityriasis.**

Deafness. *See* **Ear.**

Debility.—(Where a symptom of still active disease, the disease itself must be dealt with first.) Debility after acute disease; exhaustion after overwork or worry, *Calc. phos.* 3, gr. v. 8h. Debility after acute disease, such as diphtheria or typhoid fever, profound prostration, chilliness, desire to lie down constantly, *Psorin.* 30, 4h. General weakness, tendency to faint, loss of appetite, *Ars. iod.* 3x, gr. iii. thrice daily after food, to be continued as long as improvement continues, and omitted temporarily should pain in the body and looseness of the bowels come on. Non-febrile debility, with blueness and coldness, *Carb, v.* 6, 8h. Debility, with flushing to head or face; tired feeling in brain, *Ferr. phos.* 3, gr. v. 8h. Depression, weakness, anæmia, (1) *Helon.* φ, 8h.; (2) with constipation; earthy complexion; palpitation, *Nat. m.* 6, 8h; (3) *Cinchona rubra* φ, gtt. x. 8h. In over-wrought, nervously run-down women, *Mag. c.* 200, 4h. Irritability, weakness, loss of appetite, constipation, *Nux v.* 1, gtt. v. 8h. Nervous exhaustion, *Strych. nit.* 3x, gtt. v. 8h. Loss of vigour, timid, apprehensive, *Pip. methys.* φ—1x, gtt. x, 8h. Cardiac and general muscular depression and weakness, *Verat. alb.* 3, 6h. In fat, pale children, *Calc. c.* 6, 8h. In thin, rickety children, *Silic.* 6, 8h. From loss of blood or other animal fluids; from overwork or anxiety, *China*, 1x, 6h. With emaciation, *Iod.* 3x, 4h. *See also* **Anæmia.**

Nervous Debility.—*Ign.* 3, 6h. Failure of mental powers, tendency to perspiration, weakness without irritability, after excesses, *Phos. ac.* 1x—1, 3h. (Five drops of *Phos. ac.* 1x may be taken in a tumbler of water as a beverage with meals.) Loss of memory, apprehensive, *Anacar.* 3, 4h. Unconquerable drowsiness after meals, *Nux mosch.* 3, 2h. Nervous debility, sleeplessness; after influenza, *Scutel.* φ, gtt. v. 8h. *See* **Dyspepsia, Neurasthenia, Spermatorrhœa,** etc.

Delirium Tremens.—[Give the patient strong soup or beeftea.] *Scutel.* φ, gtt. x. in hot water. ½h. until relieved. If there is much gastric disorder, vomiting of mucus, *Ant. tart.* 3x, ¼h. In the early stage *Nux v.* 1, ½h. After it has passed its height, *Nux v.* 1, 1h. At the height of the delirium, if it is furious, with starting eyes, *Bell.* 1x, ¼h. If it is low, muttering, *Hyoscy.* 1, ¼h. Visions of animals, *Stram.* 3, ½h. *See also* **Alcohol Habit** and **Alcoholism.**

Delusions.—Things appear larger than they are, distances greater, time longer, *Cann. i.* 3, 2h. Things appear smaller than they are, *Plat.* 6, 2h.

Dengue-fever.—First paroxysm, *Acon.* 1, 1h., followed if necessary, by *Rhus t.* 3, 1h.; if bone pains very severe, *Eupator. perfol.* 1, 1h. Flushed face, rash, pains in head and eyes, low fever, drowsiness, *Echin.* φ, gtt. v. 2h. Second paroxysm, *Gels.* 1, 1h., followed, if necessary, by *Rhus t.* 3, 1h.

Dentition.—MORBID.—In pale children of soft fibre, teeth late in appearing, *Calc. phos.* 3, gr. v. 8h. In thin, irritable, cachectic children, extreme agitation and wakefulness whilst the teeth are being cut, the teeth often decaying as soon as they appear, *Kreas.* 6, 8h. With suppression of urine; child wakeful at night; screams as if frightened; startled look, clenches fingers; twitchings; picks nose; burning soreness and swelling of gums; otitis, *Tereb.* 3—30, 2h. With aphthæ, children start on any sudden noise; dread downward motion, *Borax* 30, 4h.

DISORDERS DURING.—Fever, restlessness, dry skin, *Acon.* 3, 2h. Fretfulness, with sour, green, watery diarrhœa; flushing of one cheek, *Cham.* 6, 2h. Diarrhœa, green stools, sour, *Calc. c.* 6, 2h., till relieved, then after each stool. Stools like chopped spinach, great irritability, *Mag. c.* 6, 2h. Diarrhœa, green stools, fetid, *Silic.* 6, 2h., till relieved, then after each stool. Great soreness of the gums, *Merc. sol.* 6, 2h. Nervousness and sleeplessness, *Act. r.* 3, 2h.

CONVULSIONS.—*Bell.* 1, ¼h. *See* Convulsions.

Depression of Spirits and Melancholia.—These cases often require very careful assessment and skilful homœopathic treatment along classical lines. From grief or worry; or at the change of life, *Ign.* 3, 6h. Melancholy, restlessness, irritability, anxiety, anguish, *Ars.* 3, 6h. Prostration, unappeasable restlessness, convulsive trembling, *Tarent.* 3, 6h. Religious melancholy with constipation, *Plumb. acet.* 6, 6h. Depression, with pain at the heart, *Spigel.* 3, 6h. Gloom as if a black pall were over everything; fears going crazy; suicidal; visions of rats, etc., *Act. rac.* 3, 4h. Suicidal melancholia; inquietude; hopelessness; < sunset to sunrise, *Aur. met.* 3, gr. v. 8h. Depression, timidity, taciturnity, aversion to society; from sexual causes, as enforced abstention, *Con.* 30, 6h. Sadness during the menses; depression, with palpitation on lying down at night, or after food, *Nat. m.* 6, 6h. Nymphomania, *Plat.* 3—6, 6h. With suppressed menses, *Sen. aur.* φ gtt. ii., unit doses repeated every 7 or

10 days. Acute melancholia, *Bell.* 3, 3h. Melancholia after typhus fever; and in girls at puberty, *Hell.* 3, 3h. *See also* Mania and Erotomania.

Derbyshire Neck.—*See* Goitre.

Diabetes.—INSIPIDUS (profuse flow of colourless urine containing no sugar). Night and day, *Scilla* 1, 3h. Chiefly in the night, *Phos. ac.* 1x, 3h.; failing this, *Murex purp.* 6, 3h., or *Uran. nit.* 3x—30, 8h.

MELLITUS (true diabetes, increased flow of urine containing sugar).—From nervous causes, *Phos. ac.* 1x, gtt. iii.—30, 8h. From digestive derangement, *Uran. nit.* 3x—30, gtt. v. 8h. Especially if accompanied with swollen ankles, *Arg. met.* 3, gr. v.—30, 8h. With restlessness, depression, irritation of the skin, *Cod.* 3x, 4h. In gouty persons, *Nat. sulph.* 3, gr. v. 8h. From a fall, *Arn.* 3, 6h. If these fail—(1) *Syzygium* 1x, gtt. v. 8h. (this is a good general remedy and may be given with others); (2) *Silica* 3, gr. v. 8h. Diabetic coma (acetonæmia), *Op.* 3x—30, 1h. [The proper diet will be prescribed; *see* Diet.]

Diaphragm.—Simple myalgia, *Act. r.* 1, 2h. Rheumatic inflammation, cutting pain on every breath, *Bry.* 1, 2h. Acute but non-febrile rheumatism, *Sticta pul.* 1, 2h. Rheumatism, with constrictive sensation, *Cactus* 1, 2h. Hypochondriasis with pains in the diaphragm, *Stann.* 3, gr, v. 8h.

Diarrhœa.—SUMMER DIARRHŒA.—Frequent watery stools with griping pains, *Chi.* 1, 1h. Vomiting and purging, much cutting colic, prostration, watery stools, *Verat. a.* 1—3, 1h. Watery yellow stools, early morning, *Podoph.* 6, 2h. Yellow or brown pappy or watery stools, after catarrh, much colic, causing to bend double, *Coloc.* 1, 1h. Sudden copious gushing stools, *Croton t.* 3, 1h. When the attack has been induced by wet and cold, *Dulc.* 1, 1h. When there are bilious vomiting and evacuations, *Iris v.* 1, 1h. Before and after menses, *Bovist.* 3, 2h. *See also below, under* CHRONIC *and* SPECIAL KINDS OF.

DIARRHŒA. From the use of antibiotics. *Nit. ac.* 30 or 200 is almost specific. A dose every two hours will produce rapid improvement if the remedy is well indicated.

CHRONIC DIARRHŒA.—Painless watery stools, *Chi.* 1, 4h. Watery, black or yellow, acrid stools, *Ars.* 3, 4h. *See also below, under* SPECIAL KINDS OF.

SPECIAL KINDS OF.—Camp diarrhœa, (1) *Pyro.* 30, 4h.; (2) *Bapt.* 1—30, 2h.; (3) *Liatris* 1x, 4h. Acute diarrhœa with deathly nausea and prostration, vomit at the smell or thought of food, *Colch.* 1, 1h. Abdomen seems filled with wind and water, which is explosively discharged, great weakness of sphincter, loss of confidence, *Apocy.* 3x, 1h. Lienteria, *Chi.* 1, 2h. Painless, greyish-white, watery, involuntary; evacuations not followed by feeling of weakness, *Phos. ac.* 1x—30, 1h. White, stinking, liquid, in children; copious, watery, clear-coloured, very fetid; urine high-coloured and strong-smelling, *Benz. ac.* 3x, 3h. Solid hard lumps in watery diarrhœa, *Ant. crud.* 6, 2h. In the morning, from 2 a.m. to 10 a.m., violent urging felt in hypogastrium and rectum, uncertainty, patient can scarcely retain fæces; diarrhœa alternating with pains in the head, *Aloe* 3, 2h. Sense of insecurity in rectum, uncertain whether gas or

stool will come, *Alo.* 3, 2h. Anus open, stool runs away
without patient knowing, (1) *Phos.* 30, 2h.; (2) *Phos. ac.* 30,
2h. Morning diarrhœa, urgent, yellow, *Sulph.* 3, 2h. Painless, greenish-yellow diarrhœa, gushing, occurring every
morning, *Apis* 3x, 2h. Morning diarrhœa, brown, watery,
urgent, waking patient from sleep, *Rumex c.* 6, 2h. Yellow
diarrhœa, between 4 and 5 a.m., *Nuphar l.* 3, 2h. Watery
yellow stools, without pain from 3 a.m. to 9 a.m., followed
by sensation of weakness in abdomen and especially in
rectum, *Podoph.* 6, 2h. Diarrhœa immediately *after eating
or drinking*, sensation of weakness in rectum after, *Podoph.*
6, 2h. Immediately *after eating or drinking* with great pain
in abdomen and tenesmus, stools fetid, at times bloody,
Trombid. 30, 1—2h. Brown watery stools *after eating* or
drinking, with much colic, *Coloc.* 1, 2h. Brown stools
immediately after eating, *Ars.* 3, 2h. White stools, *Dig.* 3,
2h. Black stools, *Leptandra* 1, 2h. Pappy stools *after eating*,
Chi. 1, 2h. Diarrhœa *on beginning to eat*, *Ferr.* 6, 2h. Diarrhœa
preceded by prolapse of rectum, *Podoph.* 6, 2h. Chalky
offensive stools, *Podoph.* 6, 2h. Green watery diarrhœa, with
grinding of teeth and rolling of the head (during dentition),
Podoph. 6, 2h. Dysenteric diarrhœa, with heat in the rectum
and tenesmus, *Podoph.* 6, 2h. Diarrhœa alternating with
head symptoms, *Podoph.* 6, 2h. Diarrhœa only in the daytime; < from cabbage, *Petrol.* 3, 2h. Passive mucous
diarrhœa, with little pain, chiefly at night, *Puls.* 3, 2h.
Mucous diarrhœa, green or greenish-yellow, with griping,
Ipec. 3, 2h. Sour-smelling diarrhœa, frothy, green, like the
scum of a frog-pond, *Mag. carb.* 6, 2h. Green mucus,
chopped white and yellow mucus, *Cham.* 1 or 6, 2h. Slimy,
offensive, excoriating, of various colours, *Merc. sol.* 6, 2h.

Slimy, blood-streaked, *Merc. cor.* 3, 2h. Diarrhœa in infants from artificial food disagreeing, vomiting and purging without actual inflammation, *Nux v.* 3, 2h. Frequent fæcal stools (sour), with colic and urging, *Rheum* 1, 2h. Passing intestinal sand, *Urt. ur.* φ, gtt. v. in hot water, 3 or 4h.

See also **Cholera, Cholera Infantum,** and **Cholera Nostras.**

Diet.—It is impossible to lay down rules to suit all cases: every individual case must be studied by itself. The following hints may, however, serve as useful guides to the prescriber.

IN HEALTH.—So long as digestion is performed without discomfort, and the bodily weight, strength, and activity are maintained, the less people think about their diet the better.

HOMŒOPATHIC DIETARY.—In the days when the higher dilutions were more largely given, patients under homœopathic treatment were put on much more strict dietary rules than it is now the custom to enjoin. It is an observed fact that those who live exclusively on vegetable diet are more readily acted on by medicines than those who eat meat; and, in a general way, the simpler the dietary of a person is, the more amenable he is to the action of medicines. If the person under treatment lives plainly, and the disorder is not specially connected with the digestive system, no change need be made in the dietary. If the patient is not a simple liver, the following rules should be laid down:—Avoidance of all alcoholic drinks and tobacco; also strong tea and coffee. The latter are better replaced by plain warm milk or scalded milk (a cup one-half or two-thirds full of milk filled up with boiling water). Cocoa made from the nibs, or cocoa shells, or the cocoa essences, are better than tea or coffee. Strong acids and pickles, strong spices, and very salt things and pastry, should be forbidden. There should be an interval of at least five hours between the meals; and all eating between meals should be disallowed. In cases of stomach disorder it is often advisable to take the meals dry and drink only half an hour before the meals. For the rest, breakfast may consist of porridge of some kind with milk; toast, bread, butter, and bacon, eggs, or fish. Lunch: Soup, fish, a little meat, white or red, milk pudding or stewed fruit (i.e. either the one or the other; the two should not be taken together by those whose digestion is at all delicate), and ripe fruit. Marmite may be used in place of stock for making vegetarian soups. Dinner: A variation of lunch, only a little more substantial. Among substitutes for meat, various dishes containing cheese, e.g. macaroni cheese, are the best. Cooked cheese is more digestible than raw cheese. Grated cheese added to soup improves its nutrient properties. After cheese, nut foods, lentils, peas and haricot beans are the most valuable of nitrogenous foods. (But lentils and other pulse foods contain purins and are thus no better than meats as regards gout. They are therefore only efficient meat-substitutes when gout is not in question.) It should be borne in mind that though freshly-cooked chicken, and especially boiled chicken, is very digestible, *cold* chicken is quite the reverse. The flesh of chicken, in becoming cold, sets into a hard fibre which is much more difficult to digest than cold beef.

INFANTS.—Until infants are eight months old they should have nothing but their mothers' milk; or, failing that and a wet nurse, the nearest substitute, cow's milk. As that is a little richer than human milk, it is necessary to dilute it with one eighth of water. Of course it should be warmed to blood-heat (roughly 100°F. or 37.5°C.) before it is given, but not boiled. Goat's milk is more rich than cow's, and is therefore not so suitable to the digestion of infants; but is often very good for thin, weakly children. There are many excellent milk and baby food preparations available today.

After a child is eight months old, it should be partially weaned: and cow's milk and foods made with milk and rusks, baked flour, or nursery biscuits, should be added. An excellent food for infants is made by gently simmering groats in milk. A tablespoonful of groats is put into a vessel containing a pint of milk; this is then placed in a saucepan, or other vessel, containing water, which is allowed to boil. When the milk has lost a quarter of its bulk, it should be strained, and is then ready to be given. The groats remaining behind make an excellent food for older children. At ten months it should be completely weaned, and the same food given in increasing quantity. In the second year, as the teeth develop, solid food, such as bread and butter and milk-puddings, may be given; also gravy with bread or potatoes, and later a little meat.

CORPULENCY.—Avoid the following:—All fat and fatty meats, pork, goose, duck; all fatty fish as salmon, eels, trout, etc.; soup; butter, cream, milk, sugar, sweets, pastry, puddings, farinaceous articles—as corn-flour, rice, sago, potatoes, peas, beans (except French beans), carrots, parsnips, beet-root, sweet ales, porter, stout, port wine, and all sweet wines. The following dietary is to be recommended:—Dry, toasted wheaten bread, especially brown bread, or plain hard biscuits; gluten biscuits; lean meat, poultry, game, lean ham, tongue; fish, not of the rich kinds, and eaten without rich sauce or butter, but with lemon-juice or vinegar; eggs; green vegetables, cresses, lettuces, endive; fresh fruits but not of the highly saccharine kind. During lunch and dinner no drink should be taken, but one or two glasses of dry, light wine, or a tablespoonful of whisky in water may be taken after lunch and dinner. At breakfast and tea-time, tea or black coffee without sugar.

A rapid method of reducing weight is to adopt an exclusive fruit dietary, taking no other food whatever, and no drink. This may be arranged by making a breakfast of oranges, luncheon of apples and bananas, tea of oranges, dinner of apples, tomatoes, and bananas. I have sometimes found it useful and practicable to make a modification of this, allowing a breakfast of oranges and tea of the same, with an ordinary lunch and dinner. The amount of fruit taken for a meal will depend on the individual patient. I have found three or four oranges generally suffice for a breakfast.

THINNESS AND TENDENCY TO, OR ACTUAL PRESENCE OF, CONSUMPTION.—Where it is well borne, cod-liver oil, beginning with a teaspoonful, immediately after meals; fat meats, butter, cream, milk, cocoa, chocolate, bread, potatoes, farinaceous foods, oatmeal porridge, sweets, a preparation of suet and milk (one-quarter of a pound of mutton suet cut fine and placed into two pints of milk, this is to be placed in a vessel of water and simmered down to one pint, the fat being skimmed off on rising) is often liked and well borne when cod-liver oil cannot be taken, and is especially valuable in consumptive cases.

FEVERS.—Water gruel is the ideal fever diet, but in these artificial days scarcely anybody likes it. In the fevers of short duration as febricula, simple scarlatina, measles, and German measles, a liberal supply of barley-water and plain water will often suffice till the fever is gone, and the stomach able to digest other food. Where the fever is more prolonged, as in the graver varieties of scarlatina and measles, and in typhus and typhoid, it is necessary to sustain the patient's strength. In typhoid and scarlet fevers, since the milk may have been the vehicle of contagion, it is well to have it boiled. It is also better boiled for another reason—it does not curdle in the stomach. Otherwise it may be taken as the patient likes it best; and when it is not tolerated plain, one-sixth lime-water, or one-half soda-water, will often make it acceptable. In addition to milk and milk foods in continued fevers, gruel may be given in alternation; also beef-tea—Brand's being one of the best manufactured, and home-made beef-tea being the best of all—mutton- veal- or chicken-tea, calves'-foot jelly; water and barley-water being given as much as the patient likes. Among other preparations may be mentioned the following:—

DR. SKINNER'S LIQUID BEEF.—It is made in this way (*see Homœopathic World*, vol. xxiv. p. 445): Take one pound of rump steak; remove all fat and membrane; cut into pieces the size of dice and pack into an empty pint jar with a closely-fitting lid. Before putting on the lid place a piece of calico or muslin over the bottom of it so as to ensure its being as steam-tight as possible. Place the jar in an open pot of cold water, bring it slowly to the boil, and then let it boil for half an hour: the *Liquid Beef* is now ready.

Remove the lid and pour out its contents. At first an oily yellowish fluid passes, and then a thick grumous-looking fluid. These two together constitute the *Liquid Beef*. This may be given in teaspoonful doses frequently repeated, and will sustain the strength when nothing else can be retained. After the *Liquid Beef* has been poured off, pour into the jar just sufficient hot water to cover what remains; stir well with a spoon and then pour off the liquid into a cup. This is very good beef-tea, and may be taken by itself or added to the *Liquid Beef*.

BEEF ESSENCE or COLD BEEF TEA is prepared thus: Take one pound of fresh beef, free from fat, chop it up fine, and pour over it eight ounces of soft, or distilled water, add five or six drops of hydrochloric acid, and fifty or sixty grains of common salt, stir it well and leave it for three hours in a cool place. Then pass the fluid through a hair sieve, pressing the meat slightly, and adding gradually towards the end of the straining about two more ounces of water. The liquid thus obtained is of a red colour, possessing the taste of soup. It should be taken cold, a teacupful at a time. If preferred warm it must not be put on the fire, but heated in a covered vessel placed in hot water.

THREE-MEAT TEA or INVALID BROTH.—Mince up equal parts of ham, beef, and mutton, say half a pound of each; put in an ordinary stone salt-jar, with a pinch of salt, and fill up with cold water. Put on the cover and place in a brisk oven. In one and a half hour's time pour off the broth, which is then fit for use, and refill the jar about two-thirds with warm water. Leave in the oven for another two hours. Then pour off and throw the solid residue away. To vary the flavour it is well to take equal parts of beef, mutton, and veal, or part of a fowl; a tablespoonful of jellied barley-water may be added to the broth, as it makes it softer and more pleasant to swallow.

The danger of over-feeding fever cases must be guarded against, as well as the opposite, since it is only what the patient *digests* that does him good, and not all that he can be made to swallow. During convalescence especial care must be had in typhoid cases not to allow the patient solid food until the temperature has been for some days normal night and morning. Sago, tapioca, and puddings of that kind, may be first given, then bread and butter, white fish, white meat, until the usual diet is gradually reached.

IN BRONCHIAL AFFECTIONS.—Hot milk in some saline water.

IN DYSPEPSIA.—Toast, stale bread, white fish, chicken, game, stewed mutton, floury potatoes, and rice may be taken; flatulent vegetables generally to be avoided. Ripe fruits which do not disagree with the individual. An egg broken into a wineglass, and swallowed whole with a little vinegar and pepper, or a tablespoonful of wine, is a sustaining and easily digested form of food. Peptonised foods, and the various preparations of pepsine, are of temporary value, but should not be relied on for long.

In intestinal dyspepsia the Metchnikoff sour-milk preparations are of great value. These may be given in the form of soured milk, junket or cheese; or the lactic bacilli may be given in tablets after meals. Allenbury Sauerin tablets are very convenient, also the Lacteol preparations.

ULCER OF THE STOMACH.—Milk in some form or other, if tolerated, should be the chief if not the only diet. Slippery

Elm Food will prove of great service until more substantial foods are tolerated.

DYSENTERY.—Milk, rice, eggs, white fish, and white flesh. Salted and dried meats, fruits and vegetables should be avoided. *Ulmi cortex* (Slippery Elm), used for thickening milk, is an excellent preparation. In extreme cases, patients may be kept alive on wine alone when the stomach will retain nothing else. Claret is the best in this country, and in wine-growing countries the ordinary table wine. Eight ounces may be taken daily, as much as two or three ounces being given at a time, and *extremely slowly*. Rice-milk— milk having had rice boiled in it for two or three hours, and then strained—may afterwards be given as well. A teacupful may be given two hours after the wine. Great care is required in returning to solid food, and the importunities of patients must be strenuously resisted.

GOUT.—Meat to be taken very sparingly; wines and malt liquors to be avoided altogether; except in atonic cases, when port wine may be a necessity. Tea is more irritating to the kidneys than coffee.

BRIGHT'S DISEASE.—Absolute skim-milk dietary; or a diet which is almost entirely derived from the vegetable kingdom. Eight- or ten-grain doses of *Kali citricum* (Citrate of Potash) in a wineglassful of water, two or three times a day, facilitate the action of the kidneys when skim-milk diet is being used. When the tongue becomes slimy a few grains of salt will put it right. Skim-milk diet may be persevered with for a short time; but if the strength runs down under this, a more liberal diet must be given. It must not be forgotten that it is quite possible to get rid of the albumen from the urine and starve the patient at the same time.

DIABETES.—Gluten bread, green vegetables, cream, butter, meat with fat; tea and coffee may be taken, and saccharine, mannite or glycerine used to sweeten them if necessary. Sugar-containing and starchy foods to be avoided. Sucking ice will relieve thirst, and rinsing the mouth with iced water will be as refreshing as a deep draught.

LITHIC ACID DIATHESIS AND TENDENCY TO STONE IN THE BLADDER.—Avoid milk, red meat, rich fish, sugar, starchy food, fruits (except those named below), potatoes, tea coffee, beer, wines or spirits. The dietary to consist of plain cocoa without milk or sugar, stale bread, white fish, bacon, eggs, bird (chicken or game), apples, tomatoes, and lemons.

SYPHILIS.—Alcohol and tobacco to be strictly avoided; in extreme cases a vegetarian dietary must be enjoined.

CANCER.—I have seen many cases of cancer cured in patients who are taking ordinary diet, but the evidence available of the advantage of a non-meat diet in the treatment of such cases makes its adoption a matter of simple common sense. So long as flesh foods of all descriptions are excluded patients may make out dietaries for themselves. As far as possible uncooked foods should be taken, since cooking kills certain of the vital properties of fruits and vegetables. The subjoined menus are given as suggestions.

Early morning.—The juice of two oranges and one lemon sipped slowly on waking.

Breakfast.—Uncooked pear, apple, grape-fruit, pine-apple, bananas. Followed by grated nuts—Jordan almonds, brazils, walnuts.

Or alternatively,

Weak China tea with milk and sugar to taste. Brown bread or toast with fresh butter. Lightly boiled egg. Chivers' Old English Marmalade or honey.

Lunch.—Uncooked salad selected from the following: Lettuce with grated carrots; watercress; mustard-cress; onions; chicory. A dressing may be prepared from the raw yolk of egg, olive oil, lemon-juice and half a cup of boiling water. This is to be poured on immediately before serving.

This is to be followed by dinner biscuit, fresh butter, Camembert, or cream cheese.

Dinner.—Hors d'œuvres of olives, vegetable soup served with marmite, spinach with egg, some milk pudding, preferably made with barley, tapioca or rice; dessert, sultanas and grated nuts.

Instead of the egg course, under certain circumstances white fish—whiting, sole, or plaice—may be taken with potatoes.

Bed-time—If desired, melon, grape-fruit, or pine-apple.

It was an observation of Burnett's that milk, unless cooked, should be avoided in breast cases, as it tended to favour the growth.

Here is a variorum dietary given me by a colleague for a patient whom I had referred to him. This insists on meals taken *dry*, the fluids being taken before meals.

1. *Early morning.*—A tumbler of water, hot or cold, on rising. (The same to be repeated at least half an hour before lunch and dinner, and again at bed-time.)

2. *Breakfast.*—Porridge, well-boiled, with milk. Coffee with milk, or cocoa, boiled for 2 or 3 minutes. Wholemeal bread and butter. Fruit of various kinds—apples, pears, oranges, or bananas. Honey in the comb.

3. *Luncheon.*—Green vegetables, preferably steamed, pota-toes roast or boiled in their skins, with butter. Green salad or fruit salad. Milk puddings. Cheese with bread and butter. Fresh fruit. Raisins. Nuts.

4. *Tea.*—Weak China tea. Wholemeal bread and butter (not cake). Fresh fruit.

5. *Dinner.*—Macaroni cheese, or plain cheese. Junket, or egg custard. Milk-pudding, green salad, or fruit salad. Whole-meal bread and butter. Whole fresh fruits. Ripe nuts. Sultanas. (All fruits should have the skins well washed in cold water.)

Diphtheria.—True, malignant, membranous diphtheria, (1) *Diphtherin* 30—200, 2h. (2) *Merc. cyan.* 6—30, every hour. At the same time the throat may be cleansed from time to time with a wash of *Phytol.* φ (5 drops to the ounce), a small sponge, fixed in a handle, sold by chemists, being the best means. [A teaspoonful of yeast may be given every two or three hours.] This treatment alone will suffice for the great majority of attacks. If this does not control it, *Ecchin.* φ, gtt. i.—x, 1—2h. When there is œdema of throat, *Apis* 3x, every hour. Excessive pain on swallowing, throat livid,

ulcerated, external neck swollen. prostration, *Ail. g.* 3x, 1h.
Air-passages involved, and the croup symptoms becoming
worse, *Iod.* 1, 1h. (*see* CROUP). Great prostration, the constitutional symptoms predominating much over the amount
of local affection; beginning on left side and spreading to
right, *Lach.* 6, 1h. When the affection begins on right side
and spreads to the left, *Lyc.* 6—30, 1h. Changing from side
to side, *Lac. can.* 30—200, 1—2h. When prostration is
extreme, *Ars,* 3, every ten minutes, will often restore the
patient. The greatest care must be taken not to raise the
patient from the recumbent position, as that is often of
itself sufficient to induce fatal syncope. [When tracheotomy
has been performed, the tube and the trachea should be
cleaned out from time to time with a solution of boracic
acid (gr. viii.—ʒj.). Steam from a kettle containing a few
drops of kreosote in the water may be kept playing within
the tent.]

SCARLATINAL DIPHTHERIA.—The treatment in general is the
same as above; if, however, there is much swelling in the
external glands, *Merc. bin.* 3x, gr. ii. 2h.; the throat being
cleansed, if necessary, with *Phytolacca* gargle, as above.

FEVERISH DIPHTHERIA.—With high fever, pains in the back
and limbs, but no prostration, *Phyt.* 1x, 1h. with the local
application of *Phytolacca* as above.

AFTER-EFFECTS.—Weakness, *Psorin.* 30, 4h. Paralysis, *Gels.* 1,
3h. Paralysis of vocal cords or bladder, *Caust.* 30, 2—4h.
Deafness, *Mur. ac.* 1, 2h.

Diplopia. *See* **Eyes:** SIGHT.

Distension.—After a meal with desire to loosen the clothes, *Puls.* 3, 4h. Flatulent distension of the upper part of the body, flatulence passing upwards, if at all, *Carb. v.* 6, 6h. Flatulent distension of the lower part of the body, flatulence passing downwards, *Lyc.* 6, 6h. *See also* **Flatulence.**

Dizziness. *See* **Vertigo.**

Dreams. *See* **Nightmare, Sleep.**

Dropsy.—Simple, acute, febrile dropsy, *Acon.* 1, 2h. Acute febrile dropsy with absence of thirst, *Apis* 3x, 2h. Unabsorbed effusions after inflammation of serious cavities, absence of thirst, *Apis* 3x, 2h. Dropsy of incipient Bright's disease, *Apis* 3x, 2h. Dropsy after scarlatina, with no albumen in the urine and no thirst, *Apis* 3x, 2h. Dropsy after scarlatina, with albumen in the urine, thirst, *Ars.* 3, 2h. Dropsy with hæmorrhage from the kidneys, *Tereb.* 1x, 2h. Acute dropsical swellings with suppression of urine, *Scilla* 1, 2h. Dropsy of leucocythæmia, aggravated by bathing, *Calc. c.* 6, 4h. Cerebral dropsy, *Hell. n.* 3, 1h. Dropsy with dark, scanty urine, *Hell. n.* 3, 2h. As a general remedy for dropsy, anasarca, hydrocephalus, hydrothorax, ascites, *Apocy. cannab.* 1—3, gtt. v. 2h. Dropsy from disease of the liver, *Apocy. cannab.* φ—3x, gtt. v. 3h. (This will relieve the dropsy frequently without remedying the disease of the liver. This remedy must be given carefully. In sensitive patients the φ tincture will sometimes produce vomiting and symptoms of collapse.) From syphilitic liver, *Aur.* 3, gtt. iii. 8h. Dropsy from organic disease of the heart, *Ars. iod.* 3x, gr. iii. after meals. From degenerated heart muscle with or without valvular disease; small frequent irregular pulse, dyspnœa; burning in gullet or stomach, nausea, vomiting; diarrhœa, *Stroph.* φ—3, gtt. i.—v. 4h. If the pulse is feeble, irregular, fluttering, *Digit.* 1, 2h.

Drowsiness. *See* Sleep.

Duodenum, INFLAMMATION OF.—*Arsen.* 3, 3h. If this fails after forty-eight hours, *Podoph.* 6, 3h.

ULCER OF.—(1) *Uran. nit.* 3x, gr. ii. 3h. (2) *Orinth. u.* φ, gtt. ii. in powder; unit-dose. (3) *Cad. sul.* 3 gtt. ii. 4h. From burns, *Kali bichr.* 3x, 3h.

Dupuytren's Contraction.—Recent cases, *Gels.* 1. 8h. Chronic cases, *Thiosin.* gr. ii.—3x, gr. viii. night and morning. *Calc. fluor* 30, one dose a week for six weeks has given excellent results. Repeat periodically if required.

Dysentery.—Begin in general with *Merc. cor.* 3, every hour. If there is much colic, relieved by bending double, *Coloc.* 1, 1h. Tenesmus, > after stool, *Nux v.* 1, 1h. Should these fail within two days to effect great improvement, the following may be given as indicated: Autumnal dysentery, with fatiguing tenesmus, worse at night, *Sul.* 3, gr. v. 3h. Dysenteric stools with white flocks, tenesmus, nausea, *Ipec.* 1, 2h. Heat, rawness, soreness in rectum with prolapse, *Aloe* 3, 2h. Burning and tickling in the rectum, tenesmus; pain after stool, *Nit. ac.* 1, 3h. Stool after all food or drink, much abdominal pain and straining, *Trombid.* 30, 1—2h. In very chronic cases, *Vaccinium myrtillus* φ, gtt. x, 8h. Low

typhous condition, *Rhus tox.* 1, 2h. *See also* **Diarrhœa** for
particular indications. Tenesmus after dysentery, enemata
of *Linseed tea*, *Nux v.* 1, 2h. After these, *Lil. tig.* 30, 2h.

Dysmenorrhœa. *See* **Menstruation,** PAINFUL.

Dyspepsia (INDIGESTION).—From indigestible food, tongue
brown at the back, cramping or spasmodic pain, flatulence,
vomiting, constipation; dyspepsia of drunkards, *Nux v.* 3,
3h. Flatulent dyspepsia, great belching of wind, cutting
pains in the chest, acidity, loose bowels, *Carb. v.* 6, 3h.
Feeling as of a stone at the stomach, sharp pain going
through from epigastrium to the back of the chest, pain
between the shoulders, bilious vomiting, pain across the
forehead, white tongue, constipation, *Bry.* 1, 2h. Craving
for meat, pickles, and other coarse food; gnawing, hungry,
faint feeling at epigastrium, *Abies Canad.* 3x, 4h. Sensation
of undigested hard-boiled egg in the stomach; constriction
at lower end of œsophagus; sensation as of something
lodged in the chest to be coughed up, but nothing does
come up, and coughing only aggravates; loss of appetite in
mornings, great craving for food at noon and night, *Abies
nigra* 3x, 4h. Bilious dyspepsia with great irritability and
spasms, *Cham.* φ, gtt. i., frequently. (Put about twenty
drops of the medicine in a tumbler of *hot* water, and let
the patient drink it in sips.) Bilious vomiting, black stools,
dull pain in forehead, and as if a band were tied across it,
Lept. 1, 3h. Pale flabby tongue, depraved taste, foul breath,
light stools, depression of spirits, *Merc. sol.* 6, 3h. Vomiting
from chronic catarrh of the stomach, tongue thick yellow
coat, red beneath; in beer-drinkers; weight rather than pain
after food, alternation of gastric symptoms with rheumatism,

Kali bichr. 3x, 3h. Ravenous hunger, white-coated tongue, heartburn; waterbrash; milk disagrees; swelling of epigastrium, tight clothes unbearable; abdomen distended and hard; offensive, white stools, *Calc. carb*. 6, 6h. Dry, sore tongue, white; fatty and acid risings; nausea on every inward emotion; constant feeling as if the stomach were filled with water; great sensitiveness of epigastrium; burning and sticking pain in liver; great distension of abdomen after eating a little; stitches in the chest; sick headache, *Kali. c*. 6, 6h. Yellowish-white coating of tongue, it feels burnt; longing for indefinite things; for spiced food; offensive eructations; nausea not relieved by vomiting; salivation; bitter vomiting with headache, burning, pressure or empty feeling at stomach, soreness in epigastrium, *Sang. c*. 3, 6h. Tongue blistered, dry, burning when eating; bitter taste; loss of taste, loss of all desire for tobacco in smokers; salivation; intense thirst; waterbrash; heartburn; heart-distress, palpitation, throbbing in epigastrium after food; "swashing" and fermentation in abdomen; constipation with hard, dry, unsatisfactory stools, feeling as if part remained behind, *Nat. mur*. 6, 6h. From eating fat food; mucous derangement, thickly coated, moist white tongue, nausea with little vomiting, heartburn, absence of much pain, feeling of distension, clothes have to be loosened, bowels loose or regular, *Puls*. 3, 3h. Tongue milky-white, eructation of wind and fluid tasting of food taken, *Ant. crud*. 6, 8h. Milky-white tongue, nausea, vomiting, prostration, *Ant. tart*. 6, 8h. Waterbrash, tongue coated white, flatulent distension of bowels, borborygmi, cannot bear the pressure of the clothes, constipation, gravelly urine, great sleepiness after dinner, *Lyc*. 6, 4h. Sodden-looking face, yellow slimy tongue, sour or putrid eructations, "goneness" after meals, alternate diarrhœa and constipation, *Hydrast.* 1, 3h. Vomiting, acute dyspepsia, great flatulent distension, *Carbol. ac.* 3x—3, 2h. Heartburn, flatulence coming away easily, excess of acid, heart's action disturbed by the stomach disorder, *Arg. n.* 6, 3h. Deficiency of gastric juice, *Alumina* 6, 3h. Irritative dyspepsia red tongue, loose bowels, fever, irritability, faintness, *Ars.* 3, 2h. Sense of weakness and oppression at epigastrium, oppression at the chest, acidity with heartburn and lateritious urine, lump in the throat-pit, impeding respiration and swallowing; "stomach cough," *Lobel.* 3, 2h. Inability to digest milk: vomiting of curdled milk immediately after taking it, *Æthus.* 3, 4h. Symptoms disappear during eating, and return in two hours, *Anac.* 1, 2h.

See also Diet—In Dyspepsia, Duodenum, Eructations, Stomach.

Dysphagia. *See* Swallowing, Difficult.

Dyspnœa. *See* Asthma, Croup, Heart, etc.

Dysuria. *See* Urination.

Ear.—External, Inflammation of.—Erysipelatous, *Bell.* 3, 2h. Erysipelatous and vesicular, *Rhus tox.* 3, 2h. With much swelling, *Apis* 3x, 2h. Redness, heat and itching of external ears; external meatus swollen and inflamed; stringy discharge, *Kali. bi* 3, 2h.

Eczema of.—Acute, *Rhus tox.* 3, 2h. If this fails within two or three days to effect improvement, *Croton* 3, 2h. If both these fail, *Mezer.* 1, 2h. Chronic, (1) *Psor.* 200. 3 doses given at four hourly intervals. Then wait, do not repeat under one month. (2) *Gunp.* 3x, gr. vi. 8h. (3) *Bovista* 6, 8h. After this *Arsen.* 3, 4h. Behind the ear, *Graphites* 6, 6h.; locally, glycerole of tannic acid (*Tan. ac.* ℥i., *Glycer.* ℥iv., rubbed together in a mortar, then heated until dissolved) may be used. If this fails to cause improvement in a fortnight, *Petrol.* 3, 6h.; locally, vaseline.

GLAND BEHIND, INFLAMMATION OF.—(1) *Caps.* 3, 2h. (2) *Bell.* 3, 2h.

EXTERNAL ORIFICE, INFLAMMATION OF.—*Acon.* 3, 1h., until the pain is relieved, then less frequently. Should there be no relief within five hours give *Bell.* 3, 1h., to be followed, if necessary, by *Merc. sol.* 6, 1h. Pustular, inflammation, minute boils: (1) *Calcarea picric.* 3, gtt. ii. 2h.; a plug of cotton wool saturated with glycerine will often allay the pain; or the meatus may be painted with a solution of *Hydrochlorate of Cocaine* (gr. v. to the ℥i. of distilled water). (2) *Bell.* 3, 2h.; external measures as above. Tendency to pustules in the ear, *Sul.* 3, 8h. External meatus (1.) inflamed, stringy discharge, *Kali bi.* 3, 2h. Chronic inflammation with blocking of the canal; (1) *Graph.* 6, 8h.; locally, application of a solution of *Nitrate of Silver*, one grain to the ounce. (2) *Ferr. phos.* 3, gr. v. 8h. (3) *Gunp.* 3x, gr. vi. 8h. If there is exudation, *Kali mur.* 3, gr. ii. 8h.

MIDDLE EAR (TYMPANIC CAVITY), INFLAMMATION OF.—After exposure to dry cold, at the beginning, pain, restlessness, anxiety, *Acon.* 3, ½h.; *Plantago* φ, diluted with an equal quantity of warm water, to be dropped into the ear every ten minutes or less often, according to urgency, a little cotton wool being placed in the orifice of the ear after each application. After *Acon.*, or when the local affection is decided, the pain almost making the patient beat his head against the wall, *Merc. s.* 6, ½h. Should the pain not yield readily, *Plantago* φ, 1h.; and locally, as directed above. Jerking, tearing pains as if something would be pressed out; external ear swollen, hot; pains through whole side of face, *Puls.* 3, ½h. Chronic catarrh, *Kali mur.* 3, gr. viii. 8h. When the mastoid cells are involved, *Caps.* 3, ½h. When there is distinct suppuration around the mastoid cells a free incision may be necessary. Chronic inflammation. *See* DISCHARGE.

DISCHARGE FROM.—Abnormal accumulation of wax: let the wax be softened by dropping into the ears pure olive oil for two or three nights, and then gently syringe with water at blood-heat. Occasional dropping in of oil will prevent the hardening of wax and facilitate its natural discharge when there is a tendency to accumulation. In chronic purulent discharge from the ear, whether depending on chronic inflammation of the middle ear or due to other causes, the following courses of treatment may be adopted. (But it must always be borne in mind that a discharging ear is not always an unmixed evil. Deafness *with* ear-discharge is generally less hopeless than deafness *without*. In all cases the constitution must be studied, and constitutional as well as local treatment administered. *See under* CHRONIC DISEASES.) Precise indications cannot be given, and remedies are therefore arranged in the order of the probability of their general usefulness. They should be tried for periods of not less than three weeks before being changed, and should be continued as long as there is improvement. The discharge should be allowed to flow freely from the ear at night. The local application should be used at bedtime, and the ear washed with plain warm water in the morning:—(1) *Kali mur.* 3, gr. v. 6h. (*Kali muriaticum* is the *chloride* of potassium, not the *chlorate*; it is one of Schüssler's tissue remedies.) (2) *Borax* 3, 6h.; about six grains of finely powdered *Boracic acid* to be blown into the ear at bedtime; [in place of the pure boracic acid, a mixture of *Boracic acid*, with tincture of *Plantago*, and sugar of milk may be used: thoroughly moisten a quantity of sugar of milk with *Plantago* ϕ; triturate in a mortar gradually, adding as much *Boracic acid* as there is of sugar of milk. Triturate until the powder is dry.] (3) *Hydrast.* 1, 6h.; glycerole of *Hydrastis* (*Hydrast.* ϕ, eight drops to glycerine half an ounce), to be dropped into the ear every night. (4) *Hepar sul.* 6, 8h. Ill-smelling discharge, psoric subjects, *Pso.* 30, night and morning. (5) Discharging pus, *Merc. sol.* 6, 8h.; a very dilute ointment of *Acid Nitrate of Mercury* (fifteen grains of the *Nitrate of Mercury ointment* of the British Pharmacopœia to half an ounce of vaseline) may be applied to the ear every night. Watery excoriating discharge smelling like fish-brine, *Tellur.* 6, 8h.—(N.B.—In all inflammatory and catarrhal ear affections the teeth should be examined; decayed teeth and improperly irrupted wisdom teeth will often cause trouble sympathetically in the ears. Some of the fillings used by dentists contain mercury, and in sensitive persons these may occasion disorders of the ears and hearing.)

POLYPUS.—In strumous subjects, *Calc. c.* 6—200, 8h. In others, *Thuja* 30, 6h.; the polypus may be painted with the mother-tincture of *Thuja* every night. If these measures fail, (1) *Nit. ac.* 6, 6h. (2) *Sang.* 3—30, 8h.

DEAFNESS.—From blocking of the Eustachian tube, *Merc. sol.* 3, gr. v.—6, 3h. If it does not yield after a week of this, *Hydrast.* 1, 3h. After this *Mezer.* 1, 3h. Deafness from a blow, *Chin. sulph.* 3x, 3h. Deafness of children, *Calc. c.* 30, 8h. Deafness of middle and of old age, *Mag. c.* 200, 8h. Deaf to human voice, *Phos.* 30, 8h. As from stoppage of ears, *Verbasc.* 1, 8h. Deafness, with roaring or thundering noises in the ear, the hearing being > in a noise, *Graph.* 3, gr. v.—6, 8h. Deafness, with noises and vertigo (Meniére's disease), *Nat. salicyl.* 3x—3, 6h. After this, *China.* 6, 6h. Deafness, with cold sensation in abdomen; noises in the ear on coughing; intolerance of music, which < the cough, *Ambra.* 3, 4h. Long-lasting deafness, discharge from the ears, *Elaps.* 3, 4h. Deafness as if the ears were stopped, *Mang.* 6, 4h. Deafness accompanying a morbid condition of the blood or blood-vessels ("Vascular Deafness" of Cooper); (1) *Ferrum Phos.* 3, gr. v. 8h. (2) *Ferrum picric.* 3x, gr. v. 8h. *See also* medicines recommended for **Anæmia**.

Earache.—From cold, *Acon.* 3, 1h. After *Acon.*, *Puls.* 3, 1h. Intolerance of the pain, < by warmth and at night, *Cham.* 6, 1h. Locally, one or two drops of *Mullein oil* (*Verbascum*) will generally relieve pain instantly. Or, equal parts of *Plantago* φ and water, warmed, may be dropped into the ear every hour until the pain is relieved.

Ecchymosis (EFFUSION OF BLOOD WITHIN THE TISSUES AS IN A BRUISE).—From injury, *Arn.* 1, 2h.; locally, if the skin is unbroken, arnica lotion (*Arn.* φ, gtt. v. to the ounce). *See also* **Bruise**. Isolated spots of effusion, appearance of, a bruise, *Arn.* 1, 2h.; more general, *Phos.* 3, 2h. *See also* **Purpura**.

Ecthyma.—Whole body affected; pustules large, round, with burning; or pale, livid, depressed; changing to ulcers—*Ant. tart.* 6, 4h. Pustules on face in fat people, yellowish or brownish scabs; desire for acids, *Ant. c.* 6, 4h. Confluent pustules with oozing and burning; greyish brown crusts on abdomen; pustules with scarlet redness of skin; itching, followed by painful burning; cannot bear to scratch for the pain it gives; pains > after sleep, *Crot. t.*, 12, 4h. Great sensitiveness of pustules to slightest touch, *Hep.* 6, 4h. Black pustles forming hard scabs; pustules on red base; burning and itching, < at night, and in cold, wet weather, *Rhus t.* 3, 4h. Red pimples on face, neck, shoulders, and back, some containing thickish fluid, *Juglans reg.* 3, 4h. Suppurating pustules, running together, bleed easily, itching from warmth of bed, *Merc. sol.* 6, 3h. Yellowish scabs all over body, especially scalp, always with great itching; painful to touch; < by washing, *Sulph.* 30, 4h.

Eczema.—Simple, acute, general or local, *Rhus ven.* 3, 6h. [When the eczema is general, an absolute milk diet is of great assistance to aid the cure. Sometimes a vegetarian dietary is essential to a cure. In giving *Rhus* in skin diseases it is necessary to be prepared for aggravations. Should the skin become worse, the medicine should not be changed, providing it is clearly indicated, but a single dose of a higher dilution (30) of the same medicine should be given and the result waited for. As local applications bran-baths (four pounds of bran boiled with a little carbonate of soda in one gallon of water, the liquor after straining to be added to a sufficient quantity of water to make a bath), and where the affection is local, bran water packs are useful; a solution of *Borax*, twenty grains to the pint; vaseline, when an ointment is required. Soft water should be used for washing. When crusts form, a linseed poultice should be applied to remove them.] Dry, irritative eczema, *Alumina* 5, 4h. Burning, stinging itching, *Urt. ur.* 3x, 8h. Eczema of backs of hands (bakers' and grocers' itch), *Bovista* 6, 6h. Eczema of scalp, *Oleander* 6, 6h. Of face and genitals much itching, *Croton* 3, 6h. Face; genitals; anus; severe continued itching, and after rubbing, soreness, *Ant. crud.* 6, 6h. Palms of hands, *Graph.* 6, 6h. (An ointment of *Graph.* 3x, ʒi.—ℨi. of cetacean ointment may be used at the same time.) Eczema of chin in males, *Cicut. v.* 3, 4h.

CHRONIC ECZEMA.—As a routine remedy, *Gunp.* 3x, gr. vi. 8h. Rather dry than weeping, *Ars.* 3, 6h. Dry, very irritable, gouty eczema, *Alumina* 6, 4h. Weeping, *Merc. cor.* 3, 6h. Bloody cracks, scanty discharge, *Petrol.* 3, 6h. Oozing of glutinous discharge; eczema behind the ears, *Graph.* 6, 6h. Inveterate eczema, *Hep. s.* 6, 6h.

IMPETIGINOUS ECZEMA (PUSTULAR ECZEMA).—*Rhus ven.* 3, 6h. In scrofulous children, *Merc. c.* 3, 6h. In chronic cases, *Hep. s.* 6, 6h.

ECZEMA RUBRUM.—(1) *Rhus ven.* 3, 6h. (2) *Petrol.* 3, 8h.; vaseline locally. (3) *Ars.* 3, 8h. (4) *Rad. bro.* 30 once a week.

ECZEMA CAPITIS (SCALLED HEAD, MILK CRUST).—The same remedies are useful as for simple eczema, but more particularly—(1) *Viola tric.* 1, 6h.; (2) *Vinca minor* 1, 6h.; a glycerole of *Vinca m.* φ (a drachm to the ounce of glycerine) to be applied locally. When more chronic—(1) *Sepia* 6, 6h., (2) *Hepar* 6, 6h. Dry, *Lyc.* 6, 6h.

ECZEMA MARGINATUM.—This is a parasitic disease, and is best treated by *Sul.* 3, 6h. and an application of *Sulphur* ointment or painting with *Sulphurous acid.* After these, if necessary, *Chrys. ac.* 2 gtt. ii. 8h. and paint at bedtime with *Chrys. ac.* 2.

Elephantiasis Arabum.—(Hypertrophy of the skin and areolar tissues of the lower extremities and scrotum, due to plugging of the lymphatics, and attended with fever and depraved nutrition.) (1) *Hydrocot. asiat.* φ—6, 6h. (2) *Anacard. orient.* 1x—6, 6h.

Elephantiasis Græcorum. *See* **Leprosy.**

Emaciation. *See* **Atrophy.**

Emissions.—[For the treatment of sexual disorders, firm but kindly moral counsel is required. Evil habits must be entirely abandoned. All stimulating foods and drinks, and tobacco must be avoided.] Abnormally frequent nocturnal emissions: (1) *Kali brom.* gr. ii.—30, 8h.; (2) *Dign.* 3x, gr. i. in the morning on rising. From morbid excitability of the organs; emissions induced by slight abdominal irritations, *China.* 3, 4h. Sthenic, with terrible erections and great desire, *Picric. ac.* 3x, gr. i.—30, 4h. Accompanied by strangury, *Canth.* 3, 4h. Easily excited in the presence of females, *Con.* 30, 6h.

WEAKNESS FROM.—(1) *Chin.* 3, 4h.; in nearly all cases, *Phos. ac.* 1x, gtt. v., in a tumbler of water may be given as a beverage with dinner. (2) *Calc. phos.* 3, gr. v. 6h. When there is constipation, *Nux v.* 3, 4h. Epilepsy, *Cupr. met.* 6, 4h. *See also* **Self-abuse, Spermatorrhœa.**

Emphysema.—*Lobelia* 3, 3h. *See also* **Asthma, Bronchitis, Chest,** and **Cough.**

Empyema. *See* **Pleurisy.**

Encephalitis. *See* **Brain, Meningitis.**

Encephalitis Lethargica. (*Sleepy Sickness*).—*Helleb. nig.* 1—30, 1h. This is the nearest general analogue. With typhoid conditions, loaded tongue, *Bapt.* 1—30, 1h. For special symptoms *see* **Brain** and **Meningitis.**

Enchondroma.—(1) *Sil.* 3, gr. iii. 8h. (2) *Calc. fluor.* 3, gr. v. 8h.

Endocarditis. *See* **Heart.**

Endometritis.—*Arsen.* 3, 6h. *See also* **Leucorrhœa.**

Enteralgia. *See* **Colic.**

Enteric Fever.—**Typhoid Fever.**—(Whenever there is the least suspicion of Typhoid fever all solid food should be stopped; *see* **Diet.**)—At the very commencement. *Typhoidinum* 30—200, 4h. (This may be continued throughout. When typhoid is epidemic, this may be given on the first indication of internal derangement.) Tongue coated yellow or white, flat, bitter taste, loose stools, restless, *Bapt.* φ—30, 2h. After *Bapt.* and in all cases which do not respond readily to remedies, *Pyro.* 6x—30, 4h. Sore, bleeding gums and lips; throat dark red or black; tongue like raw beef; offensive breath and discharges; exhaustion, *Ecchin.* φ, gtt. iii.—x, 2h. Low fever, shooting or jerking tearing pains in head, throat, chest, abdomen, and limbs, pains < by movement, white tongue, *Bry.* 1, 2h. Low fever, general soreness and tenderness, rheumatic pains > by movement, restlessness, *Rhus t.* 1, 2h. If the fever persists and increases, and the diagnosis is no longer doubtful, *Arsen.* 3, 2h. This medicine is of itself often sufficient from the beginning to the end of the disease. Great excitement, turgescence of face, shining eyes, *Bell.* 1, every hour until the patient is calmed. Tremor, restlessness, constant desire to get out of bed, twitching of eyeballs, *Agar.* 1, 1h., in the same way as *Bell.* Somnolence, incoherent mutterings, *Hyoscy.* 1, every hour. Flushed face, paretic weakness, tremors, sensorium less clouded than in *Hyo.*, *Gels.* 1—30, 2h. When there is slipping down to the foot of the bed, tendency to involuntary evacuations, aversion to food, copious urination, *Mur. ac.* 3x, 1h. Great prostration, profuse perspirations, involuntary evacuations, *Phos. ac.* 1x, 1h. If the lungs become inflamed, *Phos.* 3, 2h. If with the inflammation there is sharp, pleuritic pain, worse on motion, better by lying on affected side, *Bry.* 1, 1h. If there is epistaxis, or if there is blood in the stools, the blood being bright, *Ipec.* 1, 1h. for some hours, until the symptoms calling for *Ipec.* are entirely removed. If the blood is dark, *Ham.* 1, in the same way as *Ipec.* If there is tympanitis along with hæmorrhage, *Tereb.* 3, 1h.; locally, application of flannels wrung out of hot water, with a few drops of turpentine sprinkled on. When there is peritonitis or peritoneal pain, *Merc. cor.* 3, 2h. When diphtheria complicates typhoid, *Merc. cyan.* 6, 2h. Pains in tibiæ as sequela of enteric, *Lach.* 30, 8h.

Enteritis. *See* **Diarrhœa** and **Peritonitis.**

Enuresis. *See* **Urine.**

Ephelis.—*Kali c.* 6, 4h. If the face tans quickly, *Bufo* 12, 4h. [Locally, *Calc. chlor.* solution, one part to ten of distilled water, may be applied at bedtime. Or, the juice of a lemon may be applied once or twice a day.]

Epididymitis, *See* **Testicles,** INFLAMMATION OF.

Epilepsy.—(The general condition of the patient must always be considered. Epilepsy will often be removed by medicines homœopathic to the general conditions when medicines chosen according to the characteristics of the convulsions alone would have no influence. The following remedies are recommended on the supposition that the convulsions are the only, or at any rate the only serious departure from health.)

RECENT EPILEPSY.—Falls insensible, turns blue, violent convulsions; dyspnœa, *Kali cyan.* 3, 8h. Recent, in young, sanguine subjects, *Bell.* 1x—3, 6h. Epilepsy with mental hebetude; with cerebral congestion, coming on at each menstrual period. *Kali bro.* 30, 8h. Petit mal, *Absinth.* 3, 8h. Violent convulsions, frightful distortions of eyes and limbs opisthotonus, *Cic. v.* 3, 6h. Violent convulsions, rigidity, foaming at the mouth. *Œnanth. croc.* 3x, 6h. From emotional disturbance, *Ign.* 3, 6h. Recent epilepsy caused by fright; in stammerers, *Stram.* 3, 6h. Fits coming on in sleep, much drowsiness, constipation, *Op.* 3, 6h. Associated with digestive disorder, excessive belching of flatulence, *Arg. n.* 6, gtt. ii. 8h. (When the belching is premonitory of a fit, *Arg. n.* taken every half-hour will prevent it.)

CHRONIC EPILEPSY. In general, *Bufo* 6, 8h. In pale, lymphatic subjects, *Calc. c.* 6, 8h. Fits during sleep, nervous irritability,

Sil. 6, 8h. Fits in sleep, drowsiness, constipation, *Opium* 3, 8h. Very obstinate constipation, cachexia, malnutrition, unhealthy skin, *Plumb*, 30, 8h. When the "aura" is a wavy sensation in the brain, *Act. r.* 1, ½h. will ward off a fit. In subjects of sulphur type *Sulph.* 200 at bedtime, followed, if necessary, by *Pso.* 200 at bedtime. *Also* remedies named above under RECENT EPILEPSY when the symptoms correspond.

Epistaxis. *See* Nose.

Epithelioma. *See* Cancer.

Epulis.—(1) *Thuja* 1, 4h. (2) *Plumb. acet*, 6, 4h. (3) *Calc. c.* 200—cm. once a week. (4) *Lac. can.* 200 at bedtime.

Erotomania.—NYMPHOMANIA.—Lascivious furor, uncovers genitals, *Hyosc.* 1, 1h. Erotomania and inclination to suicide; great sexual excitement driving to onanism; leucorrhœa, *Origanum* 3, 1h. Nymphomania, in lying-in-women, with voluptuous tingling from genitals into abdomen. *Platina* 6, 2h. Sexual delirium, talks about lewd subjects; excessive menstrual flow; after menses, sobbing and whining, *Stram.* 3, 1h. Extreme excitement, menses too early and profuse; pains and spasms of uterus; pruritus vulvæ; leucorrhœa, *Tarentula* 3, 1h. When occurring before the monthly period, *Calc. phos.* 30, 8h. During the period, *Puls.* 30, 8h. Nymphomania; irritable condition of the organs with congestion, *Gratiola* 3—30, 4h.

SATYRIASIS.—*Picr. ac.* 3, gr. ii. 4h. Where there is local irritation, *Canth.* 3, 2h. Purely nervous cases, *Phos.* 3, 2h.

With general exalted sensitiveness, *Hydrob.* 6—30, 2h. In alcohol drinkers, *Nux v.* 3, 2h.

Eructations.—Loud, copious, painless belchings, *Arg. n.* 6, gtt. ii. 3h. Distension of the stomach; eructations tasting of food taken, with or without heartburn, *Carbo. v.* 6, 6h. After *Carbo v.*; flatulence rising up into œsophagus and causing pressure and choking, *Carb. an.* 6, 6h. With nervous dyspepsia, *Carbol. ac.* 3x—3, 2h. With sensation of painful lump at epigastrium, *Abies nig.* 3, 4h. Burning sensation rising up from pit of stomach to the throat, *Manc.* 30, 4h. Flatulence in nervous subjects, *Nux mosch.* 1—3, 2h. Eructations of particles of food very sour (rumination), *Sul.* 30, 8h. (During the attacks, *Cham.* φ, gtt. i. in hot water ½h., for three or four hours, will often give relief if the others, which may be given both in the attacks and over a length of time, fail to do so.) *See also* Dyspepsia, Flatulence.

Eruptions. *See* Acne, Eczema, Herpes, Nettle-rash, Psoriasis, etc.

SUPPRESSED.—Chronic eruptions, *Sul.* 6, 8h. Eczema, erysipelas, scarlatina, and measles, with coldness, and prostration, *Camph.* φ, gtt. i. 15m. With chest symptoms, *Bry.* 1, 1h. With oppression of the brain, *Cupr. acet.* 3x, 1h.

Erysipelas.—In simple acute cases, *China.* φ, gtt. x, 2h. (This will often cut short an attack if given at the outset.) Smooth, tense, red skin, *Bell.* 3, 1h. Much swelling, *Apis.* 3x, 1h. Vesicles and bullæ, *Rhus v.* 3, 1h. Erysipelas, commencing l. side of face and spreading to r., *Rhus t.* 3, 1—2h. Phlegmonous erysipelas (when the tissues under the skin are involved and suppuration threatens). *Verat. v.* 1x, 1h.;

Verat. v. φ to be painted on the part. When suppuration has occurred, *Hepar sulph.* 6, 1h. Where there is low fever, thirst, red tongue, anxiety, prostration, *Ars.* 3, 1h. (It may be necessary to make an incision.) Should gangrene occur, *Crotalus* 3, 1h. Erysipelas of the head striking in, *Cupr. acet.* 3x, 1h. Erysipelas of the throat with swelling, *Apis* 3x, 1h. Wandering erysipelas, spreading from r. to l., *Graph.* 6, 6h. The same, where there is great sensitiveness of the skin to the slightest touch or the least cold, *Hep. s.* 6, 6h. Œdema after erysipelas when painful, *Hep. s.* 6, 6h. When painless —(1) *Graph.* 6, 6h.; (2) *Sul.* 3, 6h.; (3) *Aur. met.* 6, 6h.; locally, *Verat. v. φ*, as paint.

CHRONIC.—*Ferrum phos.* 3, gr. v. 6h. With much œdema, *Nat. mur.* 6, 6h.

Erythema.—Simple erythema, *Bell.* 3, 2h. In old people from obstructed circulation *Mezer.* 1, 2h.

Erythema Nodosum.—*Apis* 3x, 2h. (If there is considerable fever, *Acon.* 3, 1h. should be given at the commencement.) Much rheumatic pain, *Rhus tox.* 3, 2h. After these, *Fer. phos.* 3, gr. viii, 8h.

Excitement, EFFECTS OF.—Fever and restlessness, *Acon.* 3, 1h. Headache, *Bell.* 3, 1h. Sleeplessness, *Coff.* 3, 1h. Bilious derangement, *Cham.* 6, 1h.

Excoriation.—Between the nates of infants (intertrigo). *Cham.* 6, 6h. When it recurs frequently, *Lyc.* 6, 6h. When the affected parts are very painful, *Merc. sol.* 6, 6h. Excoriations of thighs from walking, *Æthus.* 3x, 4h.

Excrescences.—Granulations in wounds (proud-flesh), *Silic.* 6, 4h.; locally finely powdered bluestone to be dusted on. *See also* **Warts.**

Exhaustion, MENTAL. *See* **Brain-fag.**

BODILY.—From over-exertion, *Arn.* 1. 1h.; a hot bath (about 102°F.) in which Arn. φ (a teaspoonful to the gallon) has been mixed. Strong beef-tea given hot.

Exophthalmic Goître. *See* **Goître.**

Exostosis.—*Calc. fluor.* 6, 8h. When occurring on the head and jaws, *Hecla* 6, 8h.; of long bones, *Phos.* 6, 8h. Syphilitic, (1) *Aur.* 30, 8h.; (2) *Merc. c.* 3, 8h.

Expectoration. *See* **Cough, Throat.**

Extremities. *See* **Hands, Feet,** etc.

Eyes.—ORBIT.—Bruised, *See* **Black Eye.**

LIDS.—Quivering. *See* **Blepharospasm.** Sebaceous cyst. *See below,* TUMOURS. Acute inflammation of the margins, *Euphras.* 1, 2h.; locally a lotion of *Euphras.* φ (ten drops to the ounce) to be used every three hours. Chronic redness and irritation of the margins (this is sometimes due to hypermetropia, and should then be treated by suitable glasses; when due to other causes), *Clem.* 1, 4h. Constitutional, *Bac.* 100, gl. v. once a week. Irritation with formation of much matter, *Hep. s.* 6, 4h. Inflammation and great redness of the margins, dry mucus on the lashes, morning agglutination, *Graph.* 6, 4h. Chronic irritation in strumous subjects, *Calc. c.* 6, 6h. Itching, biting in the margins, *Mezer.* 1, 4h. Scurf of the margins, *Ars.* 3, 4h. Simple agglutination of the lids, *Merc.* sol. 6, 6h.; locally, vaseline to be applied at night, very lightly.

INTERNAL SURFACE.—Acute inflammation.—The same treatment as for inflammation of conjunctiva of eye. *See below*, INFLAMMATION OF THE EYE. Chronic inflammation—(1) *Hep. s.* 6, 6h.; (2) cracks or soreness at commissures, *Graph.* 6, 6h.; (3) *Merc. cor.* 3, 6h.

TUMOURS.—Sebaceous. Give (1) *Staph.* 6, 8h. After this (2) *Calc. c.* 30, 6h., (3) *Benz. ac.* 3x, 8h.; locally paint at bedtime with *Benz. ac.* 3x. The treatment must be persevered with for a long time. The surgical measure usually adopted is to puncture and scrape out the cyst from within; but this does not prevent recurrence. Tarsal wart-like tumours, *Thuja* 1, 6h. *Thuja* φ painted night and morning.

PTOSIS.—(1) *Gels.* 1, 4h.; (2) *Morph.* 3, 4h. With dull frontal headache, *Sep.* 6, 4h.

ECTROPION.—*Borax* 30, 4h. *See also* medicines as indicated under LIDS.

ENTROPION.—*Borax* 30, 4h. *See also* under LIDS.

INFLAMMATION OF THE LACHRYMAL SAC.—At the commencement, *Puls.* 3, 2h. After this, *Clem.* 1, 2h. When the matter has formed, *Hep. s.* 6, 4h. If this fails to benefit speedily, *Silic.* 6, 3h.

LACHRYMAL FISTULA.—(1) *Silic.* 6, 4h.; (2) *Fluor. ac.* 6, gtt. ii. 4h.; (3) *Merc. cor.* 6, 4h. A course of *Sul.* 3, 4h. may be given with advantage as an intercurrent medicine. It may be

given for one or two weeks. The remedy originally given
may then be resumed if indicated.

INFLAMMATION OF THE EYE (CONJUNCTIVITIS.)—[N.B.—In
almost all acute inflammatory states of the eye frequent
bathing with *hot* water is advantageous.] Acute, from cold
or injury, *Acon.* 3, 1h.; lotion of *Boracic ac.* (eight grains to
the ounce) to be kept applied until the pain has subsided.
If the inflammation is not very much better within forty-
eight hours. *Euph.* 1, 1h.; lotion of *Euph.* φ (ten drops to
the ounce) to be kept applied. In unhealthy subjects, *Sulph.*
6, 2h. Pustular inflammation *Ant. tart.* 3x, 4h.; going on to
ulceration of cornea, *Merc. cor.* 3, 4h.

PURULENT INFLAMMATION OF THE EYE (EGYPTIAN OPHTHAL-
MIA).—*Acon.* 3, every hour for six hours, then, if the
symptoms are not subdued, there not being much pus,
Rhus tox. 3, every hour. If there is much pus, *Argent. nit.*
3x, every hour. The eye to be kept scrupulously clean with
a *Borax* wash (ten grains to the ounce), and a solution of
Arg. nit. (one grain to the ounce), to be dropped in every
two hours.

GONORRHŒAL INFLAMMATION OF THE EYE.—*Merc. cor.* 3, 1h.;
locally, a lotion of *Merc. cor.* 1, ten drops to the ounce,
every two hours. This should be injected under the lids
with a glass syringe, or else a solution of *Arg. nit.* 2 gr. to
the ounce, should be injected in the same way. After *Merc.
cor.*, when the acute stage has subsided, *Hep. s.* 3, gr. v.—6,
3h. If there is much pain, *Acon.* 3, ¼h., may be given intercurrently, until pain is relieved.

PURULENT INFLAMMATION OF THE EYE IN NEWBORN CHILDREN
(OPHTHALMIA   NEONATORUM).—*Hygienic   Treatment:*—
Immediately after birth the nurse must wash the infant's
eyes with the greatest possible care, removing all traces of
mucus. For this purpose a fine linen rag, dipped in clean
water, may be used. Beginning at the outer corner, the
eyelids are gently wiped from side to side, until all traces
of mucus are removed, and the eyelids remain perfectly
clean. Sponges must never be used. As soon as the child's
eyes are thus washed clean and dried, the nurse is to wash
her own hands most carefully in water with which carbolic
acid, Condy's fluid, or other disinfectant has been mixed. If
in the first few days after birth signs of inflammation
appear—redness, swelling, and sticking together of the lids
—the greatest care must be taken. If from any reason the
doctor cannot be in attendance immediately, the nurse
must herself cleanse the eyes in the following manner:—
A perfectly clean and very soft piece of linen is moistened
with tepid water; any excess of water is then squeezed out.
The muco-purulent discharge between the eyelids is wiped
off very gently—without scrubbing or scratching; special
attention being paid to the inner corner of the eyelid where
the mucus particularly accumulates. After repeatedly rinsing
the linen in clean water, the upper eyelid is gently raised
by means of the thumb placed on the eyelid immediately
above the lashes, but without making any undue pressure.
The muco-purulent matter which escapes is removed with
the rag as often as it appears. In the next place, the lower
eyelid is drawn down with the forefinger, and also wiped
with great care. If the eyelids stick together, they must be
moistened with water until separation takes place without

any effort. The water used in cleansing the eyes must be perfectly pure; no milk or soap is to be mixed with it. *Medical Treatment :*—*Arg. nit.* 3, 2h.; after well washing, a drop of a solution of *Arg. nit.* (two grains to the ounce) to be injected under the lids.

SCROFULOUS INFLAMMATION OF THE EYE (STRUMOUS OPHTH-ALMIA).—(For the photophobia, *Acon.* 3, or *Conium* 3, may be given as long as indicated intercurrently with any of the following medicines, if it should not yield readily to the latter.) (1) *Sulph.* 6, 6h.; scrupulous cleanliness. If *Sulph.* does not suffice for the cure, after a fortnight's time give *Merc. cor.* 3, 3h. If these fail, give (1) *Hepar s.* 6, 4h.; (2) *Rhus tox.* 3, 3h.; (3) in fair subjects, inclined to be fat; with cold, damp feet and hands, *Calc. c.* 6, 4h. Where the nervous element predominates, *Arsen.* 3, 3h. If the in-flammation is vesicular (phlyctenular conjunctivitis), *Ant. tart.* 3, 2h.

GRANULAR INFLAMMATION OF THE EYE (GRANULAR OPHTH-ALMIA—GRANULAR LIDS).—Lids closed, red, swollen, painful, burning, acrid flow of tears; stitching pains in eyes, photophobia, *Calc. c.* 6, 8h. If irritating lotions and applica-tions have been used, they must be omitted, and a weak *Calendula* lotion (five drops to the ounce) used three times a day. In patients of the blonde feminine type, eyes > in open air, < in warm room or near a fire, *Puls.* 3, 4h. Where there are cracks at the commissures, *Graph.* 6, 8h. Lids swollen, red, painful, stinging pains, great sensitiveness to touch, pain in brow and head proceeding from eyes, photophobia, pains < in the night, < from cold, > from warmth, *Hep.* 6, 4h. If these fail after a trial of a few weeks, *Kali bich.* 3x, gr. ii. 6h. After this, *Thuja* 12, 3h.; lotion of *Thuja* φ (five drops to the ounce) three times a day. Then *Arsen.* 3, 3h. Pterygium, *Ratanhia* 1, 3h. After four weeks, if this has no effect, *Zinc.* 6, 8h. [*Sulph.* 6 may be given for a time in all chronic eye affections, if the seemingly indicated remedies fail to respond. *Acon.* 3 may be given intercurrently with any of the above when the pain and photophobia are distressing.]

RHEUMATIC INFLAMMATION OF THE EYE.—Much pain in the eye from cold, little redness or intolerance of light, *Acon.* 3, 1h. Intense aching pains in eyeballs and behind eyes, *Act. r.* 3, 2h. If these fail to make great improvement within two days, *Spigel.* 3, 1h. Sudden attack of inflammation and pain in the eye in gouty persons (gout in the eye), *Nux v.* 6, 10m.

INFLAMMATION OF THE CORNEA (KERATITIS).—Suppurative, early stage, *Hep. s.* 6, 4h. Interstitial keratitis, cloudiness of centre of cornea, in syphilitic subjects. *Merc. cor.* 3, 3h. Should this not prove efficient, *Kali bichrom.*, 3x, gr. ii. 4h. And if this fails, *Aur. mur.* 3x, 3h. Ulceration of the cornea, deep spreading ulceration without much pain, *Merc. cor.* 3, 2h. Should this fail, *Calc. c.* 6, 4h. Numerous small ulcerations, *Arsen.* 3, 4h. Afterwards if this is not sufficient, *Sulph.* 3, 4h. Then *Hep. s.* 6, 4h. (When there is much photophobia, *Con.* 3 may be given intercurrently with any of the above.)

SCLEROTITIS.—Acute, (1) *Acon.* 1, 2h. (2) *Act. r.* 1, 2h. Chronic, *Merc. cor.* 3, 3h. When complicating keratitis, the treatment of the keratitis will answer for both.

OPACITY OF THE CORNEA.—(1) *Euphras.* 1, 6h.; (2) *Mag. c.*
30, 8h.; (3) *Calc. c.* 6, 6h.; (4) *Cann. sat.* 1, 6h.; (5) *Silic.* 6,
6h. The persistent use of lotion of *Euphras.* φ (gtt. v. to ℥i.
of water, hot or cold according to the case) two or three
times a day is of great assistance.

IRITIS.—If taken at the very beginning, slight turbidity,
sluggish action of the muscle, pain, *Acon.* 1, 1h. When
lymph is effused and adhesions threaten, *Atropine* (one
grain to the ounce; if adhesions have formed, four grains
to the ounce) must be instilled into the eye to dilate the
pupil; internally, *Merc. cor.* 3, 1h. If these prove insufficient,
Clematis, 1, 1h. In syphilitic cases, mercurial inunction
(mercurial ointment of the B. P. to be rubbed in) daily on
the inner surface of the thighs. When mercury has been
fully tried without good effect, *Kali bich.* 3x, gr. ii. 8h.;
locally, *Atropine*, as above. When the patient has already
had mercury, *Nit. ac.* 3x—12, 2h. Gonorrhœal (1) *Thuja* 1,
1h.; (2) *Clem.* 1, 1h. Serous iritis must be treated by operation, remedies suited to the constitution of the patient
being given internally, generally *Ars.* 3, 2h.

SYMPATHETIC OPHTHALMIA.—This must be treated according to the indications given in above section. The atten-
dant must consider the propriety of removing the injured
eyeball.

CHOROIDITIS.—Recent cases, with congestive headache, appearance of lights and colours, *Bell.* 3, 2h. Recent cases,
with less active symptoms, *Gels.* 1, 2h. Recent cases, with
crushing or pressing-asunder pain in eyeballs, *Pru. spi.* 1,
2h. Chronic cases, appearance of flames and colours, *Phos.*

3, 2h. Disseminated choroiditis—(1) *Kali iod.* 1, 2h.; (2) *Merc. sol.* 3, 2h. Suppurative choroditis (panophthalmitis), *Rhus t.* 3, 2h.

RETINAL HYPERÆMIA.—From cold, *Acon.* 3, 1h. From anomalies of refraction or accommodation—suitable glasses. From overstrain, *Santonine* 3, 4h., and rest. From heart disease, *Cact.* 3, 2h. From menstrual disorders, *Puls.* 3, 2h.,

RETINITIS.—Simple and recent, *Bell.* 3, 1h. More chronic, sensitiveness to the glare of a fire, *Merc. sol.* 6, 4h. Syphilitic, *Kali iod.*, gr. ii. 4h. Symptomatic of renal disease—(1) *Plumb.* 6, 4h.; (2) *Merc. cor.* 3, 4h. (The patient must be treated according to the general state.)

RETINAL HÆMORRHAGE.—From accident, *Arn.* 1, 1h. Passive, *Ham.* 1, 1h. Multiple hæmorrhages, *Phos.* 3, 2h. For re-absorption of effused blood, *Lach.* 6, 4h.

DETACHMENT OF THE RETINA.—Recent, (1) *Apis* 6, 2—4h. (2) *Gels.* 1, 2—4h.; afterwards, *Aur. mur.* 3x, 2h. *See also* SIGHT.

OPTIC NEURITIS.—In the first stage, (1) *Apis* 3x, 2h. (2) *Carbon. sul.* 3—30, 2h. (3) *Benz. dinit.* 3—30, 2h. Secondary inflammatory changes, effusion, *Arsen.* 3, gtt. i. 2h. If depending on cerebral disease, this must be treated; if of syphilitic origin, *Kali iod.*, gr. v. 4h. for four days, and longer if improvement progresses; to be followed, when the *iodide* appears to be losing its effect, by *Merc. cor.* 3, 4h.

Subsequent atrophy may be arrested by (1) *Phos.* 3, 4h; (2) *Nux v.* 1, 2h.

SCLEROSIS OF THE OPTIC NERVE.—(1) *Phos.* 3, 2h.; (2) *Nux* v. 1, 2h.; (3) *Strych. nit.* 3x, 2h.; (4) *Carb. sul.* 30, 4h.

GLAUCOMA.—(The surgeon will decide when operation is necessary.) When taken at the commencement, if the disease has not been induced by instillation of atropine, *Bell.* 3, 1h. Eye protrudes, feels sore, as if pressed out from above, *Comocl.* 1, 1—2h. Aching in upper outer portion of (r.) eyeball with hard feeling, *Coloc.* 1—30, 1—2h. Severe burning, sticking and cutting pains, extending from eye up into head and around eye; or else aching pain, going back into head, usually < at rest, at night and on stooping, > by firm pressure and on walking in a warm room, *Coloc.* 1—30, 1—2h. If atropine has been the cause, drop in *Eserine* (two grains to the ounce), and give, if the pains are burning, sticking, tearing, pressing, *Acon.* 1, 1h., to be followed, if necessary, by *Phos.* 3, 1h. If the pains are intolerably pressing and sticking, *Spigel.* 1, 1h.

CATARACT. *See page* 109.—Soft cataract, *Colch.* 1, 4h. Traumatic, *Con.* 3, 4h. Capsular opacity, *Euphras.* 3x, 4h.; lotion of *Euphras. φ* (ten drops to the ounce), three times a day. Hard cataract, in the early stage, concentric opaque laminæ—(1) *Calc. c.* 6, 4h.; (2) *Phos.* 3, 4h. Later stages, *Silic.* 6, 4h. Flickering and sparks before eyes, *Calc. fluor,* 6, 8h. [*Cin. mar. φ*, the succus, not the spirit tincture, one drop instilled in the eye four or five times a day, and continued for some months, is reputed to have cured many cases.]

SQUINT.—When due to errors of refraction or accommodation, suitable spectacles, and operation if necessary. When a sequel to convulsions, *Bell.* 3, 4h. In choreic subjects, with muscular twitchings, *Hyos.* 3, 4h. Convergent, *Cyclamen* 3, 4h. With worm symptoms—(1) *Cina* 3, 4h.; (2) *Spigel.* 3, 4h. Squint of either eye; loss of power of internal rectus, *Alumina* 6, 6h. Internal squint with right eye, *Alumen* 6, 6h. Internal squint of either eye, *Gels.* 3, 6h. Squint; staring, protruding, injected eyes; delirium, *Stram.* 3, 6h.

SIGHT—WEAK.—When due to errors of refraction or accommodation, suitable spectacles must be provided. (In children, before adopting spectacles, constitutional treatment should always be persistently followed. Great improvement, if not cure, may be effected, whilst premature recourse to spectacles fixes the imperfection.) Failure of accommodation may be helped by the following medicines:—Inability to see fine work at night, soreness of eyes, *Baptis.* 3, 6h. Ciliary overstrain, *Arn.* 3, 6h. and lotion of *Arn.* φ one drop to the ounce in *hot* water. Small objects appear large, *Oxal. ac.* 6, 6h. Everything appears too large, *Nux mosch.* 3, 6h. Hypermetropia; presbyopia; astigmatism; blurred sight, with heat in eyelids and eyes; disposition to cover or press on eyes; light painful, darkness pleasant; appearance of a veil before the sight, *Lil. t.* 30, 8h. Blurred, smoky vision; blindness, vertigo, *Gels.* 3, 8h. In rheumatic patients, when caused by exposure to dry cold, *Caust.* 3, 4h.; when caused by damp cold, *Rhus t.* 3, 4h. Simple paralysis of ocular muscles; and after diphtheria—(1) *Sant.* 3, gr. v. 4h.; (2) *Gels.* 1, 4h. In cases of nervous weakness, as from sexual excess, *Phos.* 3, 4h. Weak sight from over-use, when the external muscles are affected, causing aching on moving the eyes, *Natr. mur.* 6, 4h. Dazzling vision, smarting soreness of the eye after working a short time; eyes ache, burn and feel strained; from fine sewing or reading too much, *Ruta* 3, 4h.; lotion of *Ruta* φ (ten drops to the ounce). Short sight or myopia, *Physostigma* 3x, 4h. *See also* **Hemiopia.**

SIGHT, DISORDERS OF.—*Coloured Vision.* Red, *Bell.* 3, 4h. Print red when reading *Phos.* 6. 3 times daily for one week, then reduce to once daily. Yellow, *Sant.* 3, gr. ii. 4h. Fantastic, of overpowering brilliancy, *Anhal.* 3, 4h.; As if through a mist—(1) *Phos.* 3, 4h.; (2) *Plumb.* 6, 4h. *Double vision*, with heaviness of the eyes, giddiness, *Gels.* 3, 4h. With mental depression, *Aur. met.* 3x, gr. ii. 4h. Of horizontal objects at some distance, *Nit. ac.* 6, 4h. *See also* **Amaurosis, Amblyopia, Hemiopia.**

Face.—ACHE. *See* **Gumboil, Neuralgia, Toothache.**

COMPLEXION.—Earthy, unhealthy-looking, *Nat. m.* 6, 4h. Yellow; yellow spots; yellow saddle across the nose; yellow round the mouth, *Sep.* 6, 4h. "Liver spots," *Lyc.* 6, 4h. Blotches and roughness of the skin, produced by cold winds—(1) *Kali c.* 6, 4h.; (2) *Petrol.* 3, 6h. Scurfy eruption round the mouth, *Ars.* 3, 4h. Painful pimples on forehead, *Ambra* 3x, 6h. Painful pimples on forehead and face; also over the whole body, *Indigo* 3, 6h. *Pimples* on forehead, dry or moist; boils; much irritation, *Ledum* 6, 4h.; afterwards, if necessary, *Calc. phos.* 3, gr. v. 6h.; if this is not sufficient, *Clematis* 3x, 6h. Eruption on chin, *Cicuta* 3x, 6h. *See also* **Acne.**

FLUSHING.—At the change of life. *See* **Change of Life.** From excitement, *Acon.* 3, 1h. Whilst eating, with sweat, cold hands and feet, *Carbo an.* 6, 4h.

Facial Paralysis. *See* **Paralysis,** Facial.

Fæces. *See* **Constipation, Diarrhœa.**

Fainting.—During the attack the patient must be laid in the horizontal posture, cold water applied to the forehead, and ammoniacal smelling-salt placed under the nostrils; internally, *Moschus* 3, every five minutes.

Tendency to.—When due to disease of the heart or other constitutional disorder, the condition on which it depends is to be treated. When fainting occurs from no discoverable cause, it is often really epileptic, and must be treated as directed for **Epilepsy.** Simple fainting in nervous subjects, *Moschus* 3, 4h. From worry; hysterical fainting, *Ign.* 3, 4h. Periodical fainting in debilitated subjects, *Ars.* 3, 4h.

Faintness.—Sense of, at Pit of Stomach.—(1) *Act. r.* 3, 4h. (2) *Ign.* 3, 4h. (3) *Hydrastis* 1, 4h. At 11 a.m., *Sulph.* 3, 4h.

Falls. *See* **Bruises, Sprains.**

False Pains. *See* **Labour.**

Famine Fever. *See* **Relapsing Fever.**

Fatigue.—Fag and stasis, *Bellis p.* 1, 4h. *See* **Exhaustion.**

Fatty Degeneration.—General, (1) *Phos.* 2, 4h. (2) *Vanad.* 6, 4h.

Fatty Tumours. *See* **Tumours.**

Favus.—The crusts to be removed by poulticing, and the part kept saturated with lotion of *Dilute sulphurous acid* (one part to three of distilled water.) If after a fortnight this fails to remove the disease, a solution of *Corrosive Sublimate* (one part in five hundred) may be painted on night and morning, when the scales have been removed. Internally, *Cod-liver oil* should be given to weakly children, and *Sepia* 6, 6h. Extremely offensive odour, *Medor.* 200, gl. iv. every seven or fourteen days.

Fear or Fright.—Congestion of the head, feverish heat, restlessness, great fear; fear of death, *Acon.* 3, 1h. Continued anguish, with fear, cries, and tears, *Bell.* 3, 1h. Fears to be alone, especially evenings in bed, *Kali c.* 6, 4h. Great fear of death with sadness, *Plat.* 30, 8h. Fears to be in the dark, *Stram.* 6, 4h. Examination funk: *Arg. nit.* 30; *Æthusa* 30, these two may be combined, or given in alternation twice daily, commencing day prior, and continuing through examination period; stage-fright in musicians, *Anac.* 1, 4h.

Effects of.—Pains in the forehead, stupefaction or loss of consciousness; involuntary evacuations, *Opium* 3, 1h. Effects of fright, deep consuming grief, gastric disturbance, headache, convulsions (especially in children), *Ignat.* 3, 1h. diarrhœa caused by fear, *Puls.* 3, 1h.

Febricula. *See* **Fever.**

Feet.—Aching.—From over-walking, *Arn.* 3, 2h.; hot foot-bath with *Arnica* φ, a drachm to the gallon. A very effective alternative footbath is Muriate Ammonia, one drachm to a pint of warm water.

Burning.—*Apis* 3x, 4h. Burning in the soles, < whilst walking, *Graph.* 6, 4h. Burning in the feet at night, *Silic.* 6, 4h. Burning of the hands and feet, *Secale* 3, 4h. Heat of the feet with burning sensation in the evening in bed, followed by itching, *Sul.* 3, 4h.

CHILBLAINS. *See* Chilblains.

COLDNESS.—*Carbo v.* 6, 4h. With numbness and cramps, *Secale* 3, 4h. *See also* Circulation Cyanosis.

PAINS IN.—Painful drawing, as if sprained; heaviness and tension; stitches in the heels, as if stepping on needles; spasmodic contraction of the toes; pains < during rest, > during motion, *Rhus t.* 3, 4h. Feeling in the feet as if swollen and stiff, *Apis* 3x, 4h. Swelling and pain in the ankle, stiffness of the feet in the morning; heaviness of the feet; bruised pain under the heels; ball of right toe feels soft, thick, painful on stepping; boring in right great toe, *Led.* 6, 4h. Drawing pains in ankles, feet, and toes, *Caul.* 1, 4h.

SOLES.—Pains in, pains on stepping, *Mur. ac.* 3x, 4h. Violent spasmodic pains in the soles and heels, preventing stepping; burning in feet and soles; heels and balls of toes painful as if sore on stepping; toes sore as if ulcerated, *Phos. ac.* 1, 4h. Soles painful as if beaten; burning pain in soles, *Puls.* 3, 4h. Soles painful when walking on pavement, *Petrol.* 3, 4h. Burning in soles and heels when walking, *Graph.* 6, 4h. Burning in soles, *Sul.* 3, 4h. Cramp in the legs and feet; feet asleep and stiff, *Secale* 1, 4h. Neuralgic pain in instep and ball of toes; pain as if stepping on something hard in middle of ball of toes, *Brom.* 6, 4h.

HEELS.—Tearing in the heels, sprained pain in the ankles, boring in the great toe, *Silic.* 6, 4h. Cramps in the feet, tearing in the instep and great toe, *Colch.* 3, 4h. Tearing in the left heel and tendo Achillis, *Calc. caust.* 3, 4h. Stinging and pain in the heels, worse when sitting; sticking and weak feeling in tendo Achillis, *Valer.* 3, 4h. Acute pain in the heels; pulsative stitches in the left heel when standing, *Ran. bulb.* 3, 4h. Pain as if ulcerated, on standing, *Berb.* 1, 4h. Drawing tension in tendo Achillis; slow large stitches in tendo Achillis, *Mur. ac.* 3x, 4h.

PERSPIRATION.—Excessive and fetid (frequent washing in water containing a little Condy's fluid; stockings to be changed every day or oftener), *Silic.* 6, 4h. With tenderness of the feet, *Petrol.* 3, 4h. In persons subject to skin eruptions, *Sul.* 3, 4h. Profuse perspiration of the soles, causing soreness of the toes and balls of the feet, with sticking pains as if walking on pins, *Nit. ac.* 1, 4h. Profuse perspiration of the feet until they become sore, *Lyc.* 6, 4h.

SORENESS.—Soreness of the soles, especially towards the toes, *Silic.* 6, 4h. Swelling and heat in anterior portion of the sole, *Petrol.* 3, 4h. Sensitiveness of the soles, large horny places, *Ant. crud.* 6, 8h. Soreness, easily chafed, especially on heels, *All. cep.* 12, 8h.

Felon. *See* Whitlow.

Fester, TENDENCY OF SLIGHT WOUNDS TO.—(1) *Hep.* 6, 6h.; (2) *Gunp.* 3x, gr. vi. 6h.; (3) *Silic.* 6, 6h.; (4) *Petrol.* 6, 6h. *See also* Skin, UNHEALTHY.

Fetid Breath. *See* Breath.

Fever.—Fever from chill as sudden fall of temperature, *Aco.* 1—30, 1h. If not well relieved in twenty-four hours there is probable internal congestion development, *Sul.* φ—30, 2h. This will in most cases cut it short. If inflammation develops, see under appropriate heading. Simple ephemeral fever (febricula), *Acon.* 3, 2h. Simple continued fever with

bilious or gastric symptoms, *Baptis.* 1x, 2h. Continued
fever of a low typhoid type, (1) *Echin.* φ. 2h. (2) *Arsen.* 3,
3h. Fever of remittent type in children or adults; passing
off without perspiration, *Gels.* 3, 2h. Fever with exacerbation
every 3, 4, 12 hours or multiple of 12 hours, *Sul.* φ—30,
4h. *See also* **Hyperpyrexia**, and the various fevers under
their names.

Fibroma. (*Fibroid Tumour*).—*Silic.* 3, gr. iii. 8h. Uterine,
Secale 1, 4h. Profuse hæmorrhage, *Epihyst.* 30, once or
twice a week. Especially in women with tendency to enlarged
thyroid, *Thyroidin* 3x. gr. v. t.d. Menstruation too early and
profuse; flow bright red; *Ipec.* φ, unit doses. With cachexia,
Carcin. 100 gl. vi. once a week. Intractable bleeding from,
(1) *Ficus r.* φ—3x, 4h. (2) *Thlaspi bursa pastoris* φ, gtt. v. 4h.;
(3) *Hydrastinin mur.* 2x, gr. ii.—2, 4h. *See* **Menorrhagia**,
and **Uterus**, BLEEDING FROM.

Finger, GATHERED. *See* **Whitlow.**

Fissures. *See* **Anus, Hands, Nose,** etc.

Fistula.—Lachrymal, *Silic.* 6, 6h. Lachrymal and dental, *Fluor.
ac.* 6, gtt. ii. 6h. Anal, (1) *Sil.* 6, 8h.; locally, *Calendula*
lotion (a drachm to two ounces). (2) *Aur. mur.* 5x, 8h. In
tuberculous subjects, *Bac. test.* 30, gl. vi. every four or
seven days. After this, *Bism. trisnit.* 3x, gr. viii.—5, gtt. ii.
8h. Should these fail—(1) *Calc. phos.* 3, gr. viii. 8h.; (2)
Caust. 6, 6h.; *Calendula* lotion; (3) *Cal. fluor.* 3, gr. v. t.d.

Fits. *See* **Apoplexy, Convulsions, Epilepsy, Fainting, Hysteria.**

Flatulence.—Flatulent distension, causing frequent sighing or
belching, *Carbol. ac.* 3, 4h. Flatulence in the stomach,

coming upwards, causing oppression of the breathing, or
sharp pains about the chest, the bowels being regular or
loose, *Carb. v.* 6, 4h. Flatulence of the lower part of the
body, passing downwards if at all, constipation, *Lyc.* 6, 4h.
Pain relieved by eructations, *Lach.* 6, 4h. Wind coming away
easily, rushing upwards through the mouth, *Arg. n.* 6, gtt.
ii. 4h. Eructations, frequent, tasteless, odourless; or acid
and scalding pharynx; or tasting of food, *Sin. alb.* 3x, gtt.
v. 8h. Painful flatulence, impossible to pass it up or down,
Raph. 30, 2h. Flatulent dyspepsia, where "everything turns
to wind," *Nux mosch.* 3, 4h. Eructations empty, fetid,
bitter, putrid, causing sore pain in epigastrium and chest,
followed by sticking pain in stomach, contractive pain in
epigastrium taking away the breath; collection of wind in
epigastrium which is sensitive to touch, *Calc. i.* 3, 4h.
Flatulence and relief from eructations, *Cham.* ϕ, gtt. i. or
ii. in hot water, ½h. *See also* **Abdomen**, DISTENDED, **Distension, Dyspepsia, Eructations.**

Flooding. *See* **Labour** and **Menstruation.**

Fluor Albus. *See* **Leucorrhœa.**

Flushings of Heat. *See* **Face** and **Change of Life.**

Forehead. *See* **Face.**

Fracture.—To promote the union of, *Symph.* 1x, 4h. Where
the bones are much bruised, *Ruta* 1, 4h. In scrofulous
subjects, *Calc. phos.* 3, gr. v. 6h. In rickety subjects, *Silic.*
6, 4h.

Frambœsia, or Yaws.—(1) *Jatroph. curcas* 3x, 4h.; (2) *Merc.
nit.* 3x, 4h.

Freckles.—Dark freckles; on chest, *Nit. ac.* 1, 4h.; on hands, *Fer. magn.* 6, 4h.; on face, *Kali c.* 6, 4h.; on cheeks, *Sep.* 6, 4h. [Dilute *Citric acid* may be applied night and morning.]

Fright, Effects of. *See* **Fear.**

Frog. *See* **Aphthæ.**

Frost-bite.—Paint the part with compound tincture of *Benzoin* (Friar's balsam); if it is in the feet, and the stockings adhere, rub olive oil over the *Benzoin.* Internally (1) *Agar.* 3x, 4h.; (2) *Ferr. phos.* 3, gr. v. 4h. *See also* **Chilblains.**

Fungus. *See* **Excrescences.**

Fungus Hæmatodes. *See* **Cancer,** **Bleeding.**

Furunculus. *See* **Boil.**

Galacturia (*Chyluria*).—*Iod.* 3x, 4h.

Gall-stones. *See* **Calculus,** **Biliary.**

Ganglion.—(1) *Ruta* 1, 4h.; (2) *Benz. ac.* 3x, 4h. *Benzoic acid* lotion rubbed in night and morning (pure *benzoic acid*, fifteen grains; rectified spirit, three drachms; distilled water, eight ounces). (3) *Sulph. cm.*, once a week.

Gangrene.—Of wounds, *Lach.* 6, 2h.; lotion of *Lachesis* 6 (a drachm to two ounces) to be applied locally. Gangrenous ulcers, *Ecchin.* φ, gtt. i.—x, 2h.; locally, application of tincture, diluted with equal parts of water. Senile gangrene, *Secale* 1, 2h.; locally, an ointment of *Boracic acid*, where there is blood-poisoning from the wound. Great vital depression, coldness of extremities, blueness of the skin, burning pains, *Carb. v.* 6, 4h. Restlessness, anxiety, prostration, thirst, burning pains. *Ars.* 3, 4h. *See* **Pyæmia.**

Gastralgia. *See* **Gastrodynia.**

Gastric Catarrh. *See* **Dyspepsia, Stomach.**

Gastric Fever. *See* **Fever,** Simple Continued; **Enteric Fever.**

Gastric Ulcer.—(Rest and milk diet; if milk is not tolerated, Sanvia.) In general, especially when the ulceration is near the pyloric end of the stomach, *Uran. nit.* 3x, gr. ii. 6h. In chlorotic subjects, *Arg. nit.* 6, gtt. ii. 6h. With dry, red tongue, thirst, cachectic or typhoid condition. *Ars.* 3, 4h. After burns, *Kali bichr.* 3x, gr. ii. 6h. In elderly people with incarcerated flatulence, suspicion of cancer, *Ornith. u. φ* gtt. i. in powder, unit dose, or 3x, 8h. (For the relief of the pain which sometimes accompanies the affection, if the remedy most indicated does not suffice, *Atrop. sulph.* 2, gr. ii. may be given intercurrently.) *See also* **Duodenum.**

Hæmorrhage from.—If bright, *Ipec.* 1, every fifteen minutes. If dark, *Ham.* 1, every fifteen minutes. (Ice to suck; small pieces may be swallowed.)

Gastritis.—Acute croupous inflammation of the stomach is due to poisoning, and this must be treated by the appropriate antidote. Catarrhal, *see* **Dyspepsia, Stomach.** Degenerative inflammation of the stomach causing destruction of the peptic glands, *Phos.* 3, 4h.

Gastrodynia, Gastralgia, Pain in the Stomach.—Cramping, spasmodic pain, *Nux v.* 3, 2h. Burning pain, *Ars.* 3, 2h. Cutting pain, *Oxal. ac.* 3, 2h. Cramp-like and pressive pains in stomach, especially after eating, *Bism.* 6, 2h.

Gathering. *See* **Breast, Whitlow,** etc.

German Measles, *See* **Roseola,** Epidemic.

Giddiness. *See* **Vertigo.**

Glanders.—Begin with the nosode of the disease, *Hippoz.* 5—30, 2—4h. Copious discharge of glairy mucus, *Kali bich.* 3x—5, 1h. Intense depression, *Aur.* 3, gr. v. 2h. Restlessness, nervousness, anxiety, *Ars.* 3x, 2h. Ulceration of the mouth and skin, salivation, *Merc. c.* 3x—30, 2h. Intolerance of touch, low typhoid state, *Lach.* 6, 2h. Chronic glanders in horses, *Graph.* 3, gr. v. 4h.

Glandular Swellings, Acute.—At the commencement, *Bell.* 3, 1h. If *Bell.* fails to cut the affection short within twenty-four hours, *Baryt. c.* 6, 1h. If in submaxillary glands, *Arum tri.* 6, 2h. Bronchial glands, *Calc. c.* 6, 4h. If suppuration threatens; actual suppuration in inguinal glands, *Merc. sol.* 6, 4h.; in inguinal glands when *Merc. sol.* ceases to do good, *Nit. ac.* 1, 2h. If suppuration has actually taken place; threatening or actual suppuration in axillary glands, *Hep. s.* 6, 4h. After evacuation, *Silic.* 6, 4h. Locally *Calendula* φ lotion (a teaspoonful to two tablespoonfuls of water). *See also* **Breast, Bronchial Glands, Bubo, Hodgkin's Disease,** and **Tonsils.**

Chronic.—In all cases of scrofulous glands the treatment should be commenced with *Bacillinum* (*see under* Consumption). It should be given in doses of four or five globules of 30, 100 or 200 once a week, or less often. Other medicines may be given in the intervals, if indicated. If the condition is due to inherited syphilis, *Kali iod.* 1 or 30, every 4h. Submaxillary glands, *Arum tri.* 6—30, 4h. In pale flabby subjects, *Calc. iod.* 3x, 4h. In thin, weakly subjects, *Arsen.*

3, 4h. Should these fail—(1) *Baryt. c.* 6, 6h.; (2) *Cistus c.* 1, 4h. (3) *Plaguinum*, 30, 4h. *See also* **Goitre, Hodgkin's Disease.**

Glaucoma. *See under* **Eyes.**

Gleet.—*Thuja* 12, 4h. After *Thuja*, if necessary (1) *Nit. ac.* 12, 4h.; (2) *Cinnabar* 3x, gr. v. 4h.; (3) *Naphthalin* 3x, 4h.; (4) *Guaiac.* 3x, 8h. *Carcinosin* 30 or 200. 3 doses, at 6 hourly intervals will often cure when well indicated remedies help but fail to completely cure.

Glossitis. *See* **Tongue.**

Goitre.—Simple, soft, in general, *Thyr.* 3x, gr. ii.—30; or 1 or 2 tablets of the extract, 8h. (The action of this remedy should be carefully watched, and it should be stopped on any sign of over-action occurring). In dark-complexioned subjects, with dark eyes, *Iod.* 3x. 4h. In pale subjects, of soft fibre, cold moist feet, *Calc. c.* 6, 6h. If these fail, *Fluor. ac.* 3. gtt. ii. 6h. In old, hard goitres *Spong.* 3, 4h. persistently.

EXOPHTHALMIC.—In general *Thyrodin* 1 or 2 tablets, 8h.; or 3x, gr. ii.—30, 8h. (The action of this remedy should be carefully watched, and it should be stopped on any sign of over-action occurring.) In dark subjects, *Iod.* 3x—30, 4h.; in fair subjects, *Bell.* 3, 4h. In florid subjects, especially if chilly, *Caps.* 200, 8h. Protrusion of eyes, tumultuous action of heart, *Lycopus* 30, 8h. If there is anæmia, with full bursting headache, flushed face, *Ferr. met.* 6, 8h. In ill-nourished subjects, constipation, earthy complexion, *Nat. mur.* 6, 6h. During attacks of palpitation, *Glon.* 3, every half-hour.

Gonorrhœa.—At the commencement, during the feverish stage, *Acon.* 1, every half-hour. Thick yellow discharge, profuse, scalding, erections; when the prostrate gland is affected, *Thuja* 1—12, 1h. If there is much engorgement, with erections, *Canth.* 3x, 1h. Sudden and frequent urging to urinate, *Petrosel.* φ, gtt. v. 8h. When the acute stage is over, *Can. sat.* φ, gtt. ii. 3h. In females, *Copaiv.* 3x, gtt. v. 8h.; (2) *Sepia* 6, 2h. Chronic cases, *Naphthalin* 3x, 4h. Yellowish thick discharge; constitutional gonorrhœa, *Nat. sulph.* 3, gr. v. 8h. Suppressed gonorrhœa, headache and periodical pains from, *Sarsap.* φ, 8h. *See also* **Chordee, Gleet, Stricture.**

Gonorrhœal Rheumatism. *See* **Rheumatism,** Gonorrhœal.

Gout.—The paroxysm, (1) *Bell.* 3, ½h.; (2) *Urtica urens,* φ, gtt. v. in ʒi. of hot water, 4h. Locally, a hot compress on which several drops of *Colch.* φ have been dropped may be applied. Dejection, ill-humour, great weakness, nausea, shootings and tearings in muscles and joints < by movement < at night; tearings in legs, feet, and toes; with swelling, *Colch.* 3x—3, 2—4h. In the forming stage, *Puls.* 3, 2h. When gout flies about from joint to joint, *Puls.* 3, 2h. When it is connected with uterine disorder, *Sabina* 3, 2h. Subacute gout, *Led.* φ, 2h.

Gouty Diathesis.—Where there is tendency to skin eruptions, *Sul.* 6, 6h. Where there is constipation and copious deposit of lithates, *Lyc.* 6, 6h. *See* **Diet:** Gout.

Stored Gout.—This is Burnett's appropriate expression for sufferings localised in particular organs or tissues due to uric acid accumulations, *Urt. ur.* φ, gtt. v. in ʒi. hot water, 8h.

SUPPRESSED OR UNDECLARED.—General congestion, blueness
and coldness, *Rhus t.* 3, 2h. Coldness, earthy complexion,
constipation, *Nat. m.* 6, 6h. Congestion and pain in the
spine, *Oxal. ac.* 3, 4h.

IN THE EYE.—*Nux v.* 6, every ten minutes.

IN THE THROAT.—(1) *Guaiac.* 3x, 2h; (2) *Merc. sol.* 3, gr. v. 4h.

IN THE STOMACH.—*Nux v.* 6, every half-hour.

AT THE HEART.—Angina-like pain at the heart, coming on
suddenly in a gouty subject, *Cupr. met.* 6, every ten minutes.
See also remedies as indicated under **Angina Pectoris.**

Granulations. *See* **Excrescences.**

Gravel.—Red sandy sediment with flatulence in the abdomen
and constipation, *Lyc.* 6, 4h. Should this fail, (1) *Urtica ur.*
φ, gtt. v. 6h. (2) *Cocc. cact.* φ, gtt. v. 4h. White phosphatic
sediment, *Phos. ac.* 2x, gtt. iii. 4h. White sediment after
standing, acrid sourish odour, *Graph.* 6, 4h. Turbid urine,
white sediment; red (bloody) urine, with brick-dust sediment, *Ocim. can.* 3—30, 4h. Brick-dust or straw-yellow
granular deposit, *Chinin. sulph.* 1, 4h. White or whitish-
grey, and later, mealy reddish sediment; pain in the ureters,
Berb. φ, 4h. Pasty sediment, reddish or white, *Sep.* 6, 4h.
Oxalate of lime deposit, (1) *Nitr. mur. ac.* 1, 4h. (2) *Oxal.*
ac. 3, 4h. Turbid immediately after passing, like clay
water, much pain at end of urinating; white sand, scanty,
slimy, flaky urine, tenesmus of bladder, *Sarsa.* 6, 4h.

Green Sickness. *See* **Anæmia** and **Menstruation.**

Grief. *See* **Anxiety.**

Growing-pains.—*Guaiac.* 1, 4h.

Gum-boil.—*Merc. sol.* 6, 2h.

Gumma.—*Kali iod.*, gr. v.—xx. 8h.

Gum-rash (Red Gum).—(1) *Cham.* 6, 4h.; (2) *Ant. c.* 6, 4h.

Gums.—BLEEDING FROM.—*Merc. sol.* 6, 4h. *See also* **Purpura** and **Scurvy.**

    INFLAMED.—*Merc. sol.* 6, 4h.

    ULCERATION.—Simple ulceration—(1) *Nit. ac.* 6, 4h.; (2) *Merc. cor.* 3, 4h. With disease of the bone, (1) *Phos.* 3, 4h.; (2) *Silic.* 6, 4h.

    FALLING AWAY.—From the teeth, *Merc. sol.* 6, 4h. *See also* **Teeth** and **Toothache.**

Gutta Serena. *See* **Amaurosis.**

Hæmatemesis.—Dark blood, *Ham.* 1, every fifteen minutes. Bright blood, *Ipec.* 1, every fifteen minutes. From mechanical injury. *Arn.* 1, every fifteen minutes.

Hæmaturia.—*Tereb.* 3, 2h. Hæmaturia and hæmoglobinuria without pain or uneasiness, *Chi. sul.* 2x—30, 4h. Hæmaturia with dull renal pain, *Ham.* 1, 2h. From mechanical injury, *Arn.* 1, 2h. With red sediment, *Ocim. can.* 30, 2h. Dark, with thick urine *Thlaspi φ*, gtt. v. 4h.

Hæmoglobinuria.—(1) *Pic. ac.* 3x, gr. ii. 4h.; (2) *Phos.* 3, 4h.

Hæmoptysis. *See* **Consumption**, BLEEDING.

Hæmorrhage.—From any part if accompanied by nausea, bright-red blood and steady flow, *Ipec.* 1, 2h. FROM KIDNEYS. *See* **Hæmaturia.**

FROM BOWELS.—Dark blood, *Ham.* 1, 2h. Light-coloured blood, *Ipec.* 1, 2h. Copious, passive, painless, *Cact.* 1, 2h. Watery, not coagulating, *Sanguis.* 5, gtt. v. 8h. *See also* **Dysentery** and **Hæmorrhoids.**

LUNGS. *See* **Consumption**, BLEEDING.

NOSE. *See* **Nose.**

STOMACH. *See* **Hæmatemesis.**

UTERUS. *See* **Metrorrhagia, Labour,** and **Menstruation.**

Hæmorrhagic Diathesis.—(1) *Ham.* 1, 4h.; (2) *Phos.* 3, 4h.; (3) *Crotalus* 3, 4h.; (4) *Sanguis.* 5, gtt. v. 8h.

Hæmorrhoids or **Piles.**—Bleeding piles with open or loose bowels, *Ham.* 1—3, 4h.; locally, a lotion of *Ham.* φ, thirty drops to the half-pint of water, with which the part should be bathed night and morning; and at night a piece of lint dipped in this lotion may be placed on the tumour, or just inside the orifice. For irritation from piles, *Verbascum* ointment (*Verbascum* φ ʒi., Vaseline or Unguent. Cetac. ʒi.). Another useful local measure is the insertion at bedtime of a suppository containing, *Hamamelin* gr. ¼. Blind piles in persons of sedentary life, spare, of costive habits, *Nux v.* 3, 8h. Bleeding piles, costiveness, sinking at the stomach, especially in the forenoon; flushing; fainty spells; heat of the head with cold feet; irritable skin; < at night on getting warm in bed, and from washing, *Sulph.* 3, 8h. In sycotic subjects; swollen hæmorrhoids, pain < sitting or walking; pressing, itching and burning in hæmorrhoids; moisture at anus, *Thuj.* 1—30, 4h. Protruding hæmorrhoids, discharge of bloody mucus from anus; (follows well after *Thuja*) *Merc.*

viv. 3 gr. viii.—12, 4h. Burning, itching at anus, excoriation;
cutting pain after stool, protruding hæmorrhoids, constipation, fissure. *Nit. ac.* 5—30, 4h. Protrusion and ready
bleeding of hæmorrhoids, constipation; moisture about anus,
fissure; cramp and contraction of rectum, *Phos.* 6, 4h.
Where there is much uneasiness in the parts, pain in the
back, constipation, prolapse of rectum, generally absence of
bleeding symptoms < by walking; piles associated with
throat symptoms, *Æsch. hip.* 3x, 4h. Hard piles extremely
painful when touched, when walking, standing or sitting;
> after a stool; piles impeding stool; itching, stitching,
moist, stinging and burning; < when thinking of them; <
by touch; < when exerting voice, *Caust.* 5—30, 8h. Hæmorrhoids protruding before, during and after stool; burning
and itching in anus; < during menses, *Am. carb.* 5, 4h.
Great sensitiveness of the anus, itching, weakness of the
sphincter and tendency to prolapse, *Mur. ac.* 3x, 4h. Heat,
rawness, soreness, loose motions, prolapse, bleeding; piles
protrude like a bunch of grapes; constipation, or feeling of
insecurity of bowels, *Aloe* 1, 4h. Piles with burning and
stinging in rectum; sore and smarting; mucous discharge;
constipation, *Amm. mur.* 3x, 4h. Piles burning as if pepper
sprinkled on; tenesmus of rectum and bladder; tenacious
mucus mixed with black blood; cutting colic before stool;
tenesmus cutting and twisting during stool; after stool
tenesmus, burning, thirst, drinking causing shuddering,
drawing pains in the back; piles swollen, itching, throbbing;
soreness in anus; bleeding or blue; with mucous discharge;
with bloody mucous stools; with drawing pain in small of
back and cutting in abdomen, *Caps.* 3, 4h. Piles burn and
sting, *Carb. a.* 6, 4h. Hæmorrhoids burning, tingling;
itching and fissures in anus, *Ant. c.* 6, 4h. Soreness, itching,

moisture; piles protrude, blue suppurating and offensive; with burning; stitches in rectum, *Carb. v.* 6, 4h. Blind piles with pressure and soreness in anus and rectum; painful while sitting and standing, less while walking, though renewed and worse after taking the fresh air; prolapse of rectum from moderate exertion after stool; sharp burning pain in rectum, *Ignat.* 3, 4h. Piles with constipation from inertia of the rectum, especially when connected with uterine disorders or pregnancy, piles bleed, but only with great pressure, *Collin.* 1x—3, 4h. In blonde persons of the feminine type, bowels open or loose; mucous discharge, *Puls.* 3, 4h. Piles with much pain, bleeding and soreness; burning, biting and dryness in rectum (when persons who have piles take pneumonia), *Hyperic.* 1x, 4h. After all acute symptoms are passed, and only an insensitive swelling remains behind; external piles, *Fluor. ac.* 3, gtt. ii. 6h. [Patients should sit on wooden or cane-bottomed chairs.] *See also* Constipation.

STRANGULATED PILES.—Sometimes after a difficult stool piles become protruded, and spasm of the sphincter occurs, constricting the veins, and making return impossible, causing exquisite pain. When this occurs the best relief is obtained by applying a potato poultice. A quantity of potatoes are boiled or steamed and then mashed with plenty of unsalted butter and made into a poultice. This is placed on a triangularly folded piece of flannel and the patient made to *sit* upon it. One point of the flannel is then turned up between the thighs and the others passed round the back to meet it in the usual napkin fashion. This will give instantaneous relief, and the piles will soon find their way back of themselves. *Acon.* 1, may be given every ten minutes.

A very important measure in the management of piles is to avoid the use of paper after stool, substituting linen; and to carefully wash the parts with tepid water after each action. If possible, it should be arranged to have the action in the evening just before retiring to bed.

Hair.—DRYNESS, *Kali c.* 6, 6h. Falling off, with dryness, *Kali c.* 6, 6h. Falling off, *Fluor. ac.* 6, gtt. ii. 6h. Falling off from depressing emotions, *Phos. ac.* 1, 6h. Falling off with humid eruptions, scalp sensitive, *Nit. ac.* 30, 8h. Baldness, *Arn.* 1, 8h. Very greasy hair, *Bry.* 1, 8h.

Hands.—CHAPPED.—Application of glycerine at night. (1) *Nat. carb.* 12, night and morning; (2) *Calc. carb.* 12, night and morning. Should these not suffice *Petrol.* 3, night and morning; locally, *Sulphuros ac.* with glycerine (two drachms of *Sulphuros ac.* to an ounce and a half of *Glycerine*) to be applied at night. Failing this, paint the chaps every night with *Compound tincture of Benzoin* (Friar's Balsam) or apply Calendula cream or ointment.

BLUENESS AND COLDNESS. *See* **Chilblains.**

PAINS IN.—Drawing pains in wrist and fingers, with stiffness of fingers, *Caul.* 1, 4h. Rheumatic pains, < night, *Act. r.* 3,—30, 8h. Boring in first joints of thumbs, also tearing and sticking in the finger-joints, with tenderness of the periosteum when pressed on, *Ledum* 6, 4h. Bones in the back of the hands and wrists painful as if bruised, in rest and motion, *Ruta* 1, 4h. Sprained pains in the wrists, tearing in all the finger-joints, < at rest, *Rhus tox.* 3, 4h. Pain in r. wrist, *Act. s.* 3x—30, 4h. Pain in l. wrist, *Asc. t.* 3x—30, 4h. Spindle-shaped swelling of the fingers, stiffness and pain on

moving, *Puls.* 3, 4h. Hot, pale swelling of finger-joints, <
by motion, *Bry.* 1, 2h.

Perspiration of.—Palms constantly moist, *Fluor. ac.* 3, gtt.
ii. 6h. Cold, clammy perspiration, *Pic. ac.* 3, gtt. ii. 6h. In
Sulphur subjects, *Sul.* 200 unit dose. To be followed, if
necessary, later by *Calc. c.* 200.

Swelling.—Acute, inflammatory, *Apis.* 3x, 2h. With numbness at climacteric, *Arg. n.* 6, 4h. With flushing, *Ferr. phos.*
3, gr. ii. 6h.

Hay Asthma or Hay Fever.—In general, *Cr.k.s.* (*Chrome alum*)
3x, gr. vi.—3, 4h. This covers a large number of cases, and
is equally valuable as protective if given before the season
sets in. Violent sneezing with lachrymation, redness and
swelling of eyelids, contractive stupefying headache, *Sabad.*
3x—30, 4h.; the same dilution to be snuffed up the nostrils,
or a spray of *Sabad.* φ ʒi. to ʒiii. of water. Catarrhal symptoms < indoors, > in open air, *All. c.* 12, 1h. With fever
and prostration, *Arsen.* 3, 6h. As a prophylactic, *Ars.* 3, 8h.,
for a week or two before the hay-season begins, and a week
or two after. Constitutional, in psoric subjects, great sensitiveness to cold air, desire to lie down, *Psorin.* 30, 2—4h.
Excessive sneezing, *Gels.* 3, 4h.

Headache.—As to Character and Position.—In forehead and
temples, *fulness and throbbing*, heavy drooping eyelids, blindness or flashes of light; flushed face, hot head, sense of
burning in eyeballs; all the symptoms < by light, noise,
movement, or lying down, easiest when sitting, *Bell.* 3, 1h.
Sick headache or migraine ; drawing, tearing, pressive pains;
intolerance of light; disturbances of vision, *Kali. carb.* 6. ½h.
during an attack, 8h. during the intervals. *Pressive* headache,

as if everything would come out at the forehead; or as if
the scalp were compressed all over by a pitch cap; blind
headache; supra-orbital headache; squeezing in forehead
above root of nose; face pale or livid and anxious, *Acon.* 3,
½h. Headache over one eye, especially right; before headache comes on sight is blurred, the sight improving when
the pain begins, *Kali bich.* 5, 2h. Headache on coughing as
if the skull would burst; bursting, *full* headache; constant
pressing headache above the root of the nose, together with
some stitches through the eye and over the eye; *stitching*
headache; *throbbing* in one or other temple; *drawing, tearing*
headache, *Caps.* 3, 1—4h. Over left eye, with acidity and
eructations, *Carb. v.* 6, 4h. As if the top of the head were
opening and shutting; or as if the calvarium were being
lifted off; headache with flatulence, throbbing of occiput,
Cann. i. 3, 4h. *Heavy pressive* headache, with giddiness,
flushed face, derangement of stomach as after overeating
or drinking or smoking, constipation; increased by taking
food and on mental exertion, *Nux v.* 3, 2h. Throbbing or
pressing headache, vertex or occiput; burning heat on
vertex; < coughing; < at night in bed; < on waking; >
pressure; congestive headache with rush of blood to head;
headaches recurring once a week, *Sul.* 6—30, 4h. Periodical
every Saturday; as if head would burst and the eyes would
fall out, > by rest, by closing eyes, in open air, lying on
painful side, *Sep.* 6—30, 8h. Headache in terrific shocks;
involuntary jerking of head, *Sep.* 6—30 2h. *Sick headache*
in persons of spare build, costive habit, and sedentary life,
Nux v. 3, 1h. *Dull heavy* pains in the head, especially at the
vertex, with throbbing in the temples, drooping eyelids,
heavy eyes, giddiness, > on copious evacuation of pale
urine, *Gels.* 3, 2h. *Bursting, splitting, pressive* headache in

forehead, across the eyes, > by pressure, greatly < by
stooping, which causes a sensation as if the brain would fall
out; sick headache of right side with retching and bilious
vomiting, < from all movement, even of the eyes, *Bry.* 3,
2h. Headache from *sunstroke* or exposure to heat, violent
throbbing, made worse by every movement, flushed face;
bursting headache, *Glon.* 3, 1h. Headache from exposure to
sun, feeling of *constriction* and fullness, pressive headache at
vertex, especially with menstrual derangements, or at the
menopause, *Cact. g.* 3, 2h. Headache, as if the head were
swelling to a great size, *Bov.* 6, 2h. Heavy, *dull pressing* in
forehead, incapacitating from mental labour, *Aloe* 3, 2h.
Constant *dull frontal* headache from liver derangement.
Leptand. 1, 2h. *Pressive* headache at the vertex, *Phos. ac.* 1,
2h. Pain like a *heavy weight at the top* of the head, aching
and burning in the temples and above the eyes, pain in the
eyes, congestion, lachrymation, intolerance of light and
sound, *Phell.* 3, 4h. *Burning* sensation at the top of the
head; *supra-orbital* headache; periodical; accompanied by
debility, or *arising from debility*, red tongue, low, feverish
condition, > by wet applications and in open air, *Ars.* 3, 2h.
Supra-orbital neuralgic headache, dim vision, *Chinin. sulph.*
3, 4h. Headache coming on in the *morning* on waking, and
lasting the greater part of the day; headache brought on by
coughing, *Nat. m.* 6, 4h. *Burning vextex* headaches of the
menopause; one-sided sick headache, with pale face; headache < after sleep, *Lach.* 6, 4h. *Weight and oppression* at
vertex, with cold feet and flushing of the face; dull but
severe pain in the fore part of the side of the head, with
great depression, *Naja* 6, 2h. *Dull* headaches, with depressed
spirits and constipation, *Plumb.* 6, 4h. Headaches from loss
of sleep, mental strain, worry; *aching* at the *vertex, occiput,*

and in *eyeballs*, *Act. r.* 3, 2h. Headache *beginning in the occiput*, extending forwards and downwards, causing obscuration of sight; shooting pain up spine into head, *Pic. ac.* 3, 4h. *Constant dull* aching in the *nape* of the neck, *Hell. n.* 3, 2h. *Pressive aching* in limited spots; pressure at centre of forehead and root of nose; headache from worry, anxiety or grief; "*clavus*," pressive sick headaches, with disturbance of vision, passing off with a copious discharge of clear urine, face pale, *Ign.* 3, 2h. Headache beginning with a blur before the eyes, dull, heavy, or *throbbing and shooting* in the forehead and up the right side, with nausea, vomiting, and great depression, *Iris v.* 3, 2h. Headache on vertex, temples (mostly r.), above eyes, root of nose, < *when covered*, < at night and lying down; > in open air and from cold; < 4—8 p.m., *Lyc.* 6—30, 2—4h. *Pressive* headache on the right side and over the right eye, *Chel.* 1, 2h. (*Chel.* and *Lyc.* follow and complement each other well.) *One-sided sick headache*, pain coming from back of head, and settling in right eye, > by lying down and by sleep, accompanied by bilious vomiting; aching of teeth and in ears; pains in the limbs, electric shootings in the head, and shiverings (menses profuse), *Sang.* 1, 2h. *Sick headache*, with vomiting, as in sea-sickness, *Cocc. ind.* 3, 2h. *Sick headache*, with violent vomiting, *Zincum sulph.* 6, 2h. *Sick headache*, with coldness of the head much acid in the eructations and vomit, *Calc. acet.* 3, 2h. *Chronic headache*, with sensitiveness to pressure, noise, motion and light, > by warmth (as by wrapping the head in a shawl); chronic headache with nervousness and loss of memory from overwork, commencing low in the back of the neck with a feeling as if the muscles could not support the head, passing over to the top of the head, forehead, and at times involving the eyeballs and making them sore, *Silic.*

6, 4h. *Boring* pain at the root of the nose, *rheumatic* headache, where the pressure of the hat is not tolerated, *Hep. s.* 6, 4h. *Chronic* headaches with melancholia, *Zinc.* 6, 4h. Headache, like *neuralgia*, especially on left side, pain coming at regular intervals, spreading from the brow to the face and neck, and involving the eyes, < by the least concussion or motion, especially stooping; pale face, restlessness, palpitation, *Spig.* 3, 2h. Headache of *passive congestion* after great losses of blood, *Ferr. pyrophos.* 1x, gtt. iii. 4h. *Jerking, tearing* pains in the head; the brain beats in waves against the skull; sensitiveness, noises in the ear, made < by walking, > by lying down, *China.* 1, 2h. *Pressive drawing* pains in the head, *intolerable*, < when attention is directed to them. *Cham.* 6, 2h.

ACCORDING TO CAUSE AND OCCASION.—On *coughing*, as if the skull would burst, *Caps.* 3, 4h. Headache caused by *every cough*, *Nat. m.* 6, 4h. Headache < by *coughing;* brain racked by coughing, which causes intolerable pain, *Lob. i.* 1, 2h. Stitches in the head with *cough*, *Bry.* 1, 2h. In the occiput, on coughing, *Sul.* 6, 4h. From *over-eating or drinking*, *Nux v.* 3, 4h. Periodical headaches arising from or associated with state of *debility*, *Ars.* 3, 4h. From *sunstroke*, violent throbbing, *Glon.* 3, 1h. From *sunstroke*, as if a tight band were bound round the head, *Cact.* 3, 1h. From *liver derangement*, constant dull frontal headache, *Leptand.* 1, 4h. Alternating with diarrhœa, *Pod.* 3, 2h. Burning vertex headache of the *menopause*, *Lach.* 6, 4h. Headache after *checked menses*, (1) *Æthus. c.* 3. 4h. (2) *Sen. aur.* 1, 2h. Headache from pain in other parts; or congestion after great *losses of blood*, *Ferr. pyrophos.* 1x, gtt. iii. 4h. Pain in head on *shaking* it, *Hep.* 6, 4h. Headache of school children, (1) *Calc. ph.* 6x, gr. vi., night and morning; (2) *Nat. m.* 30, night and morning.

Head Lice.—The hair to be washed daily, and after each washing to be bathed with a lotion of *Sabadilla* φ, an ounce to the pint. Internally give *Nat. m.* 6, 4h. There are extremely effective proprietary preparations obtainable from chemists which will speedily remove this nuisance.

Hearing. *See* Ears: DEAFNESS.

Heart.—PERICARDITIS.—If taken at the very commencement, pain, oppression, anxiety, restlessness, fever, *Acon.* 3, 1h. After *Acon.*, pain sharp, worse on motion, *Bry.* 1, 3h. Little fever, much effusion, *Merc. s.* 3, gr. v. 4h. Effusion remaining behind after the acute symptoms have passed, *Arsen.* 3, 2h. Pericarditis secondary to Bright's disease, *Arsen.* 3, 2h.

ENDOCARDITIS.—Stitching pain in chest, anxiety, restlessness, fever, *Aco.* 3, 1h.; sharp, shooting pains in the region of the heart, palpitation, restlessness, *Spig.* 3, 1h. Ulcerative, *Lach.* 6, 1h. With low fever, *Echin.* φ, gtt. v. 4h. With rheumatism of joints, pains shifting much, *Kalm.* 1, 2h. In pyæmic conditions, *Gunp.* 3x, gr. iv. 2h. Valvular affections remaining after the acute stage is past, *Naja* 6, 4h.

HYPERTROPHY, SUFFERING FROM.—When the hypertrophy has been brought on by prolonged over-exertion, as in athletes, *Arn.* 3, 4h. [When the hypertrophy is secondary to valve-disease, it is really compensatory and not a morbid condition; but then it sometimes gives rise to great distress, which may be removed by treatment as indicated.] Feeling of weight at the heart, palpitation, strong beats, throbbing in the carotid and temporal arteries, *Acon.* 3, 2h. Violent palpitation, felt worse on lying on the back, increased by excitement, motion, rising up suddenly or walking; throbbing of the temporal arteries, flushed face, headache at the vertex, *Cact.* 3, 2h. Much palpitation, felt in the throat, full pulse, sleeplessness and restlessness at night, *Bell.* 3, 2h. *See also* PALPITATION.

DILATATION AND WEAKNESS OF THE HEART-MUSCLE (whether consequent on valvular disease, or due to general debility, or to primary fatty degeneration of the muscular fibres). In general, especially if co-existent with respiratory affections, *Ars. iod.* 3x, gr. ii. or gtt. ii., thrice daily, immediately after food. [If this fails to give any relief, it should be left off entirely and the medicines to be named given as indicated.] Weak heart, with or without valvular disease, dropsy, dyspnœa; nervous, irritable, melancholic, *Cratæg.* φ, gtt. v. 4—8h. Irregular, intermittent, feeble action, sudden pain in heart region, *Phaseol.* 9x, gr. ii. 6h. Great weakness, anxiety, long-lasting palpitation, *Baryt. carb.* 3x, gr. v. 6h. Slow pulse, intermittent or irregular, palpitation on the slightest movement, breathlessness, pallor and faintness on sitting up, *Dign.* 3, gr. v. 4h. Palpitation and fainting fits, worse on movement or stooping, *Thyr.* 3x, gr. iv.—30, 4h. Frequent fainting attacks, *Mosch.* 6, 1—2h. Constrictive feeling at the chest, violent palpitation, *Cact.* 3, 4h. Degeneration of heart muscle; small frequent irregular pulse; dyspnœa; œdema; nervous palpitation and arrest of breathing; loathing of food, vomiting, distaste for alcohol, *Stroph.* φ, gtt. i.—v. or 3x, 4h. Pains about the heart, followed by palpitation, "sinking" sensation at the pit of the stomach, *Act. r.* 3, 4h. Darting, stabbing, shooting, or lancinating pain at the heart, passing down the left arm, *Spigel.* 3, 4h. Pain at the heart and down the left arm, with numbness, palpitation, faintness, *Naja* 6, 4h.

FATTY HEART.—The treatment of fatty degeneration is the same as that for DILATATION. For deposit of fat about the heart as a part of general obesity, *Phos.* 3, 4h., with suitable regimen and diet. After this, *Baryt. c.* 3x, gr. v. 6h. When the symptoms are such as indicate degeneration, the medicines recommended for DILATION may be given as indicated.

NERVOUS WEAKNESS.—From excessive use of *stimulants* and *tobacco*, pain at the heart, depression, palpitation, nervousness, without any signs of structural lesion, *Spig.* 1—30, 4h. Palpitation worse on walking; when lying on left side at night; dull, heavy pains, worse by slight excitement; constriction as if heart grasped by iron hand; very acute pain, stitches that cause weeping and crying aloud, with obstruction of breathing; pricking pains at heart, impeding respiration and movements of body, *Cact.* 3, 4h. Heavy sensation; uneasiness; great pain near heart; depression, lowness; *Naja* 6, 4h. Violent beating, throbbing in carotids, felt only when lying in bed or during a siesta; hurried, pressing feeling, relieved when busy; interrupted pulsations of heart and breathing; dull, heavy or pressive pain in region of heart; heaviness; palpitation when lying on left side; pain in left side, as if the heart were suddenly gripped (or alternately grasped and relaxed), waking from sleep; pressive pains; sharp pain, *Lil. t.* 30, 8h. Pain in region of heart before and during menses; and before and during urination, *Lith. c.* 6, 8h.

PALPITATION.—[This is a symptom of most kinds of heart disease. The cases now considered are those where there is no structural disorder to be made out, or where palpitation is the chief trouble complained of.] Palpitation in a heart that retains its vigour, *Aco.* 3, 2h. From indigestion; <

after eating, flatulence after eating, constipation, *Nux v.* 3, 2h. From indigestion in females or blonde persons, acidity, bowels inclined to be loose, *Puls.* 3, 2h. With excessive flatulence in the stomach after food, > by eructations, *Carb. v.* 6, 2h. Palpitation and irregular action, *Iberis* 3, 4h. Nervous palpitation, during the paroxysm, fainting or faintness, *Mosch.* 3, every twenty minutes. Palpitation and fainting, exceedingly rapid action, *Thyr.* 2x, gr. ii.—30, 4h. Palpitation, heart-failure threatened, *Crat.* φ, gtt. v. 2h. Palpitation with irregular or intermittent action, *Dign.* 3, gr. iv. 2h. Nervous palpitation in persons of great impressionability, < at night in bed, palpitation keeping the patient awake, *Ign.* 3, 2h. Palpitation on the least excitement, especially at the change of life, *Lach.* 6, 2h. Palpitation with "sinking" sensation at the pit of the stomach, and great uneasiness, sleeplessness, *Act. r.* 3, 2h. Palpitation with tightness across the præcordia, *Cact.* 3, 2h. Palpitation with shooting, cutting pain in the region of the heart, *Spigel.* 3, 2h. Palpitation on slight exertion; with full, throbbing headache, flushed face, great sensibility to light and noise, *Bell.* 3, 2h. Palpitation when lying down in bed at night or after food, *Nat. m.* 6, 2h. *See also* **Aneurism, Angina Pectoris, Arteries, Dropsy,** Cardiac, etc.

Heartburn.—Simple, *Arg. n.* 6, 4h. With white tongue, loaded urine, flatulence and constipation, *Lyc.* 6, 4h. Sensation of fire rising from stomach to throat, *Manc.* 6, 4h. With loaded tongue, flat taste, bowels loose, *Puls.* 3, 4h. During an attack, *Caps.* 3, every fifteen minutes. When due to acidity, *see under* Acidity, *See also* **Dyspepsia.**

Heat Spots.—*Apis* 3x, 4h.

Hectic Fever.—In consumption, with moist and coated tongue
   Baptis. 1, 2h. In consumption, with dry tongue, *Ars.* 3, 2h.
   [These medicines may be given intercurrently with other
   which may be indicated by symptoms other than those o
   fever.] In cases of prolonged suppuration, *China.* 3, 2h. I
   septicæmia, *Chinin. arsen.* 3x, gr. iv. 4h.

Heels. *See* **Feet.**

Helminthiasis. *See* **Worms.**

Hemicrania. *See* **Headache.**

Hemiopia.—Vanishing of the right half of objects, *Lith. c.* 6
   4h. Vanishing of the left half, *Lyc.* 6, 4h. Vanishing o
   either vertical half, *Mur. ac.* 6, 4h. Vanishing of the uppe
   half, *Aur.* 6, 4h.

Hemiplegia. *See* **Apoplexy** and **Paralysis.**

Hepatalgia. *See* **Liver,** PAIN IN.

Hepatitis. *See* **Liver,** INFLAMMATION OF.

Hernia.—[In chronic cases, a truss will be required; in strangulation operation must not be delayed; but in the absence o
   a surgeon relief may be given by the timely internal administration of medicine. The effect of posture will, of course,
   be studied. The patient will be made to lie on the back
   with the hips raised above the level of the shoulders.] Pain
   in an old hernia, *Nux v.* 1, 4h. Threatened strangulation,
   Nux v. 1, every ten minutes (the lower part of the body to
   be raised). Hernia in children, if fat, *Calc. c.* 6, 8h.; in thin,
   rickety children, *Silic.* 6, 8h. If the child has pain in the
   hernia, *Nux v.* 3, 1h. Inguinal hernia with cutting and

neuralgic pains up right side, *Æscul. h.* 1, 4h. [In umbilical hernia a pad must be used, and the skin drawn by strips of plaster from both sides so as to make it lap over the tumour, which will then contract.] Surgical advice should always be sought when possible.

Herpes.—Of lips, *Rhus t.* 3, 2h. Of prepuce, (1) *Merc. sol.* 6, 4h. (2) *Sarsap.* 6, 4h. (3) *Nit. ac.* 12, 4h.

Herpes Circinatus, or Iris.—*Tellur.* 6, 4h.

Herpes Zoster (Shingles).—In general, *Variol.* 6, 4h. After this, if necessary, a selection may be made from the following. In persons below middle life, *Rhus t.* 3, 2h. In older persons, *Mezer.* 3, 2h. Chronic cases, *Arsen.* 3, 4h. If the pain is intractable, *Pru. spi.* 30, 3h. [Locally, in all cases, a lotion of *Canth.* 3x, ten drops to the ounce, may be kept applied on linen. Or an ointment of *Canth.* 3x, ʒi. to Ung. *Cetac.* ʒi. Another useful application is a mixture of *Zinc oxide* and *Castor Oil* in sufficient proportions to make a paste. Or the eruption may be painted over with collodion. When the eruption has disappeared and the pain persists, or when there is pain without eruption, *Plantago* φ may be painted on the part.] When the scalp is affected, *Rhus t.* 30, three times daily for three days is usually sufficient.

Hiccough.—Ordinary acute cases, *Nux v.* 3, every ten minutes. If *Nux* does not speedily relieve, *Cyclam.* 3, every ten minutes; in chronic cases every four hours. *Mag. phos.* 30 in hot water, sipped frequently, is a wonderful remedy in the absence of individual indications. After drinking, eating, or smoking, *Ign.* 3, every ten minutes. With spasm and belching, *Cicut., vir.* 3, every ten minutes. Spasmodic,

Æthus. c. 3, 4h. Violent hiccough, especially in malarial cases, *Nat. m.* 6, 4h. In hysterical cases, *Moschus* 3, every ten minutes. [The same medicines may be given three or four times a day, during the intervals between the attacks, the medicines being chosen according to the indications given.] In obstinate cases, (1) *Hydrocy. ac.* 1, 2h.; (2) *Sul. ac.* 3x, 4h.; (3) *Kali brom.* gr. ii. 4h.

Hip-joint Disease.—The same treatment as for CARIES: *see under* Bone. Rest and extension so long as the disease remains active; diet of the most nourishing kind; cod-liver oil. *Bacil.* 30—200, gl. iv. once a week. For the FEVER attending the disease, if there is restlessness, anxiety, thirst, dry skin, *Acon.* 3, 2h. If the fever is of a hectic type, *Phos. ac.* 1, 2h. If there is profuse discharge and hectic fever, *China* 1, 2h. Sharp pain from hip to knee, especially of right side, *Kali carb.* 30, 8h. Coxalgia, *Arg. met.* 3x, gr. v. 4h. *See also* Joints.

Hoarseness. *See* Voice.

Hodgkin's Disease (Lymphadenoma).—(1) *Aco.* 3, 8h.; (2) *Calc. fluor.* 6, 8h.; (3) *Kali mur.* 3, gr. v. 8h.; (4) *Pest.* 30, 8h. When the spleen is enlarged, *Nat. m.* 6, 8h. When there is fever, *Arsen.* 3, 8h. A course of *Baryt. iod., Ars. iod.* and *Ferr. iod.,* each in 3x, gr. ii., given thrice daily for one or two weeks. [The constitutional symptoms of the patient will be the best guide to the remedy in treating this affection.]

Home-sickness.—Red cheeks and sleeplessness, *Caps.* 3, 4h. Much weeping, *Mag. mur.* 6, 4h. After these *Phos. ac.* 3, 4h.

Hooping-cough. *See* Whooping-cough.

Hordeoleum. *See* Stye.

Housemaid's Knee.—Acute—(1) *Apis* 3x, 2h.; (2) *Sticta p.* 1, 2h. Chronic, *Rhus t.* 3, 4h.; locally, a lotion of the same (*Rhus t.* 3x, one drachm to the ounce). If this fails, *Kali iod.* gr. ii. 8h.; locally, a lotion of *Kali iod.* (five grains to the ounce).

Hunger. *See* **Appetite.**

Hydrocele.—Congenital, *Bry.* 3, 4h.; when arising from a blow, *Arn.* 12, 4h. In acquired hydrocele, the following medicines may be given in their order, each being tried for a few weeks before being changed—(1) *Bry.* 3, 4h.; (2) *Rhodo.* 3, 4h.; (3) *Puls.* 3, 4h.; (4) *Sil.* 6, 6h.; (5) *Aur.* 6, 4h.; (6) *Graph.* 6, 4h. [The desirability or otherwise of operation will be considered in each case.]

Hydrocephalus.—ACUTE (TUBERCULAR OR SIMPLE).—*Bacil.* 100, gl. iv. in half a tumbler of water; a teaspoonful every 4 hours; if *Bacil.* acts at all it acts rapidly; no other medicines should be given so long as improvement is progressive. Violent pains in head, stupor, delirium, bloodshot eyes, *Iodof.* 3x, 2h. Flushed face, restlessness, bright eyes, dilated pupils, boring head into pillow, rolling it from side to side; starting from sleep in fright, convulsions, hot head, cold feet, *Bell.* 3, 1h. Face flushed, or alternately flushed and pale, fontanelle open and projecting, slightest attempt to move the child makes it cry, *Bry.* 3, 1h. Hot head, perspiring, feet clammy and cold, especially in fat, flabby children, sour vomiting, sour green stools, cannot bear to be moved, *Calc. c.* 30, 1h., till relieved, then less often. Boring head in pillow, rousing from sleep with shrill, piercing cry, scanty urine, *Apis* 3x—30, 1h. After *Apis* if this is not sufficient, after suppressed eruption, child lies in stupor, cold sweat on forehead, jerking of limbs, *Sulph.* 30, 1h., till relieved.

When torpor predominates, child asks for nothing, but drinks greedily when given water, fontanelle prominent, urine suppressed, *Helleb.* 3, 1h.

CHRONIC.—After suppressed eruptions, child objects to be washed and washing aggravates, stupor, jerking of limbs, hot head, cold feet, *Sul.* 30, 8h. Acid vomiting and purging, perspiration of head and face, cold and clammy feet and legs, child cannot bear to be moved, *Calc. c.* 30, 8h. Bulging in occipital region, *Hed. hel.* φ, unit doses at long intervals.

SPURIOUS.—Arising in children from exhausting diseases, such as diarrhœa, *Phos.* 3, 2h. Should this not suffice, *Zinc. mur.* 6, 2h.

Hydrophobia.—Immediately after the bite suck the wound, and whilst sucking, press the parts around in the direction of the wound. After everything possible has been drawn from the wound, the best remedy is heat—whatever is handiest—red-hot iron or coals, or a lighted cigar, to be brought as near the wound as possible without causing violent pains and without burning the skin—as close, in fact, as the patient can bear it. Several pieces should be put in the fire so that one can be used as another cools. The skin around the wound may be smeared with oil, or fat, or soap, or saliva to protect it. All that oozes from the wound should be wiped away. The applications should be repeated three or four times a day, for an hour each time or until shuddering appears, and this should be repeated several days. Afterwards the patient should take daily one or more Turkish or Russian baths for a fortnight. *Hydrob.* 30 should be taken three times a day for a week, and then *Bell.* 3 night and morning for six months at least. If, in spite of all

precautions, the disease should show itself, the patient
should at once be removed to a Turkish bath, or placed in
a Russian bath and *kept in it*. *Bell.* 1x should be given
hypodermically every half-hour, and afterwards, should
Bell. not succeed, *Stram.* 1x—12, every half-hour in the
same way. If there is excessive sensitiveness and the patient
wants to tear the clothing away from his throat, *Lach.* 6, ½h.
If the characteristics spasm of the throat at the sight or
sound of water, bright objects or draught of air is marked,
Hydrob. 30, ½h. Other remedies are (1) *Agave* φ; 2h. (2)
Hyo. 1—30, 2h. (3) *Canth.* 3, 2h. (4) *Fagus* 1, 2h.

Hydrothorax.—Effusion left behing after inflammation, if the
inflammation has been recent, *Apis* 3x, 3h. If the effusion
is of any standing, *Sulph.* 3, 4h. When secondary to heart
disease, *Arsen. iod.* 3x, gr. ii., three times a day immediately
after food. Anxiety, thirst, chilliness, prostration, *Ars.* 3,
2h. *See also* Pleurisy.

Hyperpyrexis.—When the bodily temperature becomes so high
as of itself to threaten life (106°F. and upwards), in addition
to internal remedies, cold packing and cold bathing should
be resorted to. The cold wet-pack should be tried first.
The patient should be kept in for half an hour, and the
pack repeated every two or three hours if the temperature
again rises. Should the pack not succeed in reducing the
temperature, the patient may be sponged with ice-water. If
no amelioration follows, the patient should be put into a
bath at 95°F.; and this should be gradually cooled to 70°F.
The patient should be kept in the water for twenty minutes.
The internal remedies will be those indicated by the
patient's general state. In general, *Camphor* (Rubini's Tincture) gtt. iii. in syrup, every half-hour. If the skin is dry,

and there is restlessness and anxiety, *Acon.* 1, 15m. If the
fever is of a low type with muttering busy delirium, picking
at the bedclothes, *Agar.* φ, 2h. Quarrelsome delirium,
dilated pupils, photophobia, flushed face, perspiration, hard
full pulse, *Verat. v.* 1x, 1h. Rheumatic fever, pain in joints
of vertebræ, especially in the nape of the neck and at the
back of the head, *Act. r.* 1x, 1h. Flushed face, bright eyes,
active delirium, *Bell.* 1, ½h. *See also* **Rheumatism: ACUTE.**

Hypertension.—Pulse full, strong, hard, anxiety, restlessness,
Aco. 1, 2h. Full, hard, bounding pulse, congestive symptoms,
Ver. v. 1, 2h. In arterio-sclerosis, atheroma and gout, *Visc.
alb.* φ, gtt. v. 8h. (A French preparation of Mistletoe (*Guipsine*)
may be given in the form of pills, ii. 4 times a day for a few
days and then less often as tension lessens.

Hypochondriasis.—When secondary to disordered digestion,
with constipation, *Nux v.* 3, 4h. In unhealthy subjects,
earthy complexion, constipation, great depression, *Nat. m.*
6, 4h. In syphilitic subjects, *Aur. mur.* 3x, 4h. From spermatorrhœa, *Act. r.* 1x, 4h. As of a pall over everything, cannot attend to business, and suicidal tendency, *Act. r.* 3x—
30, 4h. Feels he is losing his senses, *Calc. c.* 200, night and
morning. Hypochondriacal monomania, as syphilophobia,
Hyo. 3, 4h. From forced sexual abstinence, *Con.* 3, 4h.
Abdominal spasms and diaphragmatic pains; intolerable
uneasiness; abdominal pains relieved by walking, which,
however, soon tires, compelling to rest, rest causing the
pains to return, *Stann.* 6, 4h. Nervousness, excitement,
sleeplessness, *Valer.* 3, 4h. Where the pains are described as
burning, red tongue, thirst, *Arsen.* 3, 4h. Anxious about
salvation, sinking at the stomach in forenoon, dejected

appearance, loss of memory, *Sul.* 6, 4h. *See also* **Depression of Spirits.**

Hysteria.—In the paroxysm, *Mosch.* 3, 15m. Great impressionability, capriciousness, rapidly alternating mental states, "lump" in the throat, effects of worry, *Ign.* 3, 4h. Outbursts of passion followed by quick repentance; hysterical laughter, *Croc.* 6, 6h. Great depression, *Plat.* 6, 4h. "Lump" in the throat, hysterical cough and asthma, distension of the body, *Asaf.* 3, 4h. With amenorrhœa, *Sen. aur.* 1, 4h. Gnawing sensation in epigastrium, unconquerable gloom, tendency to suicide, *Act. r.* 3—30, 4h. Convulsive hysteria, *Tarent.* 3, 4h. Nervous excitement and sleeplessness, *Valer* 3, 4h. *See also* **Mania** and **Melancholia.**

Hysterical Joint.—Recent, *Ign.* 3, 4h. If this does not succeed, *Cham.* 6, 4h. In more chronic cases, *Argent. met.* 3, gr. v. 4h.

Hysterical Vomiting.—*Kreas.* 3, 1h.

Hystero-Epilepsy.—During the attacks, *Moschus* 3, every five or ten minutes. During the intervals, *Zinc. valer.* 3, 4h.

Ichthyosis.—In chilly subjects, cold hands and feet, *Thyr.* gr. v., or 3x, gr. iii. or 30, 8h. Ill-nourished subjects, dry skin, thirst, anxiety, *Ars.* 3, 8h. Dry scaly skin, itching and burning in scrofulous subjects, with swelling of lymphatic glands, *Ars. i.* 3x, 8h. Skin of whole body dry, cracked; frequent, empty, sour eructations, prostration, *Nat. c.* 30, 8h. Entire absence of sweat, obstinate constipation, *Plumb.* 30, 8h. Hard, dry skin, white scales, *Pip. methyst.* 1x, gtt. v. 8h. Dirty grey, cadaverous-looking skin; wart-shaped excrescences; brittle or soft nails, *Thuj.* 30, once a day, or once a week. Vaccinal cases (1) *Vaccin.* 30, 8h.; (2) *Maland.*

30—200, once a week. Whitish scales, intolerable itching, *Hydrocot.* φ—3, 4h. Where there is sycotic history *Medorrh.* 200, once or twice a week. Where there is a history of syphilis, *Luet.* 200, once or twice a week. [Locally, Turkish bath and shampooing; friction with cod-liver oil, or with *Oleum theobromatis* or cocoa butter.]

Impetigo.—Of the face (milk crust), recent, *Viol. tric.* 3, 4h. [Locally, in all cases, only rain water, or distilled water, with a few drops of *T.C.P.* put into it, to be used for washing.] Milk crust, where there are burning pains, *Cicut. v.* 3, 4h. Pustules on inflamed base, itching, stinging, *Crot. t.* 12, 4h. Deep, inflammatory redness; moist eruption; discharge excoriates other parts, *Mez.* 30, 4h. More chronic cases, *Ant. tart.* 6, 4h. Impetigo of the head, *Calc. mur.* 1x, 4h. (*See also* Eczema of the scalp.) General impetigo, *Ant. tart.* 6, 4h.; cod-liver oil and nourishing diet.

Impotence.—When there is a history of an injury or blow, *Arn.* 3, 4h. From an injury to the spine, *Hyperic.* 1x, 4h.; locally, liniment consisting of equal parts of *Hyperic.* φ, spirit of wine and distilled water to be rubbed on the injured part night and morning. Simple impotence, *Agn. cast.* 3, 4h. Impotence with wasting of the testicles, *Kali brom.* 3x, 4h. When due to sexual excess, *Phos. ac.* 1, gtt. iv. 6h. When accompanied by general nervous depression and irritability, digestive disorders, and constipation, *Nux. v.* 3, 4h. Impotence of long standing, *Lyc.* 30, 8h. Should these not succeed, (1) *Selen.* 6, 4h. (2) *Bufo sah.* 30—200, night and morning.

Incontinence of Urine. *See* Urine.

Indigestion. *See* Dyspepsia.

Influenza (EPIDEMIC, RUSSIAN OR SIBERIAN INFLUENZA).—**As** prophylactic, let all who are exposed to infection, or when epidemics are about, take *Ars.* 3, pil. iii. 8h. Another excellent prophylatic is *Bacillinum* 30 and *Influenzinum* 30, a dose of each taken together or as a combination remedy once a week during influenza epidemic. In general, *Infl.* 30, 2—4h. Aching in all limbs, headache, pains in eyes, foul tongue, fever, restlessness, with general soreness of body, heaviness and drowsiness, *Bapt.* 3x—30, 1h. Chills in back, bone pains predominating, *Eup. perf.* 1—30, 1h. Violent throbbing, bursting headache; bursting headache with cough, *Glon.* 3—30, 1h. Headache, sore throat, teasing, tickling cough, < on lying down, delirium, neuralgia, especially on right side of head and face, inflammation of the ears, *Bell.* 3—30, 1h. After *Bell.* or when suppuration occurs, *Merc. sol.* 6—30, 1h. Chills up and down spine, red face, weakness, relaxation, no thirst, *Gels.* 1—30, 1h. With low typhoid condition, *Echin.* φ, 1—2h. Cough < by least movement, pain in head with cough; pains in limbs or body, < by movement; foul, wash-leather-like tongue; thirst, *Bry.* 3x—30, 1h. Cough, with blood-streaked expectoration, difficult to detach, cannot get breath; pains worse in right side, *Sang.* 3x—30, 1h. Teasing cough, worse at night; thirst, restlessness, anguish, fear of death, rheumatic headache, *Ars.* 3—30, 1h. Fever, restlessness, fear of death; pains in the region of heart, with pallor and faintness, fear of death, *Acon.* 3—30, 1h. (*Acon.* may be given at night intercurrently with other remedies, when there is nocturnal restlessness and sleeplessness.) Bronchitis, suspiciously like tuberculosis, *Aviare* 30, 1h. With herpetic or "diphtheritic" sore throat, *Phytol.* 1—30, 1—2h. Metastases of other symptoms to heart with pain and collapse, *Camph.* one drop

of Rubini's tincture or one pilule every 5 or 10 minutes.
Sharp pain at heart, with palpitation and weakness, inability
to lie on left side, *Spigel.* 1—30, ¼h. Pleuritic pains, worse
on coughing, cough causing pain in head; tearing cough,
heat in head, nightly perspiration, early morning diarrhœa,
Sul. 3—30, 1h. Chills in back, pulse very rapid, bed feels
too hard, all discharges offensive, *Pyrogen* 5, 2h. Morning
diarrhœa, liver derangement, *Pod.* 3—30, 1h. Copious evacuations, much pain, perspiration and cold sweat on forehead,
Ver. alb. 3—30, 1h. Sciatica (1) *Rhus t.* 3x—30, 1—2h. (2)
Arsen. sul. rub. 3—30, 1—2h. Weakness after influenza, (1)
Psorin. 30, 4h. (2) *China.* 3x—30, 2h. *See also* for complications under various headings—**Cough, Diarrhœa, Headache, Neuralgia, Pleurisy, Pneumonia, Sciatica**, etc.

Sequelæ of Influenza.—Chronic illnesses brought on by an
attack of influenza, *Tuberc. k.* 30—200, once or twice a
week. Debility after influenza, *Bapt.* 1x, 4h. Debility with
nervous symptoms of restlessness and insomnia, *Scutel. φ*,
gtt. v. 4h. Nervous debility, symptoms > by diversion of
mind, *Piper. methyst. φ*—12, 2h. Nervousness, sleeplessness,
weakness and despondency, *Cyprep.* 1, 2h. Loss of taste and
smell. *Mag. mur.* 5, 2h.

Influenza Cold. *See* **Cold.**

Infra-Mammary Pain. *See* **Breast.**

In-growing Toe Nail. *See* **Nails.**

Insanity. *See* **Mania, Melancholia.**

Intemperance. *See* **Alcohol Habit.**

Intermittent Fever.—PROPHYLACTIC.—Persons going into malarious districts should take for a short time before, *Chin. sulph.* 1x, gr. v. night and morning, and continue the same at increasing intervals during their stay. If *Quinine* is not tolerated, *Ars.* 3x should be given in the same way. In persons sensitive to the action of *Arsenic*, the third centesimal trituration may be given in place of the third decimal.

THE DISEASE.—[The remedies for intermittent fever are best given at the end of a paroxysm when it is quite over. A few doses may be given at short intervals, and this repeated at the end of the next paroxysm if it occurs in milder form or if aggravated. If it is unchanged another remedy must be selected.] Tertian or quartan fevers, thirst before or after the chill, often no thirst during chill, patient craves warmth but it does him no good, sweat profuse and debilitating, attacks usually at 5 a.m. or 5 p.m., not in the night, restless the night before an attack; darting, tearing pains in joints, adapted to lymphatic and swarthy persons, debilitated constitutions, *Chi.* 1x—3, 2h. Tertian fever; chill, heat and sweat, accompanied with thirst, pain and tenderness all down spine during chill; painfulness and swelling of varicose veins during a chill; short apyrexia with great thirst, *Chin. sul.* 3x—30, 2h. When indications not clear, *Sul.* φ or 30, 8h., may clear up the case or cure. Periodicity in intervals of 12 hours or multiples of 12; psoric subjects after suppression of exanthemata; chilliness constantly creeps from sacrum up back without subsequent heat or thirst; icy coldness of genitals; burning heat of palms of hands and soles of feet; profuse sweat at night and restless sleep; thirst, but can only drink in prodroma and apyrexia, *Sul.* φ or 30, 4h. One stage absent; heat of burning character; rapid prostration; torpid weakness; dropsical swellings;

after the abuse of quinine, *Arsen.* 3, 2h. Chronic cases;
Indian fever recurring periodically in patients who have
returned to Europe, *Urt. ur.* φ, gtt. v. in ℥i. hot water, 4h.
Clean tongue, rapid exhaustion by single paroxysm, rapid
appearance of sallow pallor, *Arsen.* 3, 2h. Dumb ague chills,
Arsen. 3, 6h. Chills towards evening, little or no sweat;
agues of damp, warm and low marshy climates, *Cedron.* 3,
2h. Chill between the shoulders, thirst with chill, sweat
with heat, no thirst in heat, < by eating and drinking, *Caps.*
3, 2h. Thirst before chill (which usually occurs in the morning), bilious vomiting during the paroxysms, scanty perspiration at the close, bone pains, *Eup. per.* 3, 2h. Irregular
advent of chills beginning in the small of the back and
running up and down, lips and nails blue, violent shaking
and comparatively little coldness; during the sweat any
attempt to move causes a chilliness to pass through the
body, *Eup. purp.* 3, 2h. Vomiting in the paroxysms, especially if they come on in the evening or night, *Ipec.* 3, 2h. (If
the symptoms are not characteristic of any remedy, a few
doses of *Ipec.* may be given after an attack. This will remove
the disease or bring out characteristic symptoms which will
indicate the remedy.) During chill, sensation as if tendons
too short; chill < on lying down; increase of cough if he
drinks water during chill. *Cimex* 30, 4h. Spots on the lips,
thirst before and during the chill, headache in the heat and
at its close as if beaten with little hammers, perspiration,
beginning in the morning; after abuse of quinine, *Nat. mur.*
6, 3h. With gastro-intestinal symptoms, the heat preceding or
mingling with the chills, *Nux v.* 3, 2h. In blonde persons
with gastro-intestinal symptoms, in chlorotic girls, *Puls.* 3,
3h. Tendency to copious diarrhœa and vomiting, prostration, faintness, coldness, and sweating, *Verat. alb.* 3, 2h.

Non-malarial cases, attack coming on in afternoon, no thirst, sensation during the chill as if the hands were dead, *Apis* 3x, 2h.

THE CACHEXIA.—Sallow pallor, clean red tongue, faintness; after abuse of quinine, *Arsen.* 3, 6h. Earthy complexion, chilliness, enlarged spleen, constipation, headaches beginning in the morning and lasting all day; after abuse of quinine, *Nat. mur.* 6, 6h. Enlarged and painful spleen, *Ceanothus,* 1, 4h.

Intertrigo. *See* Excoriation.

Intestines.—OBSTRUCTION OF.—(If not rapidly resolved; operation should not be delayed.) When due to fæces impacted in the rectum, the mass must be dug out. Until the obstruction is removed all solid food must be forbidden, also all milk food and all farinaceous food. Only clear meat soups and meat essences to be given.) Absence of pain or desire for stool, *Opium* 3x, ½h. Violent colic, > bending double, *Coloc.* 3x, ½h. Twisting, strangulating pain, *Nux v.* 3x, ½h. Cramps, drawing in of abdomen, *Plumb. ac.* 3 gtt. ii. ½h.

ULCERATION OF.—Duodenum, from burns, *Kali bich.* 3x, gr. ii. 6h. Ulceration of intestines with chronic diarrhœa, *Kali bich.* 3x, gr. ii. 6h. Ulceration of large intestine, with slimy, bloody stools; in dysentery, *Merc. cor.* 3, 3h. *See also* **Dysentery.**

Iritis. *See under* Eyes.

Irritation.—Itching, < at night, *Rad. bro.* 30, once a week. Itching, < in bed at night, scratching followed by burning, *Sul.* 3, 4h. Itching, tingling, formication, *Sul. ac.* 1, 4h. Crawling, tingling, and itching of the whole body, *Morph.* 3, 4h. Intolerable itching of the whole body, < on getting

warm in bed at night, dry skin, *Alumina* 6, 3h. Itching
coming on when the part is exposed to cold, *Rumex c.* 6,
4h. Burning itching in debilitated persons, *Ars.* 3, 4h. Itching as from crawling; after scratching, the itching reappears
elsewhere; itching of the vagina, *Mez.* 3, 4h. Itching of old
people; of the vulva, (1) *Rad. bro.* 30, once a week; (2) *Rhus
v.* 3, 4h. Itching of the urethra, after gonorrhœa; itching of
the vulva, *Nit. ac.* 1, 4h. Itching of the vulva and anus,
Ambra 6, 8h. Burning or biting itching; inflammation and
swelling of parts, *Kreas.* 3, 8h. Violent itching with exfolia-
tion of skin; psoriasis, *Petrol.* 3, 8h. Itching of genitals,
Carbol. ac. 3, 4h.; of pudenda before menses; of scrotum,
Graph. 6, 4h.; of pudenda, with swelling, *Sep.* 6, 4h. Itching
after menses, *Tarent.* 3, 8h. Itching and burning of pudenda,
with eruption on inner side of thighs during menses, *Silic.*
6, 6h. Itching of vulva in pregnancy; with constipation and
piles, *Collins.* 1, 4h. Itching of the vulva, *Calad.* 3x, 4h.
Soreness, itching, burning of female genitals, *Carb. v.* 6, 4h.
Heat, itching, and herpetic eruptions about the genitals,
Dulc. 1, 4h. With inflammation of the labia—(1) *Apis* 3x,
2h.; (2) *Cocc. cact.* 3, 2h. Itching of the mons veneris, *Berb.*
1x, 4h. Itching of the anus, *Lyc.* 6, 4h. [When the skin
becomes harsh and irritable, and especially when violent
irritation of mons veneris and pudenda sets in without
apparent cause, it may be a symptom of diabetes, and
sugar should always be tested for.] *See also* **Anus:** ITCHING.

Itch.—There are extremely effective proprietary preparations
obtainable from chemists which will speedily remove this
nuisance. In genuine cases of parasitic itch the parts affected
may be painted over with *Oil of Lavender*, or rubbed at
bedtime with *Balsam of Peru*. One or two applications will

be sufficient. If this does not suffice, inunction with *Sulphur ointment* every night; hot bath with soap, followed by change of bed- and body-linen every second night. Internally, *Sulph.* 3—30, 4h., to be followed, if necessary, with *Psor.* 30, 8h.

Jaundice.—Simple, from catarrh of the bile-ducts; pain in liver and inability to lie on right side, *Merc. sol.* 6, 4h. Sharp pains in liver, > from lying on right side, *Bry.* 3, 1h. Yellow stools pains under angle of right scapula, *Chel.* 1, 1h. From fright or a fit of anger, *Cham.* 6, 2h. With congested liver, white stools, *Chi.* 3, 4h. Malignant jaundice (as in acute yellow atrophy), *Phos.* 3, 2h. From blood disorganisation (as in yellow fever), *Crot. h.* 3, 2h. Chronic, not due to obstruction, *Iod.* 3, 2h. With much irritation; or irritation after, *Dolichos pruriens*, 3x, 1—2h.

NEONATORUM.—(1) *Cham.* 6, 2h.; (1) *Merc. s.* 6, 2h.

Jaw.—Caries or necrosis, *Phos.* 3, 4h. After *Phos.* or when from phosphorus poisoning, *Sil.* 6, 4h. Growth of bone, exostosis, *Hecl.* 6, 4h. Epulis, *see* Epulis. Easily dislocated, feeling as if dislocated, *Petr.* 3, 4h. Cracking in the joint, *Rhus t.* 3, 4h. Painful cracking in the joint, *Granat.* 3, 4h. Pain in joint as if sprained, on swallowing, *Arum. tri.* 12, 4h. (if given in a low attenuation this should be freshly prepared).

Joints.—Cracking in, on moving, *Ginseng.* 3x, 4h. In gouty subjects, *Guaiac.* 3x, 4h. In gouty subjects with high-smelling urine, *Benz. ac.* 3x, 4h.; on stretching, *Thuj.* 3x—30, 4h. Pain in, coxalgia, neuralgia, "hysterical joint," (1) *Arg. met.* 6, 4h.; (2) *Zinc.* 6, 4h. *See also* Hysterical Joint.

ACUTE SYNOVITIS.—In rheumatic subjects, fever, restlessness, anxiety, pain, *Aco.* 3, 1h. Pain < with every movement, part sensitive to touch, *Bry.* 3, 1h. In women and children, pain < by heat > by cold, *Puls.* 3, 1h. Where there is much swelling and little pain, *Apis* 3x, 2h. When suppuration has taken place, *Hep.* 6, 4h. (externally, a lotion of *Hep.* 6, a teaspoonful to a wineglassful of distilled water). Where discharge has commenced, *Sil.* 6, 4h. (externally, a lotion of *Sil.* 6, a teaspoonful to a wineglassful of distilled water).

CHRONIC SYNOVITIS.—Syphilitic or mercurial, *Kali iod.* gr. iii. 6h. Rheumatic, *Merc. sol.* 6, 4h. Of the knee, *Berb.* 1x, 4h. Of the right knee, *Benz. ac.* 3, 4h. Dropsy of the joint, *Iod.* 3x, gtt. ii. 4h.

SCROFULOUS SYNOVITIS (WHITE SWELLING).—[In all cases where it is tolerated, cod-liver oil should be given, beginning with a teaspoonful twice or three times a day immediately after food; it may be increased in quantity as toleration is established.] *Bacil.* 30—200, gl. iv. once a week. In fat subjects of soft fibre, subject to cold clammy feet, heat of the head with perspiration, *Calc. c.* 30, 8h. Early in the disease in patients of blonde type and mild disposition, pain, < by heat, *Puls.* 3, 4h. In thin rickety subjects, offensive perspiration, especially about the head or feet, symptoms > by wrapping up warmly, *Sil.* 30, 8h. After *Sil.*, emaciation, numbness of the limbs, inability to lie on left side, *Phos.* 3, 8h. In strumous subjects with enlarged tonsils, *Calc. phos.* 3x, gr. v. 6h. Where there is marked want of animal heat, *Led.* 6, 4h. Dry skin, anxiety, fever, and restlessness, *Aco.* 3, 2h. Hectic, *Phos. ac.* 1, 2h.

BURSITIS. *See* Housemaid's Knee.

GANGLION. *See* Ganglion. *See also* Gout, Rheumatism, Hip, Knee, etc.

Joy, EFFECTS OF EXCESSIVE.—*Coff.* 3, 1h.

Kala-azar (TROPICAL SPLENOMEGALY OR DUM-DUM-FEVER).— This is a very fatal disease caused by the Leishman-Donovan protozoal body. To this *Antimony* is the antidote. It is injected intra-venously in the form *Stibacetin* beginning with 0·1 grm. and working up generally to 0·8 grm. Or a colloidal preparation of *Oxide of Antimony* may be injected intra-muscularly (1-50th of a grain in 15 drops of *Glycerine* and 15 drops of *distilled water*). The same remedy may be given by the mouth in homœopathic form. Dr. Neatby says *Arsen. alb.* is especially useful in infantile kala-azar.

Kidneys.—CONGESTION.—In early stage, with feverish symptoms, flushed face, *Bell.* 3, 1h. Suppression of urine, bloody urine, after scarlatina, *Tereb.* 3, 1h.

BRIGHT'S DISEASE.—Incipient, with dropsy, *Apis* 3x, 1h. Inflammation of the kidneys with suppression of urine, as after scarlatina, *Canth.* 3, 1h. Tubular nephritis, (especially after scarlatina), albuminuria, tube-casts, dropsy, thirst for cold water, anxiety, desire for warmth, *Ars.* 3, 2h. Nephritis of pregnancy; suppurative nephritis, *Merc. c.* 3, 2h. *Chronic Bright's Disease:* Prostration, restlessness, anxiety, thirst, cool skin, internal heat, dropsy, *Ars.* 3, 4h. Pale bloated appearance, chilly, vomiting of food or passing it undigested, fulness of the head, nose-bleeding, irritable patients, *Ferr. met.* 6, 8h. Fever, headache, irritation of the bladder and frequent desire to pass water, *Ferr. Phos.* 3, gr. v. 8h. Granular degeneration, gouty kidney, pale, bloated, heavy expression, melancholy disposition, costiveness, *Plumb.* 6, 4h. Exclusive milk diet; *see* **Diet.**

See also **Hæmaturia, Urine.**

Knee.—Pain, swelling, dryness or cracking, especially of right knee, *Benz. ac.* 3, 4h. Cracking when walking, *Caust.* 6, 8h. Stiffness, soreness, pain as if beaten, swelling, *Berb.* 1x, 4h. Coldness of knees, *Agn. c.* 3, 4h. Knees cold, < at night, *Carb. v.* 6, 8h. Knees sink down from weakness, cracking in the joints, *Cocc. i.* 3, 2h. Sharp pain, weakness, grating sensation, *Dioscorea* 3, 2h. *See also* **Housemaid's Knee, Joints, Rheumatism,** etc.

Labia, INFLAMMATION OF.—Œdematous, *Apis* 3x, 2h. Heat, swelling, and inflammation, cannot bear the touch of clothing, *Cocc. c.* 3, 2h. Irritation, *see* **Irritation.**

Labour.—PREPARATORY.—In general, *Act. r.* 3, 8h. for four weeks before term. If a difficult labour is anticipated, *Arn.* 3, 6h., four weeks before the time expected. Flatulency in pregnant women; tendency to difficult labour, *Calc. fl.* 6x, gr. v. night and morning for several months before term, intermitting it for one or two weeks at a time. Inability to walk (from relaxation of ligaments of pelvis); discomfort of later weeks, *Bellis* 3x, 8h. Constipation of later months of pregnancy, *Collinsonia* 3, 8h. Spurious pains, *Cauloph.* 3, 3h.; if there is great nervousness, *Act. r.* 3, 3h.; if due to indigestion, *Puls.* 3, 3h.

DURING LABOUR.—Great relief may be obtained during the dilation of the external parts by applying from time to time a new sponge wrung out of *hot Calendula* lotion (*Calend.* φ, ʒii. to hot water Oj). The same measure will assist healing and give great comfort after labour.

RIGID OS.—If due to the condition of the cervix alone, apply a pat of fresh lard or butter and give *Caul.* 3 every fifteen minutes. Rigid os, false pains, nervousness, tremors, prostration, *Gels.* 3x—30, ¼—1h. Barnes' bags may be used for dilating if necessary. If along with rigidity the patient is restless and feverish, *Aco.* 3 every thirty minutes. If there are feeble pains as well as rigidity, *Caul.* 3, 15m. If the patient is much exhausted, a morphia suppository in the rectum will arrest the pains and give the patient time to recover strength.

FEEBLE PAINS.—If due to general debility of the patient, *China.* 3, 15m.; hot-water douche. If due to exhaustion of uterus, *Chloral* gr. v., followed in twenty minutes by a further dose of gr. x.

RETAINED PLACENTA.—The preparatory administration of *Arnica*, *Bellis*, or *Calc. fluor.* diminishes the tendency to this.

AFTER-PAINS.—*Caul.* 3, ½h.

AFTER-TREATMENT.—If nothing abnormal, *Arn.* 3, 2—4h. for 48h., assists the recovery of the parts.

HÆMORRHAGE.—Introduce the hand, clear out any clots, apply pressure from without; the uterus will contract on the hand. If this fails, inject hot water (120°).

CONVULSIONS.—Every muscle of the body twitches from the eyes to the toes, *Hyo.* 30, ½h. Convulsions excessively violent; opisthotonus, *Cic. v.* 30, ½h. Giddiness, diplopia, cramps in abdomen, tremors, convulsions, *Gels.* 30, ½h. Insensibility, convulsions, back, face, and jaws principally affected; anosicys, *Hydrocyan. acid.* 3x, 15m.

CONSTIPATION.—*Veratr. alb.* 3, 6h.

PUERPERAL FEVER.—Dry skin, heat, pain, anxiety, restlessness, *Acon.* 3, 1h. Blood-poisoning fever, *Echin.* φ, 1—2h. (This may be given alone or alternated with other remedies). A few doses of *Sulph.* 200 or 1m, in many cases, if given early, will be all that is required. Excessive tenderness, distension, bloody and slimy evacuations, *Merc. cor.* 3, 1h. Sudden stitching pains, compelling patient to cry out; < 2—4 a.m., *Kali c.* 30, 1h. Excessive sensitiveness of abdomen, symptoms < after sleep, *Lach.* 6, 1h. Pyæmic conditions, *Pyrogen.* 5, gtt. v. 4h. Hot flannels may be applied to the abdomen, if there are peritonitic symptoms. Hot injections of a dilute Condy's fluid solution, if there are offensive discharges.

PUERPERAL MANIA. *See* **Mania.**

PUERPERAL MELANCHOLIA.—*Act. r.* 3, 3h. *See* **Melancholia.**

LOCHIA.—Offensive; suppressed; or insufficient, *Sulphur* 3, gtt. i. 2h. Locally, injections of solution of *Calendula* in hot water (one teaspoonful to the pint).

Lachrymal Sac. *See under* **Eyes.**

Lactation, DISORDERS OF.—Milk fever, *Acon.* 3, 2h. Undue engorgement of breasts, *Bry.* 3, 2h. Milk late in appearing, or afterwards diminishing in quantity, *Asaf.* 3, 2h. Agalactia, *Urt. ur.* φ, gtt. v. in hot water, 4h. When the milk is poor in quality, in pale lymphatic subjects, *Calc. c.* 6, 6h. In thin rickety subjects, *Silic.* 6, 6h.; in tuberculous subjects, *Phos.* 3, 4h. To promote the flow in pregnant women who have had poor milk in previous confinements, *Calc. ph.* 3x, gr. x., h.s.s. for two or three months before term. In weaning, to prevent engorgement, *Bry.* 3, 4h. To diminish the flow of milk, *Puls.* 3, 4h. To arrest the flow on weaning, *Urt. ur.* φ gtt. v. 4h. Effects of over-lactation, *China.* 3, 2h. *See* **Breast, Inflammation of.**

Landry's Paralysis. *See* **Paralysis, Acute Ascending.**

Laryngismus Stridulus. *See* **Croup, Spasmodic.**

Laryngitis.—Acute.—Irritating hacking cough, with restlessness, anxiety, and fever, *Acon.* 3x, every half-hour, and at longer intervals as improvement takes place. If within six hours there is no improvement, the following medicines are to be given:—Barking cough, hoarseness, aphonia, *Spong.* 3, ½h. Thick, glutinous, stringy expectoration, yellowish, hard to get away, *Kali bich.* 3x—3, ½h. When the cough has become loose, but hoarseness remains, *Hep. s.* 6, 2h.

Œdema Glottidis.—*Apis* 3x, ½h.

Chronic.—Aphonia, weakness of vocal muscles, cough hard, causing urging of urine, *Caust.* 3, 3h. Stringy expectoration, difficult to get away. *Kali bichr.* 3x, 3h. Loose cough, mucous expectoration, white tongue, feeling of sickness, *Ant. t.* 6, 3h. Dry, irritable larynx, *Phos.* 3, 3h. Hoarse, dry cough, > lying down, *Mang.* 6, 3h. Dry, choking feeling in larynx, raising of yellow matter, *Hep. s.* 6, 8h. Raising of small lumps of blood and mucus, tendency to hoarseness; commencing tubercular laryngitis, *Nat. selen.* 3, 3h. Long-standing catarrhs of elderly people, low vitality, insufficiently nourished, venous capillary dilatation, *Carb. v.* 6, 3h. Chronic irritability of larynx, without much organic alteration, *Lach.* 6, 3h. Follicular laryngitis, *Iod.* 3x, 4h. Follicular laryngitis in eruptive subjects, *Sulph.* 6, 4h. Tubercular inflammation, chronic cases, *Ars. iod.* 3x, gr. ii. 8h. after food; *Bacil.*

30—200, gl. iv., 7—10 days. Tertiary syphilis, *Kali iod.* gr. v.—x., three times a day.

Laughter, UNCONTROLLABLE.—*Croc. s.* 30, 10m. Weeping interrupted by fits of laughter, *Phos.* 6, 1h.

Lead Colic.—(1) *Op.* 1x, ¼h.; (2) *Alumen* 3, 1h.

Legs, CRAMP IN. *See* **Cramp.**

PAIN IN.—Pain in legs making lame, *Diosc.* 3, 4h. Cramp in fore part of leg near tibia, when walking; gnawing pain in shin bones; painful contraction in calves when walking, *Carb. a.* 6, 4h. Pain from ankle half way up the leg, causing lameness, *Guaiac.* 3, 4h. Pain in tibia, *Badiag.* 6, 4h.; with great sensitiveness to touch, *Lach.* 6, 4h.

PARALYSIS OF. *See* **Paralysis:** PARAPLEGIA.

SWELLING OF. *See* **Dropsy.**

ULCERS OF. *See* **Ulcers.**

VARICOSE VEINS. *See* **Veins,** VARICOSE.

WHITE LEG. *See* **Phlegmasia Alba Dolens.**

Lentigo. *See* **Freckles.**

Lepra. *See* **Psoriasis.**

Leprosy.—In the treatment of this disease deeply acting remedies, and especially the nosodes, will have to be resorted to. Courses of either *Bacil.* 100, *Vaccin.* 30—200, or *Maland.* 30—200, being given once or twice a week, sometimes for several weeks. Among other remedies that may be given are (1) *Thyroidin,* one or two tablets, 8h.; (2) *Hoang-nan* φ, gtt. v. 8h.; (3) *Hydrocotyle* φ, gtt. v. 8h.; (4) *Hura* 3x—5,

8h.; (5) Numbness, feeling of pins and needles in the parts, which are cold; patches of raised, hardened skin, anæsthesia, *Anac.* 3x—30, 8h.; (6) Pricking sensations, dirty-looking tubercles, dropping off of finger and toes, enlarged glands, *Ars. i.* 3x, 8h.; (7) Offensive discharge from the nose; melancholy, suicidal, *Aur.* 3, gr. v. 8h.; (8) Tubercular leprosy; extreme debility, *Calot. g. φ*, gtt. v. 8h.; (9) Cracks discharging sticky fluid, *Graph.* 3x—30, gr. v. 8h.

Leucocythæmia.—Pain or discomfort in the region of the spleen, *Ceanothus* 1, 2h. Earthy complexion, coldness, cachexia, *Nat. m.* 6, 4h. Cold, clammy feet, dropsical swellings, worse after washing with cold water, *Calc. c.* 6, 8h. Where there is sexual excitement, *Pic. ac.* 3x, gr. i. 4h. Vertigo, foul breath; in alcoholic subjects, *Querc.* 3x, 4h. Where these fail, *Arsen. iod.* 3x, gr. iv., immediately after meals. [*Ceanothus* may be given intercurrently with any one of the other three; should it not prove sufficient of itself, it will almost always relieve the pain. Hygienic measures should be strictly enjoined in all cases—open-air exercise, nourishing diet; in chilly subjects, sponging with spirit of wine every morning.]

Leucoma. *See* Eyes: OPACITY OF CORNEA.

Leucorrhœa (Whites).—[The attempt to "cure" this affection by medicated internal douches is radically bad; and if it succeeds in its aim it inevitably entails worse ill-health for the patient. Only such measures as are required for cleanliness should be adopted.] Simple, mucous, in blonde impressionable subjects; chilly, but averse to warmth, *Puls.* 3, 4h.; copious bland leucorrhœa, with backache as if broken in two, *Calc. ovi. test.* 6—30, 8h. Leucorrhœa with enlarged or painful spleen; in patients who have had malarial fever; in those who have taken much quinine, *Cean.* 1, 4h. Like white of egg; yellow-green, leaving green spots on clothes; thick, slimy, tough, *Bov.* 3x—30, 8h. Clear, copious, albuminous, unnaturally hot, *Borax* 3—30, 8h. Greenish and thick, or profuse, watery and offensive, *Sep.* 6, 4h. Thick, corrosive, *Sabin.* 3, 4h. Yellow, offensive, acrid, causing itching, biting, and burning of pudenda, *Kreas.* 3, 4h. Burning smarting, staining linen yellow, *Carb. an.* 3x—30, 8h. Greenish yellow, < in morning, exoriating, *Carb. v.* 3x—30, 8h. Leucorrhœa, preceded by hysterical uterine or abdominal pains extending into the thighs, *Mag. mur.* 3, 4h. Leucorrhœa with constipation, earthy complexion, *Nat. mur.* 6, 4h. Inveterate cases, profuse; raised itching spots in vagina, *Alumina* 6, 4h. Yellow, tenacious, sinking sensation, coated tongue, *Hydrast.* 3, 4h. After suppressed eruptions of discharges, sinking at the pit of the stomach in the forenoon, *Sul.* 6, 4h.

IN CHILDREN.—*Calc. c.* 6, 4h.; frequent washing. If due to worms, *Cina.* 3, 4h. *See* Worms.

Lichen.—Simple, *Sulph.* 6, 4h. Prickly heat; lichen urticatus, *Apis* 3x, 2h. M'Clinton's soap is good in these cases. Lichen ruber or planus; chronic cases with burning itching, *Ars.* 3, 6h. Red pimples on face and neck; prickling, itching, *Jug. r.* 3, 4h. Red pimples, itching coming on when undressing, *Rumex c.* 30, 4h. Lichen scrofulorum, *Ars. iod.* 3x, gr. ii. immediately after meals; inunction of cod-liver oil; and cod-liver oil internally.

Lienteria.—(1) *China.* 3, 2h.; (2) *Ferr. met.* 6, 2h.; (3) *Oleand.* 3, 2h.; (4) *Abrot.* 3x, 4h. After overdosing with Iron, *Alston* 1x, 4h.

Lips.—Soreness, chaps, *Vaseline* to be applied at bed-time.
Crack in the centre, *Nat. m.* 6, 4h. Herpes (vesicles), *Nat.
m.* 6, 4h. Soreness of the commissures, *Cundurango* 1x, 4h.
Swelling of the upper lip, *Hep.* s. 6, 4h. Swelling and soreness of the upper lip, *Rhus v.* 3, 4h. Scurfiness or rawness
round the red of the lips, *Ars.* 3, 4h. Cancer (1) *Lyc.* 6, 4h.;
(2) *Sep.* 3 gr. ii.—30, 8h.; (3) *Clemat. φ,* unit doses; (4) *Ars.*
3, 4h.; locally, *Hydrastis. See* **Cancer.**

Liver.—ACUTE YELLOW ATROPHY.—(1) *Phos.* 3, 1h.; (2) *Vanad.*
6, 4h.

CANCER.—[This must be treated according to the symptoms.]
Suspicious cases, *Cholest.* 5x, gr. v. 8h. Yellow appearance,
light stools, pain under right scapula, *Chel. φ,* gtt. v.—30,
8h. For the cachexia, *Hydrastis.* 1, 4h. Sharp pains in region
of liver, *Bry.* 3, ½h.—2h.

CIRRHOSIS.—(1) *Phos.* 3, 4h.; (2) *Ars. iod.* 3x, gr. ii. after
food; (3) *China* 3, 4h.; (4) *Aur. mur.* 3x, gtt. ii. 4h.; (5)
Hydrocot. φ—6x, 4h. This may be given either alone or in
alternation with any of the others. For the dropsy, tapping
may be resorted to.

CONGESTION.—From indolent habits, with over-indulgence in
eating and drinking, *Nux v.* 3, 2h. daily. From gormandising
and coarse feeding, great nausea and heaviness, with splitting headache, *Bry.* 3, 1h.; strict diet and regimen. From
heart disease; the original disease must be treated. *See*
DERANGEMENT.

DERANGEMENT.—In bilious subjects, sudden pallor presaging
a "bilious attack" (vomiting of bile, constipation, light
stools), *Podoph.* 6, 2h. *See also* **Bilious Attack, Biliousness,**
and **Dyspepsia.** Bilious vomiting and diarrhœa, *Iris v.* 3,

½h. *See also* **Diarrhœa**. Dull or sharp pain in region of liver, tenderness, pain in right shoulder, stools either soft and bright yellow, or whitish and costive, jaundice, *Chel.* 1x, 2h. Inactive liver, *Cholest.* 5x, gr. v. 8h. Dull, aching distress in liver region, frontal headache, soreness of eyes, pain in left shoulder, jaundice, black, fetid stools, *Lept.* 3, 2h. Left-lobe of liver enlarged, spleen involved, *Card. m. φ* gtt. v. 4h. Pain and soreness of left lobe; pain extending to uterus, *Chelone φ* gr. v. 4h. Sharp pain in liver region, pain between the shoulders, constrictive or out-pressing frontal headache; white tongue, pale stools, bilious feverish attack, jaundice, *Bry.* 3, 2h. Intense headache, soreness of scalp, soreness of eyes, redness of face, nausea, prostration, soreness of liver region, constipation, high-coloured urine; bone pains, *Eup. perfol.* 3, 2h. Costive, offensive motions, loss of appetite, depression, dull pain in liver region, simple jaundice, *Merc. sol.* 6, 4h. Bilious vomiting, or bitter taste in the morning on rising, headache in one temple or over one eye, constipation, flatulence passing upwards, *Kali carb.* 6, 4h. Abdominal distress, piles constipation, after mercury, *Hep. s.* 6, 4h. Large, hard liver, jaundice, white stools, *China.* 3, 4h. Hardness and tenderness in liver region, stools in small lumps like sheeps' dung; piles, *Mag. mur.* 6, 4h. Derangement from over-indulgence in alcoholic drinks, with large blind piles, *Nux v.* 3, 2h. Acid, bitter vomiting, sinking at the pit of the stomach in the forenoon, in patients with eruptive tendency, *Sul.* 3, 8h. White tongue, vomiting of bile, diarrhœa, especially in the morning, protrusion of piles and prolapse of the bowel, *Podoph.* 6, 2h. Chronic derangement, yellow-grey or dingy sallow complexion, flatulence, constipation, loaded urine, *Lyc.* 6, 4h. "Torpid liver," with loaded urine, venous engorgement, depression, chilliness, sensitiveness to cold air, especially in females, *Sep.* 6, 4h. In chronic liver disorders, when well indicated remedies fail to appreciably benefit, or when clear indications are not available, there are three extremely useful remedies, any of which may establish curative reaction. These are Carcinosin-Adeno-Stom; Morgan (Bach); Pituitary-Whole-Gland. A single dose of which ever is preferred, in either the 30th or 200th potency—with due regard for pathological changes, and await reaction. *See also below*, PAIN IN.

FATTY LIVER.—Regimen and suitable diet; (1) *Phos.* 3, 4h. (2) *Vanad.* 6, 4h. According to symptoms, *see above*, *under* DERANGEMENT.

HYDATID CYSTS OF.—The treatment is surgical.

INFLAMMATION OF.—From cold, sharp pain, < on touch or movement, and > by lying on painful side, *Bry.* 3, 1h.; poultices. Tongue dirty yellowish white, foetid breath, skin jaundiced, liver region sore to touch, < lying on painful side, offensive perspiration, *Merc. s.* 6, 2h. Abscess, *Hep. s.* 6, 2h.; surgical treatment if necessary. Abscess following dysentery, *Ipec.* 1—3, 2h. Inflammation of gall-bladder, *Bapt.* φ—30, 2h. *See also* medicines under PAIN IN, according to symptoms.

PAIN IN (HEPATALGIA).—With great depression of spirits, intermittent stitches in functional or organic disorder, *Am. mur.* 3x, 2h. Dull, heavy, grinding pain in the liver, < when lying on right side; dull pain in region of gall bladder; aching in left blade-bone, *Diosc.* 3, 2h. Constant, severe pain over gall-bladder, < on walking; pain from right

lateral ligament to gall-bladder, *Bapt.* φ—30, 2h. Pressure
or sticking in the liver, < by pressure; sticking in gall-
bladder; drawing in shoulder-blades; pain in loins; thick
urine, *Berb.* 3, 2h. Stitches and pressure in liver and on top
of right shoulder; pain as if bruised, and tenderness of
region of liver, *Ranunc. b.* 3, 2h. Continued pressure in
region of liver, as if with a dull instrument. *Ranunc. scel.*
3, 2h. Stitching, shooting pains in liver, pain in right scapula, yellowish skin, light yellow stools, *Chel.* 1x, 2h.

SYPHILIS.—When enlargement of the liver occurs in tertiary
syphilis, *Kali i.* gr. v.—x. 8h.; if this is not sufficient it
may be followed by *Merc. bin.* 3x, gr. ii. 8h. *Luet.* 30—200
may be given, one dose every night for a few nights. Where
there is no enlargement, but derangement of the liver in
old syphilitics, with depression, *Aur. mur.* 3x, gtt. ii. 4h.

WAXY DEGENERATION.—The disease on which it depends
must be treated according to the symptoms. If there are
no special indications, *Kali iod.* gr. iii. 4h.
See also Calculus, BILIARY: Dropsy, Jaundice.

Liver-spots (*Chloasma*).—(1) *Sep.* 6, 4h.; (2) *Lyc.* 6, 4h. (3) *Bacll.*
30 gl. v. once a week.

Lochia. *See under* Labour.

Lock-jaw. *See* Tetanus.

Locomotor Ataxy.—In the early stage, especially when occurring in children, *Secale* 1, 3h. When of evidently syphilitic
origin and diagnosed early, *Kali iod.* gr. iii.—30, thrice
daily. When the first symptoms are disorder of vision, white
atrophy of the retina with absence of knee-jerk, *Phos.* 3, 2h.
Great irritability and excitability, increased sensitiveness

to all impressions, *Nux v.* 3, 2h. When periodical priapism, or clitoridean "crises" announce the disease, *Picr. ac.* 3x, gr. ii.—30, 6h. When the disease is fully established, lighting pains, urinary troubles, (1) *Med.* 200, gl. v. every third day. (2) *Fluor. ac.* 3, 2h. With symptoms of great coldness, *Helod.* 30, 4h. Symptoms < from sunset to sunrise: (1) *Luet.* 30—200, at bedtime; (2) *Aur.* 5x—30, 4h. Lightning pains, > by warmth, *Mag. phos.* 30, 2h. When there are gastric "crises" and other digestive disorders; when the pains are of a plucking character and confined to small spots, *Arg. n.* 3x, 2h. Tightness at chest, sensation as if a cord tied round the leg under the knee or the upper arm; stitches, numbness, great coldness of legs and feet, *Alumen* 6, 4h. Pain shooting from right to left in body; flatulence, colic, constipation, *Lyc.* 6, 8h. When the pains are burning, restlessness, anxiety, irritability, *Ars.* 3, 4h. Much depression, *Aur.* 30, 8h. Worried, anxious, depressed, hysterical, *Ign.* 3, 2h.

Lumbago.—Backache, as from fatigue, especially after eating and while sitting; violent sacrolumbar pain, the slightest effort to move causing retching and cold, clammy sweat; sensation of a weight hanging on coccyx and dragging downwards, *Ant. t.* 6, 6h. (I find *Ant. t.* one of the most useful of remedies in this condition and one of the most commonly indicated.) From dry cold, from a draught; pain sharp, or as if sprained; the pain excited by touch; the part sensitive, *Acon.* 3, 1h. If with the muscular pains there are restlessness and sleeplessness, *Act. r.* 1x.—3, 2h. Stiffness in the back, painful on motion; a bruised or burning pain, > during motion; from damp cold, *Rhus t.* 3, 2h. Pain excited by every motion; muscles sensitive to touch; bruised feeling

in the back when lying on it; from dry cold, *Bry.* 3, 2h.
Pain in small of back as after stooping a long while, *Dulc.*
3, 2h. Stiffness in back, pain < whilst sitting or lying, in
the morning on awakening; with urinary or rectal troubles,
Berb. 1x, 2h. From dry cold; pains < on the approach of
storms, *Rhod* 3, 2h. From an injury, *Arn.* 3, 2h. Dull backache, walking almost impossible, scarcely able to stoop, or
rise after sitting; especially with constipation and piles,
Æsc. h. 3, 2h. Dull pressure, sticking and tearing, writhing
in loins and urinary passages; < by motion, *Colch.* 3, 2h.
Pains in paroxysms; shooting at times, *Kali bichr.* 3x, 4h.
Dull, heavy, dragging pains, weakness, sexual excitement,
Pic. ac. 3x. gr. ii.—30, 4h. Violent bruised pain in small of
back and coccyx, could not walk erect, violent only when
stooping; drawing; stitches; < at night; < warmth of bed;
< when on feather bed; after heavy lifting, and taking
cold; come on during rest, go off during motion; in venous
subjects, *Sulph.* 6, 4h. Pain as if beaten, < during motion
than rest, *Nux v.* 3, 2h. Sticking in small of back on breathing; bruised pain; pains < on going to bed, banishing
sleep; better on motion, *Merc. sol.* 6, 4h. [Locally, a flannel
belt, or, still better, a belt made of pine wool, should be
worn. In acute cases, hot flannels on which a little turpentine has been sprinkled should be applied; or the part
ironed every few hours with a flat-iron through a piece of
flannel laid over the part affected.]

Lumbrici. *See* **Worms.**

Lungs.—CONGESTION. *Active:* Difficult breathing, anxiety, restlessness, hot dry skin, short hacking dry cough, *Acon.* 3,
½h. After *Acon.*, if amelioration does not follow in a few
hours, *Sul.* 30, 1—2h. Stupor, face flushed, dark rusty

expectoration, *Phos.* 3, ½h. *Passive:* From debility; rusty sputa; purpura, *Phos.* 3, 2h. Blueness, coldness, depression, *Carb. v.* 6, 2h. *Obstructive:* From heart disease, *Ars. i.* 3x, gr. ii. thrice daily immediately after food. Fluttering, irregular heart, swelling of feet, *Dig.* 1—3, 1h. (if it has not been given before). Where there is constipation, flatulence, and diminished urine, *Lyc.* 6, 2h. *See also* **Pneumonia.**

HÆMORRHAGE.—Rusty sputa, or mucous expectoration streaked with blood, *Phos.* 3, as above, under CONGESTION. In active congestion of the chest, bright red blood in some quantity, *Cact.* 3, 1h. *See* **Consumption,** BLEEDING.

INFLAMMATION. *See* **Pneumonia.**

ABSCESS.—Hot, dry skin, restlessness, anxiety, *Acon.* 3, 1h. Flushed face, headache, delirium, pains in chest, < when lying on affected side, *Bell.* 3, 1h. Chills and heats, pus evidently forming, *Hep.* 6, 2h. Low fever, anxiety, depression, *Ars.* 3, 2h. Fetid expectoration with explosive cough and fetid breath, *Caps.* 3, 2h.

GANGRENE.—*Crotal.* 3, 2h. Blueness and coldness of the patient, *Carb. v.* 6, 1h. Fetid expectoration and breath with explosive cough, *Caps.* 3, 2h. Red tongue, thirst, low fever, *Ars.* 3, 2h.

ŒDEMA.—In the course of bronchitis, *Sang. c.* 3x, 15m. Sudden attack in the course of heart affection, *Am. c.* 3—30, 10m. Following acute congestion, *Phos.* 3, 1h. If *Phos.* fails to prevent or check œdema, or when it occurs in the course of general dropsy, *Ant. tart.* 6, 2h. *See also* **Dropsy.**

ULCERATION.—*Kali c.* 6—30, 4h.

Lupus.—*Bacil.* 30—200, gl. iv. once a week. Or *Tuberc. k.* 30—200 in the same way. [Koch's *Tuberculin* has cured a number of cases in homœopathic preparations.] In sycotic subjects or those who have been affected by vaccination, *Thuj.* 6, night and morning. (I have found this remedy with *Tub. k.* 6, twice a week, very effective.) After these, *Rad. bro.* 6—30, once or twice a week. In persons subject to skin affections, sinking sensation in the forenoon, acidity, cold feet, miserable dejected feeling, *Sul.* 6, 8h. In pale, stout subjects, who have heat and perspiration of the head, cold clammy hands and feet, acidity, *Calc. c.* 6, 8h. Great sensitiveness of the affected part, chilly, desire to be covered, *Hep.* 6, 8h. Recent cases, yellow coated tongue, constipation, faint sinking sensation at the stomach, *Hydrast.* 3, 4h.; externally, application of glycerole of *Hydrastis* (*Hydrast.* φ, ʒi., *Glycer.* ʒss.). Great debility, restlessness, anxious temperament, > from heat, < from cold, *Ars.* 3, 4h. When there is great despondency, syphilitic taint, *Aur. mur.* 3x, 4h. Afterwards *Kali bichrom.* 3x, 4h.; externally, application of the same medicine in the same attenuation; or *Hydrocotyle* φ—6, 4h.; application of glycerole of *Hydrocotyle* (*Hydroc.* φ, ʒi., *Glycer.* ʒss.). [Some excellent cures have been made with X Rays, Radium rays, and also with the Solar cautery.]

Lymphatic Glands. *See* **Glands;** *also* **Breast, Bubo, Tonsils, Hodgkin's Disease.**

Malignant Pustule (*called also* **Woolsorter's Disease,** or **Charbon**). (When so situated that it is within the reach of surgical measures, the advisability of excision must be considered, but with homœopathy it should be possible to avoid this; and in all cases internal medication will be of assistance.) *Anthracin*. 30, 1—2h. Excessive sensitiveness, purple coloration, of the parts, fear to be touched or approached, irritability of temper, *Lach*. 6, gtt. ii. 1h.; locally, a compress of the same (ʒi.—ʒii.); burning pain, great thirst, restlessness, anguish, *Ars*. 3, 1h. If there is much fever, dry, hot skin, thirst, restlessness, anxiety, and fear of death, *Acon*. 3, ½h. If there is delirium and flushed face, *Bell*. 3, ½h. *See also* **Carbuncle**, when the symptoms correspond.

Mammary Abscess. *See* **Breast.**

Mania (Insanity with Delirium).—Simple mania in a subdued form, without hyperæmia; vivacious talkativeness, with hallucinations of the senses, or spiteful, quarrelsome moodiness; muscular twitchings and restlessness of the eyeballs; suspicious, thinks is being poisoned; nymphomania (with great tendency to uncover); hypochondriacal monomania as syphilophobia, *Hyo*. 3, 1h. In every form of mania as soon as sexual desire is increased, *Bar. mur*. 6, 4h. Great depression fears he is losing his senses, *Calc. c*. 200 at bed-time. Settled melancholy, gloom over everything, suicidal, *Act. r*. 3x—30, 4h. Acute mania without symptoms of hyperæmia, *Stram*. 3, 1h. Acute mania with furious delirium, red face, large staring eyes, dilated pupils, *Bell*. 3, ½h. Mania with exalted ideas, time and space seem infinite, *Can. ind*. 3, 4h. Incontrollable laughter; outbursts of fury, rapidly alternating with fits of repentance, *Croc. s*. 3, 4h. With anguish, religious melancholy, depression, cold sweat on forehead, *Verat. a*. 3, 2h. Violent delirium with absence of menses, *Cupr. ac*. 3x, gtt. v. or *Cupr*. 30, 4h. *See also* **Melancholia.**

Marasmus. *See* **Atrophy.**

Masturbation. *See* **Self-abuse.**

Measles.—PROPHYLACTIC. When measles breaks out in a house, let all those infected take *Acon.* 3 and *Puls.* 3, each twice daily; or else *Morbil.* 12, twice daily.

THE FEVER.—*Morbil.* 12—30, 2—4h. This may be given from the first and all through, either alone or alternated with other medicines as indicated. At the commencement, catarrhal symptoms, chilly, with restlessness, dry skin, thirst at night, *Acon.* 3, 1h. Sore throat, swollen face, headache, dry cough, *Bell.* 3, 1h. When there is much digestive catarrh and diarrhœa, patients cannot bear to be warmly covered, *Puls.* 3, 1h. Great restlessness, soreness all over, and rheumatic pains, *Rhus t.* 3, 1h. Should the eruption recede or fail to appear, and oppression of the brain follow, *Camph.* 1x, gtt. ii. ½h. until reaction sets in; at the same time a hot-air bath should be given, or the patient should be placed in a hot pack. Should the retrocession of the eruption be followed by convulsive symptoms, *Cupr. acet.* 3, ½h.; the hot-air bath, or pack, in the same way. If the coryza is very distressing, the eyes should be bathed every few hours with a lotion of *Euphrasia* (*Euph.* φ, half a teaspoonful to half a teacupful of water). When the cough is a very distressing feature, the larynx being affected, cough dry, constant, irritating, *Aco.* 3, 1h. Hoarseness, phlegm difficult to raise, coming in long tough strings, *Kali bichr.* 3x, 2h. After the fever, if catarrh remains, *Merc. s.* 6. 3h.; *Euphras.* locally as above if there is coryza. Night-sweats and general weakness, *Ars. i.* 3x, gr. iv. thrice daily after meals. Hyperpyrexia, *see* **Hyperpyrexia.**

SEQUELAE.—In general, in scrofulous subjects, glandular enlargements, (1) *Bacil.* 30—100, gl. iv. once a week. (2) *Sulph.* 30, 4h. Constipation after, *Opium* 3, 2h. Conjunctival irritation, *Ars.* 3, 4h. Patients who have "never been well since an attack of measles," *Morbil.* 100 two or three times a week at bedtime. Inflammation and ulceration of the mouth, *Merc. c.* 6, 2h.; wash of borax (a piece the size of a filbert dissolved in half a teacupful of water). *See also* **Bronchitis, Cough, Diphtheria, Ears, Eyes.**

Megrim, or Migraine. *See* **Headache.**

Melancholia.—Recent, traceable to worry, grief, fright or disappointment; especially at the menopause, *Ign.* 3, 3h. Melancholy with nervousness, restlessness, and sleeplessness, unconquerable gloom, tendency to suicide, *Act. r.* 3, 3h. Anguish, vital depression, great coldness of the skin, cold sweat on forehead, *Verat. alb.* 3, 3h. Melancholy, nervousness, drowsiness, with constipation, *Op.* 3, 3h. Religious or other melancholy with very obstinate constipation, *Plumb. acet.* 6, 3h. Fears losing his senses, *Calc. c.* 200, 8h. Suicidal melancholy, especially in men, *Aur. mur.* 3x, 4h. Suicidal melancholy, especially in women; puerperal melancholia; haughtiness; objects and people seem small, *Plat.* 6, 3h. Suicidal melancholy with arrested menses, *Sen. aur.* φ unit doses; or 3x, 8h. Restless, anguished depression, *Ars.* 3, 4h. Fretful irritability, *Merc. sol.* 6, 4h. Discouragement, loss of spirits, emaciation, hungry craving, *Iod.* 3x, 4h. Worried about philosophic or religious subjects; aversion to washing; < at night and from warmth, *Sul.* 30, 4h. *See also* **Hypochondriasis, Hysteria, Mania.**

Melanoderma. *See* **Ephelis,** and **Freckles.**

Memory, LOSS OF, OR WEAK.—*Anacard.* 3x, 4h. For words and names, *Sul.* 6, 4h. With inattention, heavy listless mood, absent-mindedness, *Baryt. c.* 6, 4h. With soporous condition

of mind; mental operations difficult, *Zinc. m.* 6, 4h. Mind
distracted; easily worried, *Cocc. i.* 3, 4h. Thinking difficult,
forgetting everything, *Dig.* 3, 4h. Inability to fix attention,
Æthus. 6, 4h. Forgetfulness whilst talking; sudden disap-
pearance of thoughts, *Rhod.* 3, 4h. Loss of memory after
catalepsy, *Camph.* 3, 4h.

Ménière's Disease (Auditory Nerve Vertigo).—Giddiness
and noises in the ears with deafness)—(1) *Nat. salicyl.* 3,
4h.; (2) *China.* 3, 4h.; (3) *Chin. sul.* 3x, gr. ii. 4h. Coming on
during, or < after sleep, *Lach.* 6, 4h.

Meningitis.—Cerebral.—When caused by a blow, at the beginning, *Arn.* 1, 1h. When fever comes on, with restlessness,
anxiety, fearfulness, dry skin, thirst, *Aco.* 3, 1h. When there
is delirium, patient tries to escape, flushed face, dilated
pupils, *Bell.* 3, 1h. If there is little delirium, but much pain,
white tongue, nausea; when effusion appears to have taken
place, depression and stupor coming on, *Bry.* 3, 1h. Great
depression, much pain in the back of the head and neck,
Hell. n. 3, ½h. Shrill cries in sleep, nervous fidgetiness, *Apis*
3x, 1h. After *Apis* and other medicines, hot head, cold feet
in those subject to eruptions, *Sul.* 6, 1h. Tubercular, *Bacil.*
30—200, a single dose of four globules, dry on the tongue
or dissolved in a little water. When the fever has subsided,
if the original cause has been concussion, and after *Apis* or
Bry. has been given, *Arn.* 1, 2h. After the fever, when *Bell.*
or *Helleb.* has been given, *Zinc. met.* 6, 2h. *See also* **Encephalitis Lethargica.**

Spinal.—Acute, with fever, restlessness, fear, dry skin, *Aco.*
3, 1h. With complete prostration, numbness, tremor, *Gels.*
1—30, 1h. Pains in various parts, < on the least attempt at

movement, *Bry.* 3, 1h. Stiffness and paralysis of the lower
limbs, *Oxal. ac.* 3x, 1h.

CEREBRO-SPINAL ("TYPHOID MENINGITIS." "SPOTTED FEVER")
—(1) *Meningococcin.* 6—30, 4h. (2) *Cicuta virosa* 3, 1h.
When the fever is of a low typhoid kind and symptoms of
blood-poisoning predominate, *Crotal.* 3, 1h. Intense pain
below and behind ears (< 1.) extending to nape and
occiput, *Am. c.* 200, 2—4h. Should other remedies fail to
relieve the spasm, *Act. r.* 3, ¼h. during the spasms. After-
effects, paralysis, *Gelsem.* 1, 2h.; deafness—(1) *Silic.* 6, 4h.;
(2) *Sulph.* 6, 4h.

TUBERCULAR. *See* Hydrocephalus.

Menopause. *See* Change of Life.

Menorrhagia. *See* Menstruation, EXCESSIVE.

Menstruation.
[In all disorders of the menstrual functions hygienic measures
are important. Regular meals and regular open-air exercises
should be enjoined; but the exercise must not be taken
when the patient is in any way fatigued with exertion of
other kinds either mental or bodily. Bathing should be
omitted during the period.]

SYMPTOMS BEFORE MENSES.—Colic; leucorrhœa with weeping
mood; bleeding of present ulcers; swelling of gums and
cheeks, *Phos.* 3, 4h. Feels faint, has sourish taste in mouth
and spits a little blood, *Nat. m.* 6, 4h. Breasts painful,
menses profuse and early, *Calc. c.* 6, 4h. Breasts painful,
menses scanty, *Con.* 3, 4h. Stitches in breasts; nipples burn
and are sore and painful, *Sang.* 1, 4h. Cough, *Sul.* 3, 4h.
Itching in pudenda, *Graph.* 6, 4h. Nausea or diarrhœa

before, *Verat. a.* 3, 4h. Restless and irritable some days before, *Kreas.* 3, 4h. Very irritable the day before, *Magnes. mur.* 6, 4h. Attack of depression before, *Sep.* 6, 4h. Cross and melancholic, *Lyc.* 6, 4h. Sees the dark side of everything, *Caust.* 6, 4h. At the beginning ill-humoured, *Cham.* 6, 4h.

BEFORE AND DURING.—Dry cough and perspiration, *Graph.* 6, 4h. Pain at heart, *Lith. c.* 6, 4h.

DURING.—Hoarseness and febrile coryza; trembling, *Graph.* 6, 4h. Pains in groins during, *Borax* 6, 4h.

AMENORRHŒA (ABSENCE OF MENSTRUAL FLOW).—When the menses do not appear at puberty, there being no local or constitutional disease to account for the absence, especially in blonde, mild-tempered, impressionable subjects, > in open air, *Puls.* 3, 8h. In blondes who are sad and depressed and who are < in open air; with giddiness, headache, and visual disturbances, *Cycl.* 6—30, 8h. When due to anæmia or tubercular diathesis, *see* **Anæmia, Tuberculosis.** When suppressed from a chill, *Acon.* 3, 2h. for a few days, to be followed, if necessary, by *Puls.* 3, 8h., which may be continued for a month or longer. If there is no appearance of the flow at the time that the next period is due, *Sulph.* 3—30, 8h., especially if there is a sinking sensation at 11 a.m., flushes of heat, hot head, cold extremities. If there is headache on waking, chilliness, depression, constipation, *Nat. mur.* 6, 4h. When *Nat. m.*, though apparently indicated, fails, *Kali. c.* 6, 4h.

CESSATION OF.—Sufferings from, *see* **Change of Life.**

DELAYED AND SCANTY.—Delayed, defective, irregular; patients pale, languid, chilly, complain of headache, *Puls.* 3, 4h. Menses delayed, always after the proper time, constipation;

tendency to skin eruptions, flushings, faint sinking sensation in the forenoon, *Sulph.* 6, 6h. Delayed; itching in pudenda before, *Graph.* 6, 4h. Scanty with constipation; earthy complexion, *Nat. m.* 6, 6h. Scanty, delaying, dark, pitchy, *Mag. c.* 6, 6h. Scanty, late, irregular, painful, *Senec.* φ, 6h.

EXCESSIVE.—Too early and too profuse; with colic and nausea, *Borax* 6, 4h. Too early and excessive, especially in pale subjects, inclined to stoutness, troubled with cold, damp feet, *Calc. c.* 6, 4h. Too early, too profuse, too long lasting, with bearing down, prolapse, rectal urging, *Aloe* 3x, 4h. Simple increase of normal flow, *Ferrum met.* 6, 4h. Menorrhagia, dark, especially if accompanied with ovarian irritation, *Hamam.* 3, 4h. Menorrhagia, black lumps, *China.* 1, 4h. Black, clotted, pitchy, clots, in rags, or like leeches, *Croc. s.* 3, 4h. Severe hæmorrhage, with colic and clots, debility not recovered from between the periods, *Thlaspi. b. past.* φ, gtt. v. 8h. When due to disturbing emotions, accompanied with great irritability, the flow dark and clotted, *Cham.* 6, 4h. When the flow is sanious, dark, and fluid, especially in thin, cachectic subjects, *Secale* 1, 4h. Menorrhagia, the flow being < during the night, *Mag. c.* 6, 4h. The blood being bright red, the flow profuse and paroxysmal; < when walking or standing, *Sabin.* 3, 4h. Bright red blood, profuse, bearing down in lower abdomen, *Fic. r.* 1x, 4h. Bright red flow, with head symptoms; flow hot, feels like hot sealing-wax; flow between periods, *Bell.* 3, 4h. Simple menorrhagia, profuse, bright red discharge with or without nausea, *Ipec.* 3, 4h. Menorrhagia after abortion or dysmenorrhœa; at the climacteric; great downward pressure in the pelvis; pain in the back and thighs; offensive urine, of odour like

horses'; restlessness after midnight, *Nir. ac.* 1, 4h. Chronic
menorrhagia; thin corrosive, burning leucorrhœa, *Ars.* 3,
4h. Discharge of blood between the periods from slight
causes, *Ambra* 3, 4h. Coming on too soon and returning soon
after; violent cramps, bearing-down pain; irritable green
leucorrhœa; great irritation, *Nit. ac.* 5, 4h. Flow excessive,
preceded and followed by discharge of non-menstrual
blood, *Ustilago* 3, 4h.

PAINFUL (DYSMENORRHŒA).—[The frequency of repetition of
dose refers to the period when there is pain; the same
medicine may be given twice or thrice daily during the
intervals.]—Spasmodic, severe abdominal pains, *Caul.* 3,
1h. Stout, plethoric women, pains unendurable, *Aco.* 30,
1h. When the patient is nervous, restless, and melancholy,
Act. r. 3, 1h. With horrible pains, causing her to cry aloud;
great prostration, *Cact.* 3, 2h. With great impressionability
and fretfulness, *Cham.* 6, 1h. Spasmodic Dysmenorrhœa is
often relieved by *Cham.* φ twenty drops in half a tumbler of
water. Give one teaspoon each hour until relieved. Pain in
paroxysms, relieved by hot applications, *Magnes. phos.* 6x,
gr. ii. in a tablespoonful of hot water every ten minutes.
Pain in groins, *Borax* 6, 4h. Violent pains dragging, towards
genitals, *Mag. c.* 6, 4h. When accompanied by sickness
and giddiness, like sea-sickness, *Cocc. i.* 3, 1h. Simple dysmenorrhœa, with headache, *Gels.* 3, 1h. Simple spasmodic dysmenorrhœa; with cramps, *Viburnum op.* 3, 1h. When the
flow is scanty, black, and clotted, *Puls.* 3, 1h. When the flow
is insufficient, *Sep.* 6, 1h. When the flow is profuse and before
the time, dreadful distress and pain, especially in spare,
nervous, and delicate women, *Xanthox.* 1x—3, 1h. From
ovarian irritation, *Ham.* 1, gtt. ii. 3h. With ovarian irritation,

offensive menstrual and leucorrhœal discharge, *Bell.* 3, 1h.
Membranous dysmenorrhœa, *Borax* gr. v. thrice daily.

SUPPRESSED. *See* AMENORRHŒA.

VICARIOUS.—In general, *Ham.* 1, 2h. When it takes the form
of epistaxis, *Bry.* 1, 2h.

[N.B.—As a rule, the best time to give medicines for menstrual
irregularities is when the period is just over. They may be
continued during the next period if the symptoms are
urgent.]

Mentagra. *See* **Beard.**

Mental Weakness.—(1) *Phos. ac.* 1x, 4h.; (2) *Anacard.* 1, 4h.;
(3) after brain disorder, *Zinc.* 6, 4h. *See also* **Hysteria,
Hypochondriasis, Mania, Melancholia, Memory, LOSS
OF.**

Mesenteric Disorder. *See* **Tabes Mesenterica.**

Metritis. *See* **Uterus.**

Metrorrhagia. *See* **Uterus, HÆMORRHAGE FROM.**

Migraine. *See* **Headache.**

Miliaria.—*Acon.* 3, 1h. When oppression at the heart is very
distressing, *Cact.* 3, 1h. Sweating excessively profuse,
Jaborandi, 3, 1h.

Milk. *See* **Lactation.**

Milk-crust. *See* **Eczema Capitis.**

Milk Fever. *See* **Lactation.**

Milk Leg. *See* **Phlegmasia Alba Dolens.**

Millar's Asthma. *See* **Croup,** Spasmodic.

Mind.—Affections of.—Calls things by wrong names, *Diosc.*
30, 8h. Proud and suspicious to friends, *Lach.* 6, 8h. In-
different to friends, *Sep.* 6, 8h. Ill-treats friends, *Hyo.* 3, 4h.
See also **Melancholia, Mental Weakness, Hypochondriasis, Mania, Memory,** Loss of.

Symptoms of.—[When mental symptoms occur (especially if
unusual to the patient) as concomitants with bodily ailments
it is of the first importance to select a remedy which has a
corresponding mental state. For this a repertory is necessary;
but I will name a few of the more characteristic mental
states, indicating some leading remedies.] Agitation, anguish, sadness, fear of death, *Acon.* Gloom as of a black pall
over everything, *Act. r.* Jealousy, *Apis.* Anguish, driving
one out of bed at night; fear of being alone; despair, inclined to suicide; or excessive fear of death, *Ars.* Melancholy
with inquietude and desire to die, *Aur.* Over-sensitiveness;
spiteful, sudden, or uncivil irritability, *Cham.* Insane jealousy; irritability; ill-humour; malice, *Lach.* Sensitive; cries
when thanked; sad, desponding; weeps all day, *Lyc.* Silent
melancholy; sighs and sobs; desires to be alone; changeable
disposition, *Ign.* Sad, weeping mood without cause; < by
consolation, *Nat. m.* Irritable; morose, sullen; quarrelsome
if disturbed; malicious, *Nux v.* Proud, disdainful, *Plat.*
Mild, bashful, tearful; easily bursts into tears; can hardly
tell her symptoms for weeping; seeks consolation, *Puls.*
Suspicious, *Hyo.* Melancholy mood, weeps without cause;
foolish happiness, thinks himself possessed of beautiful
things; even rags seem beautiful; religious insanity, *Sul.*

Miner's Elbow. *See* **Bunion.**

Miscarriage.—THREATENED. When there is fever, restlessness, thirst, dry skin, anxiety, fear of death, *Acon.* 3, 1h. About the third month, *Act. r.* 3x, 3h. About the fifth or seventh month, *Sep.* 30, 4h. Tendency to miscarry, sensitiveness of genitals, *Zinc.* 30, 4h. In the earlier half of pregnancy, *Sabin.* 3, 1h.; in the latter half, *Secale* 3, 1h. With crampy, colicky pains, *Vib. op.* 3, 4h. (In women who habitually miscarry at a certain period of pregnancy *Vib. op.* should be given for some time before.) When arising from an accident, *Arn.* 3, 1h. When due to emotional disturbance, *Cham.* 6, 1h. *For repeated occurrence of abortion:*—When due to syphilis in mother or child, give (1) *Luet.* 30 gl. iv. twice a week throughout pregnancy, or else (2) *Merc. cor.* 6, 8h., to be continued throughout pregnancy, with occasional intermissions. When either parent is scrofulous, *Calc. c.* 6, 8h. throughout pregnancy, with occasional intermissions. When either parent is consumptive, *Bacill.* 100, gl. v. once a week. When there is eruptive tendency, *Sul.* 6, 8h. on alternate fortnights throughout pregnancy. When either parent is rickety, or when previous children have been so, *Sil.* 6, 8h. throughout pregnancy, with occasional intermissions. [When particular symptoms on the part of the mother indicate other medicines than those mentioned, these must be given; the deeply acting medicines of the *Chronic Diseases* of Hahnemann will be found most frequently called for. The greatest safety for the child lies in the health of the mother.]

Mole. *See* **Nævus.**

Mollities Ossium.—(1) *Phos.* 3, 4h.; (2) *Calc. iod.* 3x. 4h.

Molluscum Contagiosum.—(1) *Calc. c.* 6, 4h.; (2) *Sil.* 6, 4h.

Molluscum Fibrosum.—*Silic.* 6, 4h.

Morbus Coxæ. *See* **Hip-joint Disease.**

Morning Sickness. *See* **Pregnancy.**

Morphinism or Opium Habit.—For the nervous depression occasioned in those who wish to leave off the drug, *Avena* φ, gtt. v.—x. 8h. Irritability, crossness, extreme sensitiveness, *Cham.* 6, 2h. Constipation, *Æsc. h.* 1, 2h. Illusions, *Can. ind.* 1x—30, 4h.

Morphœa or Scleroderma.—(1) *Silic.* 6, 8h.; (2) *Phos.* 3, 4h.; (3) *Ars.* 3, 4h.; (4) *Thyroid.* gr. iv.—30, 8h. [Locally, inunction with simple ointment; friction of the skin; vapour-bath followed by inunction: electricity.]

Morvan's Disease (*Analgesic paresis with panaritiæ*).—Erysipelatous swelling of finger-tips and fingers; nails discoloured; twitchings and pains in arms and sensation of deadness, *Thuj.* 30, 4h. Felons with violent pains; nails discoloured; ulcers about them; shooting pains; atrophy of affected parts; restlessness and irritability, *Sil.* 6, 2h. Panaritium, bluish swelling, necrosis, *Lach.* 6, 2h. *See also* **Whitlow.**

Mountain Sickness.—*Coca* φ, 1h. This can be synonymous with air-hunger at high altitude and *Carb. v. b.* 12 or 30 may be required every ½ or 1h. until marked improvement is obtained.

Mouth.—Dry, red, burning, *Bell.* 3, 1h. Simple exudative inflammation of the mouth.—(1) *Caps.* 3, 2h.; (2) *Nat. mur.* 6, 2h. Sore mouth, cracks in the commissures of the lips, foul odour *Nit. ac.* 6, 2h. Scurfy patches at mouth corners, pimples on chin, *Hep.* 6, 8h. Ulcerative inflammation of the mouth, *Merc. cor.* 3, 2h. When due to mercury—(1)

Nit. ac. 6, 2h.; (2) *Hep.* 6, 2h. Mouth sore, red, inflamed, glazed, salivation, *Nit. ac.* 6, 2h. Apthous mouth, psoriasis of tongue, recurring ulcer, *Mur. ac.* 6, 2h. Very sore feeling in the mouth, redness of tongue, elevated papillæ, lips and corners of mouth cracked, nose sore, *Arum. tri.* 12, 2h. (If given in a low attenuation, this must be freshly prepared.) Mouth covered with offensive mucus after sleeping, *Rheum* 3, 4h.

ULCERS.—(1) *Merc. cor.* 3, 3h.; locally, *Muriate of Hydrastin* lotion (*Hydrast. mur.* gr. iii. distilled water, three ounces). (2) *Hydrastinin mur.* 5 gtt. viii. night and morning. (3) *Carcin.* 100, gl. vi. once a week.

CANKER. *See* **Cancrum Oris.**

Mucous Colitis.—Membranous discharges, flatulence and constipation, pains in splenic flexure of colon, *Arg. n.* 5—30, 4h. Almost gelatinous stools, cutting pains in bowels and kidneys, *Cadm. s.* 5—30, 4h. Stools like scrapings of intestines, burning pains, thirst, nausea and vomiting, *Canth.* 3, 4h. Membranous stools, colic with tearing pains, much nausea, < by sight or smell of food, *Colch.* 3, 4h. Acute crises of pain, > moving about, *Diosc.* 1—30, 1h. Spasms of pain > by pressure and bending double, *Coloc.* 1—30, 1h. There are many factors to be considered in this condition and the best results will be obtained by prescribing on individual indications, in the classical manner.

Mucous Patches.—*Nit. ac.* 6, 4h.; locally to be painted night and morning with *Thuja* φ. *See* **Condylomata, Syphilis.**

Mumps.—Fever, thirst, restlessness, anxiety, pain, *Acon.* 3, 1h. After *Acon.*, when the fever has subsided, *Mer. cor.* 3, 1h.

Dry mouth, copious salivation, *Jabor.* 1, 2h. If the testicles become affected, *Puls.* 3x, 2h. Mania coming on after mumps, *Bell.* 3, 2h. As prophylactic *Parotidinum* 30, 8h. (This may also be given as a remedy every two or three hours, when the disease is declared, either alone or in alternation with the other remedies named.)

Muscæ Volitantes (*Specks floating about before the sight*).—This affection is generally dependent on some disturbance of general health, or error of refraction in the eye. When the latter is the case, spectacles will be required; when the former, the medicine best suited to the general state. From general weakness after illness or exhausting discharges, *China.* 3, 4h. From liver disorder, *Nit. ac.* 6, 4h. From sexual excess, *Phos.* 3, 4h. From alcoholic excess, *Nux v.* 3, 2h. *See* Eyes: SIGHT.

Muscles, PAIN IN. *See* Myalgia.

Muscular Rheumatism. *See* Rheumatism, Muscular; Myalgia, Diaphragm, Lumbago, Stiff-neck.

Myalgia.—From a chill, numbness, pain excited by touch, *Aco.* 3, 2h. From exposure to dry cold, pain < by every movement, *Bry.* 3, 2h. From getting cold and wet, *Dulc.* 3, 2h. In general, *Macrotin* 3x, gr. iv. 3h. Dull pain in head, back, and limbs, with fever, drawing, aching, jerking, deep-seated pain in the limbs, weakness of the legs, *Gels.* 3, 2h. Weakness of the whole muscular system, drawing pain and cramps in the limbs and joints; crawling, thrilling, aching in the back, *Verat. v.* 3, 2h. Darting, tearing, jerking pains, which come and go, disappear suddenly, *Valer.* 3, 2h. Prostration and weariness in all the limbs, tearing in all the limbs and joints; tearing, drawing, rheumatic or bruised sensation; pain in the back after eating, and while sitting; rheumatic pain in the lumbar region in the morning, *Ant. t.* 6, 4h. Jerking and pains in all the limbs; pain in r. foot and l. arm; violent paralytic pain in the arms; jerking drawing in the shoulders, cramps, tearing in the hips and legs, *Colch.* 3, 2h. Stiffness and weakness of and pressure on the shoulder, uneasiness in the limbs; last an hour in bed in the morning; tearing in all the limbs; weakness and trembling, paralytic heaviness, intolerable uneasiness, *Caust.* 6, 2h. *See also* Diaphragm, Lumbago, Rheumatism, MUSCULAR; Stiffneck.

Myelitis (*Inflammation of the spinal cord*).—ACUTE.—Violent pain along the spine, tetanic spasms, fever, fear, *Aco.* 3, 1h. Tetanic spasms, sensitiveness to all external impressions. *Nux v.* 3, 1h. Violent convulsions, piercing cries, *Cic. v.* 3, 1h.

CHRONIC.—Great rigidity of the lower limbs, pain, chilliness, *Oxal. ac.* 3x, 2h. Cramps and spasms in the limbs, *Strych.* 6, 2h. Restlessness, cramps, and contraction of paralysed limbs, loss of sensibility to everything except cold, which excites or aggravates the symptoms, neuralgia, pains affecting hands and feet especially, restlessness, *Ars.* 3, 2h. Chronic spinal paralysis, *Plumb.* 6, 4h.

Myopia.—*Physostig.* 3x, 4h.

Myxœdema.—*Thyr.*, one or two tablets of the extract, or 3x, gr. v. 8h. Great chilliness, scaly skin, restlessness, anxiety, *Arsen.* 200, 8h.

Nævus.—VASCULAR.—[When surgical treatment is not advisable, the following medicines may be of service.] (1) *Thuja*

1—30, 6h., locally, *Thuja* φ, painted on night and morning;
(2) *Rad. bro.* 30, gl. vi. once a week; (3) *Calc. c.* 6, 6h.;
(4) *Phos.* 3—6.; (5) *Lyc.* 6, 6h.; (6) *Vaccin* 200, twice a week.

Nails.—Brittle and powdery when cut, rough and yellow, *Sil.*
6, 6h. Crippled, discoloured, crumbling off, *Thuj.* 6, 8h.
Panaritium and brittle nails, lancinating pains and tendency
to ulceration of finger tips; brittle nails and brittle skin on
tips of fingers; nails brittle, thick, spots on nails, *Alumina*
6, 8h. Slow growth, skin under nails painfully sensitive:
horny growth under nails; horny warts on hands, *Ant. crud.*
6, 8h. Pains under nails, *Sep.* 6, 4h. Cracked, *Ars.* 3, 6h.
Thickened or corrugated, *Graph.* 6, 6h. Ulcers around,
Phos. 3, 4h. Degeneration of pulp; nails separate from
matrix and leave a granulating surface, *Secal.* 3, 4h. When
there is inflammation in the base and sides of the nails,
Vetterin is a good application to apply at night.

INFLAMMATION OF PULP (ONYCHIA).—*Sil.* 6, 6h.; locally—(1)
Calend. φ (two teaspoonfuls to the half-cupful of water);
(2) *Boracic acid* (one drachm dissolved in half a teacupful of
water).

INGROWING TOE-NAIL.—(1) *Magnet. p. aust.* 30—200, 4h.;
(2) *Nit. ac.* 6, 4h.; locally, ointment of *Hydrastis* φ (one
drachm to the ounce of vaseline or simple ointment, or
Vetterin). [Surgical measures may be necessary, though for
many years I have not had necessity to have recourse to it.
The first-named medicine has cured nearly all my cases.
When the nail has to be divided in the centre, and a V-
shaped piece excised, the operation may be greatly facili-
tated by keeping the nail saturated with glycerine for two or
three days previously.]

Nausea. *See* Dyspepsia, Vomiting.

Neck. Stiffness, crick-in-the-neck. *See* Stiff-neck.

Necrosis. *See* Bone.

Nephritis. *See* Kidney.

Nervous Debility. *See* Debility, Spermatorrhœa, etc.

Nervousness. *See* Hysteria, Hypochondriasis.

Nettle-Rash (URTICARIA).—RECENT.—*Apis* 3x, 2h. Should this fail to cause improvement in a day or two, *Chloral Hydrate* 3x, 8h. When due to gastric disorder, with loaded tongue, *Ant. crud.* 3, gr. iv. 4h. From chill and wetting, *Dulc.* 1, 2h. When associated with liver affections, *Ast. fl.* 6, 4h. Stinging sensations, great irritation, *Urt. ur.* 3x, 4h. "Hives" (the American name for urticarial rashes of various kinds), *Hydrast.* 1, 4h.

CHRONIC.—*Astacus fluviatilis*, 6, 4h. When the irritation comes on at night when warm in bed, *Sulph.* 3, 6h. In weakly subjects, red tongue, thirst, much burning, *Ars.* 3, 4h. Inveterate cases, with constipation; earthy complexion, *Nat. mur.* 6, 8h.

Neuralgia.—[In severe and recent attacks the medicines may be given at first every quarter of an hour until relief is obtained.] Facial or sciatic, from cold draughts, congestive with numbness, *Aco.* 3, 2h. Recent in the young, hyperæmia, hyperæsthesia, facial, especially on r. side, *Bell.* 3, 2h. From cold and damp, tearing pains of face going into the eye; joints affected; in r. testis, *Coloc.* 3, 2h. Facial and supra-orbital, especially of the l. side, the pains coming at regular intervals jerking and tearing; spreading to the neck, involving the eyes; < by the least concussion or motion, diminished by firm pressure; pale face, restlessness, perspiration, *Spig.* 3, 2h. Pure neuralgia, pain burning, agonising, accompanied with restlessness and anguish; intermittent; periodic; at first relieved, but afterwards < by cold applications; < by rest, > by exercise, and by warmth; gastralgia; malarial neuralgia; especially when associated with debility, *Ars.* 3, 2h. Malarial neuralgia; supra-orbital neuralgia; with gravelly urine, *Chinin. s.* 3, 2h. Neuralgia of clock-like periodicity, *Cedr.* 3, 2h. Periodical neuralgia coming on about midday or midnight, *Sulph.* φ, 6h. Supraorbital, of gastric origin, *Kali bich.* 3x, gr. iv. 4h. Sudden pains, especially if r. side of face and head, < least movement or touch, eating or speaking; < 4 to 8 p.m. *Lyc.*, 6—30, 4h. After *Lyc.*; brow, face and neck, especially of r. side; intercostal, *Chel.* 1, 2h. (*Chel.* and *Lyc.* are complementary, and help out each other's action.) Eyes protrude (< r.) and are very painful, *Como.* 1, 1—2h. Intercostal and supraorbital of r. side, *Ran. b.* 3, 2h. Right side of face, and down right arm, followed by numbness, slow pulse, *Kalm.* 3, 2h. Facial neuralgia, tic, throbbing, *Glon.* 3, 1h. Tic, *Staph.* 3, 1h. With great nervousness, pains utterly intolerable, < at night and by warmth; accompanied with great thirst, heat and redness of the face, hot sweat on head and scalp; toothache, earache, neuralgia of face and neck, *Cham.* 6, 1h. Excessive sensitiveness of the surface, diffused sensitiveness, *Kali i.* 30, 2—4h. Pain excited by merely moving the affected part, rising to a fearful height; recurring; increased by touching, or, if the pain has subsided for a time, brought on again by touching and it soon becomes intolerable; > by hard pressure; in exhausted subjects, *China.* 1x—30, 2h. Drawing pressing pain, commencing lightly, increasing gradually to a very high degree, and decreasing slowly; supra orbital, *Stan.* 6, 2h. Right sided, paroxysmal, relieved by heat, *Magn. phos.* 6x, gr. iv.—30, 1—4h. Facial: intolerable drawing in the ear; pain in flashes excited by the least movement (clenching the teeth or touching them with the tongue); face red, acid eructations, *Verbasc.* 3, 2h. Supra- and infra-orbital neuralgia, *Arg. n.* 6, 2h. Left infra-orbital neuralgia extending into temple; syphilitic, *Mez.* 3, 2h. Rheumatic, < on the approach of storms, *Rhod.* 3, 2h. In the bones with swellings, *Phyt.* 3, 2h. Inveterate; syphilitic, *Kali iod.* gr. iii. three times a day. Pain, as if a nerve were put on the stretch and suddenly let go, < in warm room, > in cool air, *Puls.* 3, 2h. Cramping pains associated with coldness and numbness, *Plat.* 6, 2h. Tearing pains in the face; drawing, jerking in the jaws; caries, *Phos.* 3, 2h. General frontal headache, accompanied by stabs of pain darting from before backward to the occipital region, intracranial, no disturbance of sensation of the scalp, *Zinc. phos.* 3x, gr. ii. 2h. *Plantago major* φ is very useful in almost all kinds of neuralgia as a local application. It may be painted on the part as often as necessary. *See also* **Headache, Hemicrania, Lumbago, Sciatica, Toothache.**

Neurasthenia.—Emaciation, loss of appetite and sleep, hysterical symptoms. [Absolute rest in bed; constant feeding with nourishing and easily digested food, milk in some form being the most important. This may be given a wineglassful every hour. The Metchnikoff preparations have an advantage over ordinary milk in many cases. In addition recourse may be had to Swedish exercises, massage and (when suitable) electricity.] The following medicines will be found of great service:—Hysterical, erratic, contradictory symptoms; clavus; indigestion, and craving for indigestible articles; weeping mood, *Ign.* 6, 2h. Flatulence, constipation, mucus in stools, *Arg. n.* 30, night and morning. Loss of weight, depression, no appetite, pruritus, *Rad. bro.* 30, once a week. Great weakness, tremors, giddiness, neuralgias, *Gels.* 3, 2h. Nervous, sensitive, melancholic; all symptoms < after sleep, *Lach.* 6, 2h. Brain-fag, every attempt at mental labour causes severe throbbing headache at base of brain; weakness of back; sexual excitement, *Pic. ac.* 30, 2h. Irritability, cannot concentrate, *Scutel.* φ, 4h. Satyriasis or nymphomania with notions of grandeur and pride, *Plat.* 6, 2h. *See also* **Debility, Hysteria.**

Neuritis.—From exposure to dry cold, with intolerable pains in debilitated subjects, *Ars.* 3—30, 1—2h. Especially of the brachial nerves, with numbness of hands and arms, *Xanth.* φ—30, 1—2h. After influenza, *Tub. k.* 30, once in four days. Symptoms < after sleep, *Lach.* 6, 4h. Pressing, cramping, tearing, throbbing pain from periphery to centre, often with red streaks, *Bell.* 1—30, 1h. In exhausted, anæmic persons; alcoholic neuritis, *Ars.* 3—30, 2h. *Kali mur.* 12 or 30 may be regarded as a basic remedy in neuritis and sciatica and may be given either alone in the absence of clear prescribing symptoms or alternated with other medicines as indicated. A dose three or four times daily for several days, depending on the acuteness and severity of case. *See also* **Beri-Beri, Neuralgia, Sciatica.**

Nicotism. *See* **Tobacco Habit.**

Nightmare.—When due to indiscretion in diet, *Nux v.* 3, 4h. (diet must be regulated). When not traceable to obvious cause—(1) *Kali brom.* 1x, gr. v. at bed-time; (2) *Pæonia* 1, 4h.

Night Screaming in Children. *See* **Screaming.**

Night-Sweat. *See* **Hectic Fever, Perspiration.**

Nipples.—SORE.—(1) *Calendula* lotion (a teaspoonful to half a teacupful of water); (2) *Arnica* lotion (*Arn.* φ, gtt. xx. to a pint of water); (3) *Hamamelis* lotion (*Ham.* φ, gtt. xx. to a pint of water); (4) Glycerole of *Hydrastis* (one teaspoonful of *Hydrastis* φ to a tablespoonful of glycerine); (5) Lotion of *Benzoic acid* [fifteen grains of pure *Benzoic acid*, three drachms (teaspoonfuls) of rectified spirit of wine, eight ounces of distilled water—the acid to be dissolved in the spirit, and the water added and well shaken.]—The lotions to be used and the glycerole applied after each application of the child; the nipples to be washed before the child is again applied. This must be particularly attended to. I have recorded a case in which the use of *Calendula* to the nipples apparently gave rise to poisoning of the infant (*Homœopathic World*, Aug., 1891, p. 355).

PAINFUL.—Pain felt after each application of the child, *Phell.* 3, 4h. Neuralgic pain shooting from the point of the nipple through to the shoulder-blade, *Croton. t.* 3, 4h.

Nodes.—On the bones of the skull, *Kali bich.* 3x, gr. ii. 1h. Soft, non-syphilitic nodes, *Sil.* 6, 8h. Syphilitic nodes, *Kali iod.* gr. v.—30, 8h. *See also* **Exostosis.**

Noma Pudendi.—*Ars.* 3, 4h.

Noises in the Head.—Chronic cases, *Kali iod.* 30, a single dose to be allowed to act. Buzzing, roaring, singing, or hissing, *Chinin. sul.* 3x, gr. ii. 8h. Buzzing, whistling, hissing, singing, *Dig.* 3, 4h. Roaring with giddiness and difficult hearing, *Nat. salicyl.* 3x, 4h. Ringing, tingling, with deafness, as if ear stopped, *Carbon. sul.* 3, 4h. Roaring, thundering, with deafness, the hearing being better in a noise, *Graph.* 6, 4h. When due to recent catarrh of Eustachian tube, (1) *Hydrast.* 3, 4h.; (2) *Mer. sol.* 6, 4h. *See* **Ménière's Disease.**

Nose.—BLEEDING FROM.—In general, *Mill.* 30, ½h. From a blow, *Arn.* 30, ¼h. With throbbing headache and flushed face, *Bell.* 3, ¼h. Bright red blood, on getting up in the morning, *Bry.* 3, ¼h., in the attack, and thrice daily as a preventive. Discharge of clotted blood on the morning, *Nux v.* 3, ¼h., and thrice daily. Dark, stringy blood, *Croc.* 3, ¼h. Frequent and profuse, hæmorrhagic diathesis, *Phos.* 6, ¼h.—4h. Dark fluid, frequent, hæmorrhagic diathesis, *Ham.* 3, ¼h.—4h. Nose-bleed following a rush of blood to the head; flushed face, *Graph.* 30, 4h. With intense redness of face, *Meli. alb.* 3, 4h. Tendency to bleeding, with constipation and piles, *Sul.* 3, 6h. Recurrent bleeding without appreciable cause, *Ferr. phos.* 3, gr. iv. 8h. Recurrent bleeding in old people, *Carbo v.* 6, 8h. When preceding or accompanying symptoms of biliousness, *Chel.* 3, 4h. [When the bleeding is very violent, cold applications to the spine and, failing this, to the genitals, will almost always stop the flow temporarily. If this fails and life is in danger, it may be necessary to plug the nostrils.]

FLUSHING.—Redness of the nose after meals, *Apis* 3x, 4h. Redness in young women, *Borax* 3, 4h.

INFLAMMATION (*of external nose*).—Acute erysipelatous, *Bell.* 1, 2h. Sub-acute, *Sul.* 3x, 4h. Chronic—(1) *Aur. mur.* 3x, gtt. ii. 4h.; (2) *Fluor. ac.* 5x, gtt. ii. 4h.

PUSTULE ON NOSE.—*Petrol.* 3, 4h.

ROOT OF NOSE.—Pressure at, *Kali. bich.* 3, 4h. Pressive headache at the root of nose, *Caps.* 3, 4h.

TIP OF NOSE.—Pimple, *Am. carb.* 3, 1h. Pustule, *Kali brom.*
3x, 8h. Soreness, boil, *Borax* 3, 4h. Redness; heat in evenings, *Caps.* 3, 4h. Redness and itching, *Sil.* 6, 4h. Burning,
Oxal. ac. 3, 4h. Tension, itching, *Carb. a.* 6, 4h. Ulcer or
vesicle, *Caust.* 30, 8h.

SORENESS OF.—*Graphites* 6, 8h.; locally, vaseline at bedtime.
Suppurating nostrils, soreness, pustulation, *Kali bich.* 3x,
gr. i. 4h. *See* **Chaps**; *see also* **Catarrh, Cold, Hay Asthma,
Ozæna, Polypus.**

Nostalgia. *See* **Home Sickness.**

Numbness.—Numbness and tingling, *Aco.* 3, 2h. Numbness
of the whole body, accompanied by pricking: numbness and
insensibility of arms and legs, *Phos.* 3, 3h. A numb pain all
over one side; numbing, creeping sensation in hands and
feet, *Ars.* 3, 3h. Numbness of hands and feet, *Xanth.* 1, 3h.
Sensitive, numb sensation here and there, especially on the
head, always in small spots; numbness and rigidity, especially in the evening in bed; tense, numb sensation in forehead; in zygomatic and malar processes, as if bones of the
head were being screwed together; benumbing pressure
above r. orbit; cramp-like sensation of numbless in l. malar
bone; in l. lower teeth; crawling in the tongue; numbness
in coccyx whilst sitting, *Plat.* 6, 3h. Crawling sensation <
by heat; numbness of fingers and pricking in their tips;
numbness, insensibility, and coldness, *Secal.* 3, 3h. Parts
cold and blue; dead feeling as if frozen, *Agar.* 3, 3h. Numbness in back and limbs; numbness and sensation of swelling

in ball of thumb, *Oxal. acid.* 3x, 3h. Deadness and insensibility, numbness of all r. side, *Plumb.* 6, 3h. Limbs benumbed, with paralysis; deadness, going to sleep, numbness, coldness of hands, numbness of the whole body, *Cicut. v.* 3, 3h. Numb feeling over the whole body, *Con.* 3, 3h. Numbness of hands and feet; pricking and numb sensations in various parts of the body; morbid sensitiveness of the skin to the touch, *Codeia* 3, 3h. Numbness of hands and soles of feet, *Raph.* 3, 3h. Numb deadness of ball of heel whilst walking, *Ign.* 3, 3h.

Nyctalopia (*Night Blindness*).—(1) *Bell.* 3, 4h. (2) *Hell. n.* 3, 4h.

Nymphomania. *See* **Erotomania.**

Obesity. *See* **Corpulence,** and **Diet.**

Odour of Body.—Abominable, *Kali iod.* gr. 1, 8h. Fetid, washing makes no difference, *Pso.* 30, 8h. Offensive, with perspiration, *Merc. sol.* 6, 8h. Like garlic, *Phos.* 3, 8h. *See also under* **Perspiration.**

Œdema. *See* **Dropsy, Laryngitis:** ŒDEMA GLOTTIDIS.

Œsophagus.—Spasmodic stricture, dryness, *Naja* 6, 2h. Food arrested at cardiac end of gullet, *Ign.* 3, 2h. Strangling on attempt to swallow; throat feels as if it were closed, *Cicut.* 30, 4h. Spasm preventing swallowing, *Verat. v.* 3, 2h. Burning < by pressure; constriction; difficulty in swallowing, *Merc. cor.* 3, 4h. Burning and pain, *Phos.* 3, 4h. Burning, spasmodic contraction, and cramp-like pain, *Gels.* 3, 2h.

Offensive Breath. *See* **Breath:** FETID.

Onanism. *See* **Self-abuse, Spermatorrhœa.**

Onychia. *See* **Nails.**

Ophthalmia. *See* Eyes: INFLAMMATION.

Opisthotonus. *See* Tetanus.

Opium Habit. *See* Morphinism.

Optic Neuritis. *See* Eyes: OPTIC NEURITIS.

Orchitis. *See* Testicles.

Osteitis Deformans.—Hypertrophy of cranial bones, (1) *Sil.* 3, gr. v. 8h.; (2) *Aur.* 3. gr. v. 8h. (3) *Hecla* 5, gr. v. 8h.

Osteo-myelitis.—*Gunp.* 3x, gr. iv. 4h.

Otorrhœa. *See* Ears.

Ovaries.—Pain in ovaries at puberty, *Act. r.* 3, 2h. Neuralgic pain, with colic, *Coloc.* 3, 2h. Violent cramping pain, *Naja* 6, 2h. Stinging pain; inflammation, *Apis* 3x, 1h. Burning pain in, with urinary symptoms, *Canth.* 3, 2h. Pain, swelling and tenderness of ovaries, < at menses, with menorrhagia, pregnancy, or gonorrhœa, *Ham.* 3, 1h. Pain in ovaries, especially l., extending down thigh, bearing-down pains in uterus; great sexual excitement and loss of moral control, *Lil. t.* 30, 2h. Pain and inflammation with scanty or suppressed menstruation, *Puls.* 3, 2h. Chronic induration, *Aur. mur. nat.* 3x, gr. v. 8h. Chronic affections, with scanty menstruation and slow conception, *Con.* 3, 4h. Chronic induration with late returning and scanty menses, *Graph.* 6, 6h. Chronic irritation or induration, with menorrhagia, *Plat.* 6, 6h. Pain in r. ovary > by pressure, *Pallad.* 6, 4h. Pain in ovaries, especially left, labour-like pains in uterus, os feels open, *Lach.* 6, 2h. Pain in ovaries with excessive sensitiveness, *Hep.* 6, 2h.

Tumours.—(1) *Iod.* 1, 4h.; (2) *Kali brom.* gr. i. 4h.; (3) *Secale* 1, 4h.; (4) *Apis* 3x, 4h.; with colicky pain compelling patient to bend double, *Coloc.* 3x—30, 8h.

Oxaluria.—(Diet to be regulated; open-air exercise; cold bathing or sponging in morning, followed by brisk rubbing.) With severe backache, *Oxal. ac.* 6, 8h. After this, (1) *Nit. mur. ac.* 6, 4h.; (2) *Senna* 6, gtt. v. twice a day. With severe colic or irritation of urinary passages, *Berb.* 1x, gtt. ii. 4h. The following diet has proved effective: May take meats, fowl, game, fish, bread, rice and other farinaceous foods, potatoes, peas, beans, coffee and apples (sparingly). Forbidden articles: Milk, tea, cocoa, green and root vegetables, fruits, eggs, jellies and rhubarb. (Apples are the only oxalate-free fruit). Copious draughts of water. Vittel and Contrexeville waters are especially valuable in these cases.

Ozæna.—(1) *Cad. sul.*, 3x, gr. ii.—30, 8h.; (2) *Luet.* 30—200 at bed-time; (3) *Hydrastis* 3, 4h.; locally, spray of a solution of *Muriate of Hydrastia*, one grain to the ounce; (4) *Hippoz.* 6, 4h. In strumous subjects, *Iod.* 3x, 4h. In strumous and syphilitic subjects, with or without caries, *Aur. met.* 6, 6h. In psoric subjects, *Psor.* 30, 4h. From overdosing with mercury, *Nit. ac.* 6, 4h. With discharge of thick plugs, *Kali bich.* 3x, gr. ii.—30, 4h. [Spray of Condy's fluid solution is sometimes useful to remove the odour.]

Pains.—Characteristic pains occurring in any part of the body will often lead to the correct remedy. The following list is given as a selection of the most distinctive:—*Arnica :* Bruised pains, as from blows. *Arsen. :* Burning pains, with fear of death. *Aurum :* Bone pains *Bellad. :* Congestive throbbing pains. *Bryonia :* Pains < by slightest motion; > lying on painful side. *Cactus :* Constrictive pains. *Capsicum :*

Burning pains. *Colocynth*: Severe tearing pains > pressure. *Cuprum*: Convulsive, spasmodic pains, cramps. *Dioscorea*: Colicky pains, cramps. *Eupat. perf.*: Bone pains. *Hypericum*: Pains from injured nerves, blows to spine; pains shoot up spine. *Ledum*: Pain as from punctures; pains shoot upwards. *Kali bich.*: Pains in small spots; changing place; diagonal. *Kali carb.*: Stitching, darting pains; < 3 a.m.; < by rest; < lying on painful side. *Kalmia*: Neuralgic, rheumatic pains; pains in heart. *Lachesis*: Congestive pains < after sleep, < left side; beginning l. side and extending to r. *Lycopodium*: Sudden pains, r. sided < when covered, < lying on painful side, < 4—8 p.m. *Magnes. phos.*: Neuralgic, spasmodic pains, < r. side, > heat and pressure. *Puls.*: Wandering pains, < by heat, > slow motion. *Rhust*: rheumatic pains from cold and damp, > motion. *Sepia*: Bearing-down pains, abdominal and uterine. *Spigelia*: Shooting, tearing, stabbing.

Painters' Colic. *See* **Lead Colic.**

Palpitation. *See under* **Heart.**

Pancreatitis.—(1) *Kali iod.* gr. ii. 4h.; (2) *Merc. sol* 6, 4h.; (3) *Iris v.* 3, 2h.; (4) *Atrop. sul.* 3x, gr. ii. 4h. White or fatty stools, *Iod.* 3x—30, 4h.

Paralysis.—ACUTE ASCENDING (LANDRY'S PARALYSIS).—(1) *Gelsem.* 3x, 1h.; (2) *Con.* 3—30, 1h., *Hydrophob.* 3—30, 2h.

AGITANS.—*Merc. viv.* 3x—30, 4h. When the paralysis is of mercurial origin, or should the action of *Merc.* need supplementing, *Hyos.* 3, 4h.; Chronic tremor of head and hands, *Ant. t.* 30, 4h.; with tired feeling, cold sensation; l. side most affected, *Helod.*, 30, 8h. Thickly loaded white tongue, *Ant. c.* 3, 8h.

FACIAL.—When from cold, at first, *Acon.* 3, 1h. If it does not
yield soon, *Caustic.* 6, 2h. After these, or from the beginning
when there is tenderness of the part affected, *Kali chlor.* 3,
2h. With swelling; sensation as of a cobweb on the face,
Graph. 6, 4h.

GENERAL PARALYSIS OF THE INSANE.—In the early stages, restlessness, excitement, *Bell.* 3, 2h. Exalted notions, hilarity
followed by depression, confusion, imbecility, *Agar.* 30, 8h.
Much tremor of the limbs, *Merc. c.* 3, 2h. Fibrillary twitching, *Phos.* 3, 4h. When the exaltation of ideas is very marked,
Can. ind. 3, 2h.

HEMIPLEGIA.—Especially in old men; mental and bodily weakness, *Baryt. c.* 6, 4h. With digestive disorder; when it has
come on after over-eating or drinking, *Nux v.* 3, 1h. With
rigidity, *Strych.* 30, 4h. Aching in occiput, numbness,
tremor, speech difficult, *Gels.* 30, 4h. Speech slow, *Lach.*
30, 4h. Speech unintelligible, *Hyo.* 30, 4h. With great despondency and inclination to weep, *Aur. met.* 12, 2h. If
rigidity threatens, the limbs must be kept very warm,
active and passive movements practised, high-frequency
electricity used two or three times a day for fifteen minutes;
the current should not be strong; internally, *Secale* 1, 4h.
See also **Aphasia, Apoplexy.**

HEREDITARY (FRIEDREICH'S) ATAXIA.—Tremor, diplopia,
ptosis, *Gels.* 3—30, 4h. More developed paralysis, *Curar.*
3—200, 4h.

HYSTERICAL.—(1) *Ign.* 3, 2h.; (2) especially of muscles of neck,
Cocc. ind. 3, 2h.

INFANTILE.—At the beginning, coldness of the limbs; the
child cannot bear to be covered, *Secale* 3, 4h. Later,

especially when there is obstinate constipation, *Plumb*. 6, 4h. [In all cales the limbs must be kept warm, allowed to remain in a hot bath (110°F.) for fifteen minutes night and morning; rubbed, massaged, and exercised regularly. High-frequency electricity is very valuable in these cases.]

LABIO-GLOSSO-PHARYNGEAL.—(1) *Bell*. 3, 2h.; (2) *Plumb*. 6, 4h.; (3) *Caust*. 6, 4h.

LANDRY'S. *See* ACUTE ASCENDING.

LEAD.—(1) *Opium* 1x, 2h. Persistent faradisation, a weak current, fifteen minutes three times a day. The patient must persevere in attempts to use his muscles. *Sulph. ac*. 2x—3x, gtt. v.—10 in a tumbler of water taken as a beverage at meals; (2) *Alumen* 5, 4h.; (3) *Cupr*. 6, 4h.

LOCAL.—Drop-hand or drop-foot (when not due to lead-poisoning), *Plumb*. 6, 4h. Paralysis of the eye muscles, *Con*. 3, 4h. Of the muscles of the neck, head cannot be supported, *Cocc. ind*. 3, 4h. Of the sphincters—(1) *Physostig*. 3, 4h.; (2) especially when there is expulsion of urine and fæces, on coughing, laughing, etc., *Caust*. 6, 4h. Writers' cramp— (1) *Gels*. 1, 4h.; (2) *Cupr*. 6, 4h.

OF LARYNX. *See* VOICE.
[The use of electricity must be taken advantage of in most local paralyses. In lead-poisoning a gentle faradic current, and in writers' cramp the continuous current must be used persistently; massage, and active and passive movements should also be used as occasion requires.]

PARAPLEGIA.—From accident, *Arn*. 3, 2h.; locally, the spine to be rubbed and liniment consisting of *Arn*. 1x, a drachm, spirit of wine one ounce, distilled water to three ounces.

This to be used night and morning, and to be rubbed on for eight minutes with the hand. If this fails to bring about improvement in one or two weeks, *Hyperic. φ*—30, 2h., and a liniment of *Hypericum φ* in the same proportions to be applied in the same way. Afterwards, *Gels.* 1, 4h. From exhaustion; from contusion; sexual excess; post-diphtheritic, *Arg. n.* 6, 4h. With rigidity, *Oxal. ac.* 3, 4h. With rigidity, spasm, and exaggerated reflexes, *Lathyrus sativus* 3x, 4h.; after *Lathyrus*, *Secale* 1, 4h. If there is syphilitic history, or if the others fail, (1) *Kali iod.* gr. iii. 4h.; (2) *Merc. cor.* 3x, gtt. i. 4h. Spasmodic paralysis with wasting of muscles, *Cupr.* 6, 4h. Paraplegia from rheumatism, with restlessness and desire to keep moving about, *Rhus t.* 3, 4h. Great weakness of the muscles, especially of lower limbs, heaviness, weariness, hands and feet go to sleep, pains, numbness; great sexual excitement, *Pic. ac.* 30, 6h.

POST-DIPHTHERITIC.—(1) *Gels.* 1, 2h.; (2) *Cocc. i.* 3, 2h.; (3) *Diphth.* 200, 4h. Paraplegia, *Arg. n.* 6, 4h.

PROGRESSIVE MUSCULAR ATROPHY.—(1) *Phos.* 3, 4h.; (2) *Plumb.* 6, 4h.

PSEUDO-HYPERTROPHIC PARALYSIS.—(1) *Phos.* 3, 4h.; (2) *Curar.* 200, 4h.

SPASTIC PARALYSIS.—(1) *Lath. s.* 3x, 4h.; (2) *Nux v.* 3—30, 4h.; (3) *Hyperic.* 1x—30, 4h.; (4) *Strych. nit.* 3x, gtt. v. 8h.

SYRINGOMYELIA.—With muscular atrophy, *Phos.* 30, 4h. With analgesia, *Gels.* 30, 4h.

Parametritis.—(*Inflammation of the cellular tissue of the pelvis.*) —Throbbing, swelling, pain, *Bell.* 3, 1h. If it does not soon yield to this, *Merc. sol.* 6, 1h. If, in spite of this, it goes on to suppuration, *Hep.* 6, 2h. After it has discharged, if the discharge is thin, *Silic.* 6, 4h. Thick discharge, *Hydrocot.* φ, 8h. *See also* Abscess.

Paraphimosis.—*Jac. car.* 3x, 4h. Anoint with *Vaseline cold cream.* If it does not yield quickly, operation must be performed.

Parturition. *See* Labour.

Pediculosis.—[The first thing to be done in these cases is to observe strict cleanliness and destroy the living lice as far as possible, with their eggs. For this purpose, when the head is the seat of infection, the hair should be cut short and a paraffin lotion applied. In the case of body-lice, the clothing should be boiled, and, if necessary, burned. The best application for destroying lice, whether of the head or the hairy parts of the body (pubes, axillæ, eyebrows, in which regions the crab-lice are found) is a strong lotion of *Staphis.* φ, one or two table-spoonfuls to the half-pint. A few applications of this will kill living lice, and as the nits are hatched it may have to be repeated. But pediculosis is not always a disease of uncleanliness. Sometimes the most scrupulous care will fail to get rid of the affection; and sometimes only one in a large family will be affected, though all are subjected to the same conditions. In these cases constitutional treatment is required in addition and is very effectual.] In subjects of consumptive family, *Bacill.* 100 once or twice a week. In chilly subjects, unhealthy complexion, constipation, subject to catarrh, *Nat. m.* 30, 4h. Or *Staph.* 30 may be given internally when the lotion is being used.

Peliosus Rheumatica. *See* Purpura.

Pellagra.—(1) *Ars. sul. rub.* 3x, gr. iv. 4h.; (2) Erysipeloid condition, *Rhust.* 1, 2h.; (3) Spongy gums, tremors, *Merc. s.* 3x, gr. iv. 2—4h.

Pelvic Cellulitis. *See* **Parametritis.**

Pelvic Hæmatocele.—When bleeding is still going on, *Ham.* 1, ½h. For absorption—(1) *Arn.* 1, 2h.; (2) *Sul.* 1, 4h.

Pelvic Peritonitis. *See* **Perimetritis.**

Pemphigus.—Acute, *Rhus t.* 3, 2h. Chronic, *Arsen.* 3, 2h. Syphilitic, *Merc. c.* 3, 2h.

Pericarditis. *See under* **Heart.**

Perichondritis.—[The following refer especially to affections of the rib-cartilages; for other cartilages, *see under* **Joints.**] Burning; corroding, gnawing; pressive shooting, *Bell.* 3, 2h. Gnawing, pricking, biting, or burning, *Ruta* 3, 2h. Stitches, tenderness, burning, aching, *Oleand.* 3, 2h. Painful sensitiveness even to slightest touch, *Angust.* 3, gr. iv. 4h. Great sensitiveness; sticking or dull pressive pain, *Plumb. met.* 6, 4h. Stitches worse on inspiration, *Cham.* 6, 2h. Lancinations in cartilages of lower ribs, worse by inspiration, *Act. r.* 3, 2h. Intermittent dull stitches in cartilages of last true ribs, l. side, *Arg. met.* 6, 4h. *See also* **Bones: PERIOSTITIS.**

Perimetritis.—Pain, tenderness, *Merc. cor.* 3, 1h. Swelling, *Bell.* 3, 1h. *See also* **Peritonitis.**

Periostitis. *See* **Bones: PERIOSTITIS.**

Peritonitis.—*Acute*—At the commencement, soon after a chill has been taken, when there is fever, anxiety, and abdominal pain, *Aco.* 3, 1h. If *Aco.* does not effect decided amelioration in twenty-four hours, *Sulph.* 3—30, 1—4h. When effusion has taken place, much pain, not much fever, *Canth.* 3, 1h. Considerable fever, violent sharp pain, much effusion, *Bry.* 3, 2h. Griping cutting pains, abdomen much swollen, excessively tender, tenesmus, *Merc. cor.* 3, 1h. When there is much tympanites and colic, *Coloc.* 3, ½h. A feeling as if a spot were gripped with the nails; the transverse colon standing out like a pad, *Bell.* 3, 1h. [Locally, light poultices, on which, if there is distension, a few drops of turpentine should be sprinkled, may be applied for half an hour at a time, and left off for half an hour, the body being covered with flannel during the intervals between the poultices.] *Chronic.*—The same measure as in acute peritonitis, according to symptoms. When there is much plastic effusion, *Merc. dulc.* 3x, gr. v. 6h. When there is much distension with constipation and flatulence, pains shooting from right to left, *Lyc.* 3, gr. v. 6h. [The desirability of performing laparotomy and washing out the cavity of the peritoneum must be considered.] When there is diarrhœa, *see* **Diarrhœa.**

Dropsy remaining after.—*Apis* 3x, 2h. *See* **Dropsy.**

Puerperal.—Pain, fever, anxiety, restlessness, *Aco.* 3, 1h. Sharp, cutting pains < by the least motion or pressure, > by lying on affected side, *Bry.* 3, 1h. [Locally, flannels rung out of hot water, with a few drops of turpentine sprinkled on, may be kept applied to the body. Hot vaginal douche of Condy's solution (red, two teaspoonfuls to the pint) three times a day.]

Tubercular.—*Bacil.* 30—200, gl. iv. once a week. For acute symptoms, cutting pain in bowels and inguinal regions; delirium; typhoid condition, *Iodof.* 3x—30, 2h. Restlessness, burning thirst, anxiety, *Ars.* 3, 2h. Hard, swollen abdomen;

swelling and induration of mesenteric glands, *Calc. c.* 30, 2h. Intercurrently, if the reaction is slow, these medicines being omitted for a week, *Sul.* 3, 4h. Hectic fever, *China.* 3, 2h. Much emaciation, *Abrot.* 30, 4h.

Perityphlitis. *See* Appendicitis.

Pernicious Anæmia. *See under* Anæmia.

Perspiration.—From debility after exhausting diseases, *China.* 3, 4h. Profuse perspiration all over, especially on the genitals; night-sweat, *Phos. ac.* 1, 4h. Exhausting perspiration all over: perspiration after waking; profuse night-sweat; on head; forehead; head and chest; head and hands, *Phos.* 3, 4h. Bloody sweat: hysterical, *Nux m.* 30, 2h.; in low conditions, *Lach.* 6, 4h. Disorders of perspiration in persons subject to skin diseases, and scrofulous subjects, and from repercussion of eruptions; hot, sweaty feet, *Sul.* 3—30, 8h. Sweat offensive; odour of bad eggs, *Staph.* 3, 8h. Excessive perspiration with nervous depression; with flushes of the menopause; in phthisis; unilateral, *Jaborandi* 3, 4h. Offensive night sweat, *Carb. a.* 6, 4h. Urinous odour, *Nit. ac.* 12, 8h. Perspiration of the head, especially at 3 a.m., not offensive, *Calc. c.* 6, 4h. Offensive perspiration of head or feet, *Sil.* 6, 4h. Glutinous or sour perspiration; moist palms, *Fluor. ac.* 3, 6h. Excessive; viscid; of strong odour; at night; in fevers; "hidrosis pedum." *Merc. sol.* 6, 4h. Fetid perspiration in arm-pits; tender feet with perspiration more or less offensive, *Petr.* 3, 4h. Perspiration on waking, dry heat during sleep (cold hands and feet), *Samb.* 3, 4h. Absence of sweat *see* Anidrosis.

Pertussis. *See* Whooping-cough.

Petit Mal. *See* Epilepsy.

Pharyngitis. *See* Throat.

Phimosis.—*Congenital.*—Forcible dilatation or circumcision. *Acquired*—(1) *Merc. sol.* 6, 4h.; locally, *Hamamelis* lotion (ten drops to the half-pint) to be kept applied on linen; (2) *Jac. car.* 3x, 4h.; (3) *Guaiac.* 3x, gtt. v. t.d. The same operation as for congenital phimosis may be required. When there is irritation or inflammation of the prepuce it should be withdrawn and washed daily and anointed with *Vaseline cold cream.*

Phlebitis. *See* Veins.

Phlegmasia Alba Dolens.—Pain, fever, restlessness, anxiety, *Aco.* 3, 1h. Pain and tenderness along the vein trunks, chilly, but does not like to be covered, *Puls.* 3, 1h. [Locally, the limb must be swathed in cotton-wool and kept moist. If there is fetid discharge, a vaginal douche of a hot Condy solution (a teaspoonful to a pint) given twice daily.] If *Puls.* does not appear to do good, *Ham.* 1, 1h. After both have been tried, *Bism.* 1, gr. iv. 3h.

Photophobia. *See* Eyes: SIGHT.

Phrenitis. *See* Brain, CONGESTION OF.

Phthisis Pulmonalis. *See* Consumption.

Physometra (*Air in the Uterine Passages*). (1) *Brom.* 3, 4h.; (2) *Phos. ac.* 1, 4h.

Piles. *See* Hæmorrhoids.

Pimples. *See* Acne.

Pityriasis (*Scurf*).—In debilitated subjects; patients with fair skins, *Ars.* 3, 4h.; much irritation, *Rad. bro.* 30, once a week. Dry, scurfy, irritable scalp; falling off of hair, *Fluor. ac.* 3, 4h. With loss of hair and great itching, *Mezer.* 3, 4h. Moist scurf of the head, *Sep.* 6, 4h. Scalp scaly, with distressing itching, humid, falling off of hair, *Graph.* 6, 4h.

Pityriasis Rubra.—With anxiety, restlessness, thirst, *Ars.* 3, 8h. Fiery redness, burning and pain *Rad. bro.* 30, once a week. Squamous eruptions, scales thin, white, leaving reddened skin. If scales remain, they cause itching, < when warm from exercise, *Nat. ars.* 3, 8h.

Pityriasis Versicolor (Chromophytosis, Tinea Versicolor, Phytosis Versicolor).—This disease is closely allied to Ringworm and the treatment is similar. (1) *Bacill.* 30—200, once a week; (2) *Sep.* 30, 4h.; (3) *Tellur.* 30, 4h. Locally, the patches may be painted with *Sulphurous acid.* (4) *Chrys. ac.* 2, 4h. The parts to be painted with tincture of *Chrys. ac.* 2, once or twice a day. *See also* **Ringworm.**

Placenta, RETAINED. *See* **Labour:** RETAINED PLACENTA.

Plague.—*Pest.* 6—30, 4h. Inter-currently other remedies may be given as indicated. Early stage, marked delirium, *Bell.* 3x, ½h. Yellow sclerotica, great prostration, restlessness, sore, bruised feeling all over, *Laches.* 6, ½—1h. (In India preparations of the fresh virus of *Naja,* 3x—6, are preferable, and Deane has obtained better results by administering by subcutaneous injection than by the mouth. In plague absorption is apparently paralysed.) In pneumonic cases, *Phos.* 3—6, 1—2h. With intestinal symptoms, *Ars.* 3, 1h. Collapse, *Hydroc. ac.* 3x, ½—1h. Cramps or spasms, *Cupr. ac.* 3x—3, ½—1h.

Plethora.—Spare diet, abstinence from alcohol and red meat, active open-air exercise, *Ars.* 6, 8h.

Pleurisy.—At the commencement, before effusion has occurred, heat, restlessness, anxiety, *Aco.* 3, 1h. When plastic effusion has taken place, sharp cutting pains making all motion painful, *Sulph.* 3, 1h. Fluid effusion, not much fever, *Canth.* 3, 1h. Much fever, violent pain in the side, much effusion, pain > by lying on painful side, < by least movement, *Bry.* 3, 1h. High fever, flushed face, pain < lying on painful side, *Bell.* 3, 1h. Effusion persistent, *Sul.* 3x—30, 4h. When the pleurisy has become chronic, with formation of pus and tendency to set up phthisis, *Hep. s.* 6, 4h. If the effusion is excessive, tapping must be considered, the indications being—threatening asphyxia, danger of fainting, and no evidence of improvement. If the fluid is long in being absorbed, after the acute stage is passed, *Ars.* 3, 4h.; if this fails, *Apis* 3x, 2h. *Asclepias tuberosa* φ, 15 drops every hour, in a little water, has been found a useful remedy in many cases of pleurisy.

EMPYEMA.—(1) *Hep. s.* 6, 2h.; (2) *Sil.* 6, 2h.; (3) *Ferr. mur.* 3x, gtt. v. 2h. When there is great prostration and hectic fever, *China.* 3, 2h. Tapping may be required.

HYDROTHORAX.—(1) *Apis* 3x, 2h.; (2) *Ars.* 3, 3h. *See* **Dropsy.**

Pleurodynia.—At the commencement, from a chill, fever, restlessness, pain on motion, *Aco.* 3, 1h. Cutting pain in chest; evening, after lying down; stitches in sides on inspiration, *Kali c.* 3—30, 2h. Afterwards, if muscular, pain, depression, *Act. r.* 3, 1h. If from over-exertion, *Arn.* 3, 1h. If the seat of pain is on the right side, *Chel.* 1, 1h.; after *Chel.*, *Asclep. tub.* 1, 1h. When on the left side, *Ranunc. bulb.* 1, 1h. When purely neuralgic, if symptomatic of uterine disorder, or in hysterical girls, *Act. rac.* 3, 1h. In others, *Ars.* 3, 2h. *See also* **Neuralgia.**

Plica Polonica.—(The hair must be cut as close to the scalp as possible, and scrupulous cleanliness observed.)—(1) *Lyc.* 6, 4h.; (2) *Vinc. m.* 3, 4h.; (3) *Viol. t.* 3, 4h.

Pneumonia.—ACUTE.—At the commencement, after a chill as from sudden lowering of temperature at sundown on high altitudes; before physical signs are pronounced, pain, fever, anxiety, *Acon.* 3, 1h. If the fever does not yield in 24—48h., *Sul.* 1—30, 2h. With much congestion, *Ver. v.* 1—3, 1h. When exudation has already occurred rusty sputa, (1) *Phos.* 3, 1h.; (2) *Tuberc. koch.* 6—30, 4h. Typhoid pneumonia, great nervous depression; pneumonia coming on during the course of fever, *Phos.* 3, 1h. Great prostration, thirst, anxiety, restlessness, *Ars.* 3, 1h. Dry cough with concussion of whole chest; oppression; aching pain at night when waking; dull stitches and burning pains l. half of chest, *Seneg.* 1x—30, 2h. Pneumonia of one or both bases, gasping for breath, unable to lie down; mind confused, typhoid condition, *Carb. ac.* 1x—30, 1—2h. Pneumonia of delirium tremens; catarrhal pneumonia; broncho-pneumonia in children and old persons, *Ant. tart.* 3, 2h. Pleuro-pneumonia, sharp pains caused by the least motion, > by lying on affected side, *Bry.* 3, 1h. Pneumonia with liver involvement, jaundiced hue, bile-stained sputa, *Chel.* 1, 1h. Right-side pneumonia, troublesome cough, difficult expectoration, short breath, *Sang.* 1, 1h. Rusty expectoration, weakness, trembling, numbness of extremities, *Phos.* 3, 1h. When the cough is especially troublesome at night, disturbing sleep, a few doses of *Hyoscy.* 3 may be given at half-hour intervals. When a cough lingers after physical signs have disappeared, *Sulph.* 3, 4h.

CHRONIC.—Intercurrent doses of *Bacil.* 30—200 will help the other remedies. When the lung does not clear after the acute stage is passed. *Ars. iod.* 3x, gr. ii. immediately after food three times a day. If the sputa are rusty, *Phos.* 3, 4h. If there are sharp pains in chest on breathing or motion, *Bry.* 3, 4h. If the expectoration becomes purulent, *Hepar* 6, 3h. Yellowish-green expectoration, depression, unpleasant taste in the mouth, sluggish circulation, coldness, *Lyc.* 6, 2h. Pneumonia in persons who suffer from bleeding hæmorrhoids, *Hyper.* 1x, 2h. *See also* Consumption.

Polypus.—OF NOSE.—(1) *Thuja* 30, 6h.; locally, *Thuja* φ, to be used as paint night and morning; (2) *Formica* 3x, gtt. v. 8h.; (3) *Calc. c.* 30, 6h., *Thuja* φ locally; (4) *Kali nit.* 5x, gr. x. h.s.s.; (5) *Kali bichr.* 3x, gr. ii. 6h.; locally, the polypi to be painted with a solution of *Kali bichr.* (gr. ii.—ℨi.) night and morning; (6) *Nit. ac.* 6, 6h.; (7) *Teucr.* 1x, 6h.; locally, *Teucrium* snuff, or paint with *Teucr.* φ. When accompanied with asthmatic rose-cold symptoms, or sick headache, *Sang.* 3, 8h. Tightness at root of nose, tension in nose, offensive discharge, *Cad. ms.* 3—30, 8h. Polypus bleeding easily by touch; green or yellow mucus from nose, *Phos.* 3, 8h. Chronic nasopharyngeal discharge, chilliness, debility, *Psor.* 30, 6h.

OF EARS. *See under* Ears.

OF UTERUS. *See* Fibroma.

Polyuria. *See* Diabetes, Urine.

Porrigo. *See* Eczema: CAPITIS.

Pott's Disease. *See under* Spine.

Pregnancy. DISORDERS OF:—

BACKACHE—With sense of weakness and dragging in the loins, *Kali c*. 6, 4h. With lameness, bruised sensation, and inability to walk, (1) *Bellis* 3x—30, 4h.; (2) *Arn*. 3x, 4h.

BLADDER TROUBLES.—Sympathetic tenesmus.—(1) *Bell*. 3, 4h.; (2) *Nux v*. 3, 4h.; (3) *Puls*. 3, 4h. With burning and scalding, *Canth*. 3, 4h. Incontinence of urine, expelled by slightest exertion, coughing or sneezing, *Caust*. 6, 4h.

BREASTS.—Painful—(1) *Conium* 3, 2h.; (2) *Bry*. 3, 2h.

COUGH.—With oppression of breathing, *Nux v*. 3, 2h. Morning cough, *Bry*. 3, 2h. Hoarse or hollow cough with expulsion of urine, *Caust*. 6, 2h.

CRAMPS.—(1) *Verat. a*. 3, 4h.; (2) *Nux v*. 3, 2h; (3) *Led*. 3, 3 times daily for several days will often give prolonged relief. (4) *Mag. Phos*. 6x, is a very useful general remedy 3 or 4 times daily taken dissolved in hot water.

DIGESTIVE DISORDERS:—

   Toothache.—If there is caries, *Kreas*. 3, 2h. If there is no caries—(1) *Mag. c*. 6, 2h.; (2) *Sep*. 6, 2h.

   Salivation.—(1) *Jaborandi* 3x, 4h.; (2) *Merc. sol*. 6, 4h.; (3) *Sul*. 3, 4h.

   Depraved Appetite.—(1) (as for chalk), *Calc. c*. 6, 4h.; (2) (as for cinders), *Carb. v*. 6, 4h. For dry food, as oatmeal, etc., *Alumina* 6—30, 4h.

   Heartburn.—With acidity, *Calc. c*. 6, 4h. Without acidity —(1) *Puls*. 3, 4h.; (2) *Capsic*. 3, 3h.

   Morning Sickness.—With moist white tongue, *Puls*. 3, 2h. With brown tongue; in spare dark subjects, *Nux v*. 3, 2h. Food rejected as soon as taken—(1) *Ipec*. 3, 2h.; (2) *Nux v*.

1, 2h. Almost purely sympathetic—(1) *Apomorph.* 3, 2h.;
(2) *Kreas.* 3, 2h. Deathly nausea; vomiting continuous,
violent retching; smell or thought of food intolerable,
Symphoricarpus racemoscus 200, 2h. (This is a good all-
round remedy and has cured some desperate cases.) *Medor-
rhinum* 10m. a few doses only, will cure a great number of
cases. Continued sick feeling, day and night, without vomiting, *Tabac.* 3, 2h. Incessant nausea with or without vomiting,
Petrol. 3, 2h. With much flatulence, *Calc. fl.* 3x—6x, gr.
iv.—6, 8h. *Calc. fl.* is an excellent remedy in digestive
troubles of pregnancy and given in the later months, facili-
tates delivery. [Food should be taken frequently, in small
quantities, and the medicines given about a quarter of an
hour before food. The patient should endeavour to eat
immediately after vomiting has taken place.]

Constipation.—*Collins.* 1x—30, 3h.

Diarrhœa.—Stools chiefly at night, *Puls.* 3, 4h. With
prostration and loss of flesh, *Phos. ac.* 1, gtt. ii. 4h.

FALSE PAINS.—(1) *Secale* 3, 2h.; (2) *Caulo.* 3, 2h.

LIVER SPOTS.—*Sep.* 6, 4h.

MENTAL DISTURBANCES.—Irritability or depression, *Act. r.* 3,
3h. Crossness, *Cham.* 6, 3h. Febrile sleeplessness, *Aco.* 3,
2h. "Fidgets," *Cham.* 6, 3h.

PRURITUS VULVÆ.—*Ambra* 6, 4h.

See also under general headings, Back, Bladder, Cough,
Constipation, etc.; *also* Miscarriage and Labour.

Presbyopia. *See* Eyes: SIGHT.

Prickly Heat. *See* Lichen.

Proctalgia. *See* Rectum, Pain in.

Proctitis.—Acute, with tenesmus—(1) *Aloe* 3, 1h.; (2) *Podoph.* 6, 1h. Subacute with passage of much mucus, *Colch.* 3, 2h. Chronic, purulent discharge, tendency to stricture—(1) (especially if syphilitic) *Nit. ac.* 6, 4h.; (2) *Phos.* 3, 4h.

Progressive Muscular Atrophy.—(1) *Phos.* 3, 4h.; (2) *Plumb.* 6, 4h.

Prolapse. Of anus and uterus. *See* **Anus, Uterus.**

Prosopalgia. *See* **Toothache, Neuralgia.**

Prostate.—DISEASE OF.—Acute inflammation, as from gonorrhœa, (1) *Thuja* 3, 2h. (2) *Puls.* 3, 2h. Subacute, *Kali iod.* gr. 1, 4h. Hæmaturia with prostatic affections, or prostatic piles, *Ocim. can.* 3—200, 4h. Sensation in anal region as if sitting on a ball, (1) *Can. i.* 1—30, 4h.; (2) *Chim. umb.* 1, 4h. Chronic or acute enlargement, difficulty in passing urine or burning whilst urinating, *Sabal serrul,* 3x, 2—4h. Chronic enlargement, *Solidago, virg.-aur.*, 3x, 2—4h. Chronic irritation after an acute attack, *Staphis.* 3, 4h. Inflammation in scrofulous or tuberculous subjects, *Iod.* 3x, 4h. When suppuration has occurred, *Merc. sol.* 6, 3h. Chronic suppuration, *Nit. ac.* 6, 4h. Chronic enlargement in old men, (1) *Arg. mur.* 5, 8h. (2) *Arg. nit.* 3x, 4h. (3) *Fer. pic.* 3, gr. vi. 8h.

Proud Flesh. *See* **Excrescences.**

Prurigo.—*Rad. bro.* 30, once a week. *See* **Irritation.**

Pruritus Ani.—*Rad. bro.* 30, once a week. *See* **Anus: ITCHING.** and **Irritation.**

Pruritus Vulvæ.—*Rad. bro.* 30, once a week. *See* **Irritation.**

Psilosis (SPRUE) (1) *Fragar. v. φ*, gtt. v. 4h. (2) *Calc. lact.* 3x, gr. viii. 4h.

Psoriasis.—General, acute or chronic, *Ars.* 3x—30, 4h. When there is irritation, *Rad. bro.* 30, once a week. Especially in chilly subjects; anæmic, *Thyr.* 3x—30, 4h. In young girls, *Cupr. m.* 3, gr. ii. 4h. In scrofulous subjects, *Æth. ant.* 5, 6h.; worse from cold and in winter, *Petrol.* 3, 4h. Vaccinal or sycotic. *Thuj.* 1—30, 8h. Syphilitic (and also non-syphilitic), *Merc. bin.* 3x—30, 8h. After these, *Chrys. ac.* 3x, gr. i. 8h. Behind the ears; palms or backs of the hands; syphilitic psoriasis, *Graph.* 6, 6h. Spots having a burning pain when touched; much irritation; eruption on the ears, *Cicut. v.* 3, 4h. [In all cases alcohol should be abstained from.]

Pterygium. *See under* **Eyes:** GRANULAR INFLAMMATION.

Ptomaine Poisoning.—If taken early enough administer mustard emetic. Follow with strong, black coffee. Sausage poisoning, *Bell.* 3x, 1h. From bad fish, *Carb. v.* 6, 1h. From bad meat, *Ars.* 3x—3, 1h.

Ptosis. *See under* **Eyes.**

Ptyalism. *See* **Salivation.**

Puerperal Convulsions. *See* **Labour.**

Puerperal Fever. *See* **Labour.**

Puerperal Mania. *See* **Labour.**

Purging. *See* **Diarrhœa.**

Purpura.—*Simple non-febrile.*—Bruised sensation and bruised appearance, *Arn.* 3, 2h. Hæmorrhagic diathesis, *Phos.* 3, 2h. Where the blood-vessels are specially at fault, *Ham.* 3, 2h.

Rheumatic Purpura—with fever, pains in the limbs and stiffness, *Acon.* 3, 1h. Sensitive to heat or cold, pains < at night, *Merc. sol.* 6, 1h. Restlessness, general soreness, pains < at rest, *Rhus v.* 3, 2h. When the fever is of a low type, *Ars.* 3, 2h. *Hæmorrhagic Purpura*—where bleeding takes place from the nose, gums and other surfaces, palpitation, paleness of skin and mucous membranes, slight wounds bleed easily, *Phos.* 3, 4h. Intolerable itching, restlessness, debility, soreness, stiffness, affections of the joints, *Rhus v.* 3, 2h. Varicose diathesis, passive hæmorrhages, bruised and tired feeling all over the body, *Ham.* 3, 2h. With general sensitiveness of the surface; in rheumatic or syphilitic subjects; emaciation and debility, *Kali iod.* 30, 2h. Spongy gums, fetid odour from mouth, muscles flabby, swelling of ankles, *Merc. viv.* 6, 2h. Aggravation of all symptoms after sleep, dryness of throat without thirst, external throat very sensitive to touch, great physical and mental exhaustion, icy coldness of feet, *Lach.* 6, 4h. With great nervous depression, *Phos. ac.* 1x, gtt. ii. 2h. Disorganization of the blood, *Crotal*, 3, 2h.

Purulent Ophthalmia. *See* Eyes: OPHTHALMIA.

Pustule, Malignant. *See* **Malignant Pustule.**

Pyæmia.—After wounds or surgical operations, *Arn.* 3, 1h.; locally a lotion of *Arn.* 3x, two drachms to the half-pint of distilled water. After infection with purulent material (as dissecting wound) or exposure to foul emanations, *Lach.* 6, 1h.; locally, a compress of the same, one drachm to two ounces. Fever, *Pyrogen.* 6—30, 4h. Blood-poisoning, intolerable stench, *Echin.* φ, gtt. i.—v. 1h. Chronic blood-poisoning, with low fever, red tongue, *Ars.* 3, 4h. With fever of the hectic type, *Chin. sul.* 3x, 4h. When the joints become affected, restlessness, pain relieved by motion, *Rhus t.* 3, 2h. When effusion takes place; pain < by touch or motion, *Bry.* 1, 2h. Where suppuration occurs, *Merc. sol.* 6, 2h. [The symptoms of chronic blood-poisoning are exceedingly varied, and each case must be treated according to its leading characteristics. *See also* **Dysentery, Joints, Throat, Heart,** etc.]

Pyelitis.—Acute, *Uva ursi φ*, 1h. Where the patient is very low, *Ars.* 3, 2h.

Pylorus.—Thickening and constriction, recent, *Nux v.* 3, 3h. More chronic, *Phos.* 3, 4h. When there is pain, swelling, tenderness and signs of abscess, *Hep.* 6, 2h. Chronic suppuration, *Sil.* 6, 4h. Exhaustion from excessive discharge, *China.* 3, 2h. [Medicines must be prescribed according to the symptoms. *See under* **Duodenum, Dyspepsia,** etc.]

Pyorrhœa.—Spongy gums, bad odour from mouth, *Merc. s.* 3x, gr. iv.—30, 4h. All teeth loose; bad smell from teeth, *Kali c.* 6—30, 4h. Painful inflammation < by cold or hot things, gumboils, *Sil.* 6, 4h. Scorbutic gums, easily bleeding, putrid, *Cist.* 1—30, 4h. Free suppuration, *Gunp.* 3x, gr. iv. 4h. [A mouthwash of *Peroxide of Hydrogen*, one teaspoonful to three or four of water used night and morning is a useful accessory.]

Pyrosis. *See* **Dyspepsia, Heartburn, Waterbrash.**

Quinsy (*Simple Acute Inflammation of the Tonsils.*)—Initial chill and fever, anxiety and restlessness, with pain and soreness in throat, *Acon.* 3, 1h. After *Acon.*, if the local action is more pronounced, *Baryta c.* 6, 1h. Severe tonsillitis, pricking pains, *Sil.* 12x. trit., gr. iv. 2h. Acute tonsillitis, r. tonsil much swollen, dark red, constant aching pains, sharp stitches toward ear or swelling, *Guaiac.* 3x, 2h. With eruption of vesicles on mucous membrane, *Phytol.* 3, 1h. gargle of *Phyt.* φ, gtt. x. to Oss. Commencing r. side, spreading to l., *Lyc.* 6, 2h. Commencing l. spreading to r. side, *Lach.* 6, 2h. When suppuration is inevitable, *Hep. s.* 6, 1h. Septic tonsillitis, *Gunp.* 3x, gr. iv. 4h. [This may be alternated with *Baryt. c.* 6.]

Rabies. *See* **Hydrophobia.**

Rachitis. *See* **Rickets.**

Ranula.—(1) *Thuja* 3, 2h.; (2) *Merc. sol.* 6, 4h.; (3) *Calc. c.* 6, 4h.; (4) *Ambr.* 6, 4h. Returning periodically, with dry mouth, *Hydrob.*, 12, 8h.

Rash. *See* **Eruptions, Itching, Nettle-rash, Roseola.**

Raynaud's Disease.—*Bacill.* 30 once a week and *Fer. ph.* 6x, gr. viii. 8h. This may be followed by *Sec.* 3, gr. viii.—30, 8h.

Rectum, INFLAMMATION OF. *See* **Proctitis.**

PAIN IN.—Tenesmus, burning, violent pain, *Caps.* 3, 4h. Lancinations shooting upwards, *Phos.* 6, 4h. Contractive pain, shooting and smarting in rectum, *Ign.* 1, 4h.

PROLAPSE. *See* **Anus.**

STRICTURE OF.—Cancerous, (1) *Hydrast.* 1, 4h.; locally, injection of *Hydrastis* lotion (φ ʒii.—ʒviii.) night and morning; (2) *Ruta* φ, unit doses. Cancerous or simple, *Nit. ac.* 6, 4h.

STRAINING. *See* **Tenesmus.**

ULCERATION.—(1) *Nit. ac.* 6, 4h.; (2) *Graph.* 6, 4h.; (3) *Sul.* 3, 4h.; locally, *Hydrastis* injection (φ, ʒii.—ʒviii.) night and morning.

Red-gum (*Lichen strophulus.*)—With great irritability; during dentition; child wants to be carried about, *Cham.* 6, 2h. With intolerable itching, < at night; < by warmth, *Apis* 3x, 2h. With disordered digestion, loaded tongue, *Ant. crud.* 6, 6h. Intolerable itching all over, < at night, < in cold air, *Rhus t.* 3, 2h. In psoric subjects; hot head, cold feet; < when warm in bed at night, *Sul.* 6, 4h. To be powdered with fullers' earth, and when washed Barilla soap should be used. *See under* Lichen.

Relapsing Fever.—When the pains are increased by movement, *Bry.* φ—3, 2h. Thirst, restlessness, anxiety, *Ars.* 3x—3, 2h. When the patients are restless and constantly moving, *Rhus t.* 3, 2h. When gastric symptoms predominate, *Bapt.* 3, 2h. When the bone-pains are very distressing, *Eupat. perf.* 3, 2h.

Remittent Fever.—During the attack, *Acon.* 1x, 2h. During the remission, if the fever is not of a typhoid type, *Chin. sul.* 1x, gtt. i.—v. 3h. If the fever is of a low type, and the patient very weak, *Ars.* 3x, 3h. If there is much sickness, *Ipec.* 1x—3, ½h. (a few doses intercurrently). Children's remittents, *Gels.* 1, 2h. Bilious remittents, *Crot. h.* 3x, 1h.

Respiration.—As if breathing through a sponge, *Phyt.* 3, 4h. As if a fly in the throat, *Brom.* 3, 4h. Cheyne-Stokes breathing; wakes up feeling respiration has stopped, *Grind.* 30, 2h. Dyspnœa on falling asleep; stertorous breathing and puffing out of cheeks, *China.* 30, 2h.

Retching. *See* Vomiting.

Retinitis. *See under* Eyes.

Rhagades. *See* Cracks.

Rheumatic Fever. *See* Rheumatism, ACUTE.

Rheumatic Gout (Chronic Rheumatic Arthritis, Rheumatoid Arthritis).—Digestion disordered; in females, menses scanty; melancholia; spindle-shaped swelling of the fingers, *Puls.* 3, 4h. Accompanying uterine disorder or coming on at the change of life, the pains < at night, and in wet, windy weather, *Act. r.* 3, 2h. When the pains are worst in the small joints, *Caulo.* 3, 2h. When the affection of the joints is decidedly inflammatory; especially in females if there is menorrhagia, *Sabin.* 3, 4h. In gouty persons, dark hair; tendency to warts or corns, *Fer. pic.* 3x—3, gr. ii. 8h. Shooting and tearing pains and contraction of parts affected, < by the least movement, stiffness of the parts, *Guaiac.* 3x, gtt. v. 8h. Deep constitutional remedies, especially *Carcinosin* and *Bacillinum*, will help these cases. I have found *Strychninum* also very valuable and the administration of *Strych.* 6, gtt. viii. in a wineglass of water on rising and *Carcin.* 100, twenty-four numbered powders, of which numbers 1, 11 and 17 have six globules of the remedy, one to be taken at bed-time in numerical order, very effective in many cases. Pain, heat, swelling of joints, < on touch or motion, great loss of flesh, ravenous appetite, *Iod.* 3x, 2h. Pains worse in cold, damp weather, low fever, restlessness, anxiety, *Ars.* 3, 2h. The medicines already named and those advised below under **Rheumatism, CHRONIC**, may be given according to particular indications.

[The diet should be unstimulating. Wines and malt liquors and strongly-spiced food should be avoided. A warm, dry climate, if practicable, is to be advised.]

Rheumatism.—Acute and Subacute (Rheumatic Fever).—
Fever, restlessness, anxiety, pain in joints, *Acon.* 1—3, 1h.
Pain and swelling of joints, < at night; profuse sweat
which gives no relief, sometimes oily or offensive; pericar-
dial complications, *Merc. v.* 12, 2h. (I have cured many
cases with this alone.) After *Acon.*, when the pains are < at
night, and by warmth, sinking sensation, *Sul.* 1—30, 2h
After *Acon.* much pain in the joints, the least motion is
unendurable, *Bry.* 3, 1h. When there is great restlessness,
the pain being > by moving about, *Rhus t.* 1—3, 1h. Heat
and sweat of head, cold clammy feet and hands, violent
perspiration at 3 a.m., pains < by every movement; after
bathing, or working in water, *Calc. carb.* 30, 2h. When the
pain attacks the back, back of the neck, and back of the
head, with restlessness, and pain in the eyes, *Act. r.* 1, 1h.
Shifting rheumatic pains in all parts with soreness, < by
motion, with pains in liver, *Stell. med.* 2x, 2h. (Locally,
Stell. med. φ, ʒi—Olive oil, ʒi.) Subacute rheumatism from
getting cold and wet, *Dulc.* 3, 1h. Subacute—knees, ankles,
and small joints of hands and feet affected; shifting about,
coming on with faulty digestion; the pains < at night, in a
warm room and by rest, > in the open air and by motion,
Puls. 3, 2h. Similar pains when the patient hugs the fire
and desires warm wraps, *Ars.* 3, 4h. Acute, non-febrile
rheumatism of the joints, the pains shifting much, *Kalm.* 3,
2h. When the urine is strong-smelling and high coloured,
Benz. ac. 1x—3x, 2h. Pains < in north-east winds, larger
joints chiefly affected, slightest movement sets up inflammation, *Arbut. andr.* φ, single doses, or 3x, 4h. Pericarditis.
(*See under* Heart.) Endocarditis. (*See under* Heart.) For
pain, swelling, and joint-weakness remaining after an attack,
Sul. 3—30, 6h., and at increasing intervals. Muscular pains

and stiffness after, *Arn.* 3, 2h. Weakness after—(1) *Chin. sul.* 3x, gr. iv. 4h., (2) *Calc. phos.* 3, gr. iv. 8h.

HYPERPYREXIA.—When due to affection of the brain and its meninges, intense pain in back of the head and along the spine, *Act. r.* 1x, 1h. When due to supervention of meningitis, *see* Meningitis. Simple hyperpyrexia, *see* Hyperpyrexia.

GONORRHŒAL.—Great pains, fever, restlessness, anxiety, *Acon.* 3, 1h. [An occasional dose of *Medor.* 30—200 will often restore a suppressed gonorrhœa and cure the rheumatic symptoms, or it may be repeated every four hours.] After *Acon.*, if there is swelling of joints, perspiration, discharge, *Merc. s.* 6, 1h. Swelling and pains in joints, gastric disturbances and flatulence, *Arg. n.* 3—30, 2h. Gonorrhœa suppressed, pains flying from joint to joint, *Puls.* 3, 1h. Much pain at the conclusion of passing water, *Sarsa.* 6, 2h. The same medicines as advised for acute and subacute rheumatism may be given in gonorrhœal, according to indications. [A course of *Thuja* 30, 8h., for a few days may be given as an intercurrent remedy when the case does not respond readily. In psoric patients, *Sul.* 30, 8h., given in the same way will assist in clearing up a case.]

SYPHILITIC.—Periosteal rheumatism, syphilitic or mercurial, *Kali iod.* gr. ii.—30, 6h. Depression, pain in cranial bones, *Stilling.* 1, 6h. Periosteal rheumatism, when the patient is sensitive to cold, and has not been treated with mercurials, *Merc. sol.* 6, 6h. Pains < from sunset to sunrise, *Luet.* 200 once a day. With great despondency, pains < from sunset to sunrise; after mercury, *Aur.* 3, gr. iv.—30, 4h. Swelling on the bones—(1) *Kali bichr.* 3x, gr. ii. 6h.; (2) *Phytolacca* 3, 2h. *See also* Bones: PERIOSTITIS.

MUSCULAR AND LOCAL.—Stiff-neck from cold; rheumatic ophthalmia, *Aco.* 3, 2h. Acute muscular pains, *Macrotin* 3x, gr. ii. 2h. [Turkish or Russian baths.] Stiffness, rheumatic pains, jerking, spasms, *Ant. t.* 6, 2h. Bruised pain in back; weakness and weariness of all the limbs; tremors; pains worse on motion, come on worse just when falling asleep and wake the patient, *Merc. sol.* 6, 4h. *See also* **Ankle, Back, Diaphragm, Jaw, Joints, Knees, Lumbago, Myalgia, Stiff-neck,** etc.

CHRONIC.—[In all cases of acute rheumatism, when the symptoms of active inflammation have subsided, great attention must be paid to the joints. They must not be allowed to become stiff. Movement must be insisted on; and if the patient is unable to move the joint himself, passive movements must be given. The joint must be kept warm; and some stimulating oleaginous liniment, such as one of equal parts of *Tinct. of Capsicum* φ and *Glycerine*, should be rubbed in for fifteen minutes three times a day. Medicines according to their indications may be given as recommended above under **Rheumatism:** ACUTE and SUBACUTE. The patient's constitution must be carefully studied, and where any definite taint exists nosodes like *Carcin.* and *Bacil.* should be prescribed. Also the following medicines may be given as indicated.] In patients subject to skin eruptions; acidity; sinking at the pit of the stomach worse in the forenoon, pains worst at night, *Sul.* 6, 8h. Persons who suffer from acidity, cold clammy feet and hands, heat of head and perspiration, pains < by motion, *Calc. c.* 6, 8h.; the joints to be rubbed every night with *Pine Oil* and wrapped in Pine Wool. Silk or woollen undergarments, or else garments made of Pine Wool, are a necessity. For stiffened or almost immovable joints, with thickening of surrounding tissues, *Iod.* 3x, gtt. v. 6h. Tearing, darting pains, "doughy" swelling of joints, stiffness and extreme soreness; pains < at night, *Kali iod.* gr. 1—30, 4h. In "bilious" persons of dark hair and complexion; the pain shooting and tearing, < by motion; from exposure to dry cold, *Bry.* 3, 2h. From exposure to dry cold; < in stormy weather; muscular and fibrous tissues affected, *Rhod.* 3, 2h. Pain, stiffness, paralytic or numb sensation; no synovial effusion; restlessness, pain worst during rest; coldness; from getting wet, *Rhus t.* 3, 2h. [With the application of the *Capsicum* and *Glycerine* liniment, and dry heat, as from a bag of hot salt.] From exposure to cold, damp weather, *Dulc.* 3, 2h. Joints and neighbouring bones painful; cold, non-inflammatory affections; especially wrists and ankles, *Ruta* 3, 2h. Great coldness and depression of animal heat, in gouty subjects, *Ledum.* 3, 2h. Chronic rheumatism, tearing pains about the joints, *Kali bichr.* 3x, gr. ii. 6h. Synovial affections; the pain < towards evening and at night, at rest, and in a warm room; better by motion and in the open air, *Puls.* 3, 3h. When the right knee is most affected, *Benz. ac.* 3x, 3h. Chronic joint affections, especially of the knees, connected with urinary difficulties, *Berb.* 3, 3h. When the small joints of the hands and feet are affected, *Caulo.* 3, 2h. Small joints of hands, symptoms going from right to left, *Lyc.* 6—30, 4h. Tearing pains, in warm weather superficial, in cold weather deeper, worse at night, *Colch.* 3, 3h. Pains and swelling of joints, which are reddened; feel hot to the touch; < by motion and heat of the bed; < at night; false anchylosis; suppuration; patients very sensitive to cold, *Merc. viv.* 6, 4h. (The best mineral water treatment for chronic rheumatism is to be had at Aix-les-Bains, abroad, and at Bath, Buxton, Harrogate,

Strethpeffer and Woodhall Spa, in this country.) *See also* **Lumbago, Myalgia, Stiff-neck,** etc.

Rickets.—In fat children of soft fibre, *Calc. phos.* 3, gr. v. 8h. In thin, puny children, *Ars.* 3, 4h. Rickety children, thin, puny, perspiring head and feet, *Silic.* 6, 4h. Where there is tubercular family history, (1) *Bacil.* 30—200, gl. iv. once a week (a course of this will benefit most cases); (2) *Phos.* 3—30, 4h. In vaccinal cases, *Thuj.* 6—30, night and morning. Scurvy-Rickets, *see* **Scurvy.**

Rigors. *See* **Shiverings.**

Ringworm.—*Of the Scalp and Hairy Parts.*—Cut the hair short over a small space surrounding the part affected, wash well with soap, rinse the soap off thoroughly afterwards, dab on a little spirit to still further cleanse away all grease, then rub on a little cod-liver oil. This may be done every fourth night. Internally *Bacil.* 30—200 gl. iv. once a week. If there is disorder of stomach and acidity, retching, loss of appetite, restlessness at night, cold feet, hot head, *Sul.* 6, 4h. After *Sul.*, *Sep.* 6, 4h.; locally (after washing the head with soap and water and cutting short the hair) a paste of *Sepia* 1x, moistened with water, to be applied every night. In plethoric persons, pale, lymphatic, cold, moist hands and feet, *Calc. c.* 30, night and morning. If the local measures advised above prove insufficient, paint night and morning with tinct. *Chrys. ac.* 2. *Chrysophan. ac.* has a specific relation to ringworm, and I have frequently seen cases cleared up in a few days by the application of the ointment (gr. iv. to ʒi. of vaseline or Cetacean ointment). The intense staining properties of the ointment are a drawback. The No. 2 tincture, which is also very effective, has

the advantage of not staining the clothes. If there is general
debility, *Ars.* 3, 8h.

Of the Body.—Tellur. 6, 4h. If it does not speedily yield
to this, local measures may be adopted as recommended for
ringworm of the scalp.

Roseola (*Rose Rash*).—*Bell.* 3, 2h. If the fever is sharp, *Aco.* 3,
1h.

EPIDEMIC (*Rötheln, Rubella, German Measles*).—*Aco.* 3, 1h.,
followed if necessary by *Bell.* 3, 1h. The complications and
sequelæ are the same as those of measles and scarlatina, and
must be treated in the same way, according to indications.
See **Measles, Scarlatina.**

Rötheln. *See* **Roseola,** EPIDEMIC.

Rubella, *See* **Roseola,** EPIDEMIC.

Rumbling. *See* **Borborygmi.**

Rupia.—(1) *Kali iod.* gr. v.—30, 6h. (2) *Luet.* 200 gl., v. two or
three times a week. (3) *Æthiops ant.* 5. gtt. v. 8h. (Avoid
removing the crusts.)

Rupture. *See* **Hernia.**

Sacrum.—Violent pain in, aching, bruised, dragging, or pressing; < by lying, sitting, or stooping; with rectal troubles,
Berb. 3, 6h. Aching < by walking or standing, with constipation and blind piles; sacro-iliac articulation, *Æsc. h.* 3, 4h.
Drawing and heaviness, < in evening, with bleeding piles
and diarrhœa, *Aloe* 3, 4h. Pressing or bruised pain, stabs on
motion, < by coughing, laughing, stooping, or rising from
a seat; shooting upward or through the great ischiatic
foramen and down the thighs, *Tellur.* 6, 4h. Stitches, aching,

bruised sensation, pressure and weight, *Agar.* 3, 2h. Dragging pain; with uterine disorders, or loaded urine, *Sep.* 6, 4h.

Saint Vitus' Dance. *See* **Chorea.**

Salivation.—Simple, with sore gums and mouth; during pregnancy, *Merc. s.* 6, 4h. In mercurial salivation; in pregnancy (after *Merc. s.*), *Iod.* 3x, 2h. Failing *Iodine* in mercurial cases, *Nit. ac.* 6, 4h. Accompanying nervous headache, *Iris v.* 3, 2h. Copious flow of saliva after eating, *All. sat.* 3, 4h. From nervous causes; in pregnancy, *Jabor.* 3x, 2h.

Sarcinæ: VOMITING OF. *See* **Vomiting.**

Sarcocele (*Solid enlargement of Testes*). *See* **Testes.**

Satyriasis. *See* **Erotomania.**

Scabies. *See* **Itch.**

Scalds. *See* **Burns.**

Scalp.—Violent itching, moist, *Oleand.* 3, 4h. *See also* **Dandruff** and **Pityriasis.**

Scalled-head. *See* **Eczema:** CAPITIS.

Scapula.—Pain in right, *Juglans c.* 3, 4h. Pain under point of right, *Chel.* 1—30, 4h. Pain in left, *Cact.* 3, 4h.

Scarlatina, or Scarlet Fever:—

PROPHYLACTIC.—When there is scarlatina in a family, put 20 drops of *Bell.* 3 into a tumbler of water, and let each member of the household take a spoonful night and morning.

SCARLATINA SIMPLEX (*Simple Scarlet Fever*).—Sore throat, restlessness, dry skin, fever, *Aco.* 3, 1h. When the rash is pronounced, delirium, sore, red throat, *Bell.* 3, 1h. When the fever is gone, *Ars.* 3, 4h. (*Scarlatinin* 30, 8h., may be given in any stage of the disease, either alone or inter-currently with other indicated remedies.)

SCARLATINA ANGINOSA (*Scarlet Fever with Throat Complications*).—Fauces much swollen, stinging pain, *Apis* 3x, 1h. Ulceration of the throat and swelling of the external glands of the neck, *Crotalus* 3, 1h. Septic cases, with symptoms of strangulation; enlarged or suppurating glands, *Echin.* φ, gtt. i—v, 1—2h. Ulceration of the throat, with acrid discharge from the nose and soreness of the nostrils, *Arum tri,* 12, 1—2h. (This medicine, if given in low attenuation, must be freshly prepared, or have been specially preserved.) Throat diphtheritic, *see* **Diphtheria**. *See also below:* SCARLATINA MALIGNA.

SCARLATINA MALIGNA (*Malignant Scarlet Fever*).—Profound depression, rash delayed, fever high. Wet pack; giving at the same time—if there is great mental depression, *Cuprum acet.* 3x, ¼h. If the disease sets in with livid, rapidly swelling throat, patchy, dark-coloured eruption, quick, feeble pulse, and oppressed brain, *Ailanthus* 1x, ¼h. When the shock of the invasion of the disease is safely past, should throat symptoms become the most prominent feature, the treatment will be as above for SCARLATINA ANGINOSA.

SCARLATINA RHEUMATICA.—When the patient is restless, constantly moving about, *Rhus t.* 3, 2h. Effusion into joints and serous cavities, pains worse by every movement, *Bry.* 3, 1h. Heart complications, sharp pains, palpitations, *Spigel.* 3, 1h. *See* **Rheumatism**, ACUTE.

HYPERPYREXIA. *See* **Hyperpyrexia**.

Sequelæ.—*Strangury.*—*Canth.* 3x, 1h.

Albuminuria and Dropsy.—*Arsen.* 3, 2h. Bleeding from the kidneys, *Terebinth.* 3, 2h. Pack. *See* **Kidney**: Inflammation.

Glandular Enlargement in Neck.—*Lachesis* 6, 3h. If suppuration is inevitable, *Hep. sul.* 6, 3h.

Deafness and Discharge from the Ear.—*Mur. ac.* 1, gtt. ii. 3h. *See* **Ears**: Deafness.

Rheumatic Affections and Heart Disease. See **Rheumatism, Heart.**

Scars. *See* Cicatrix.

Sciatica.—In young people, and from cold draughts; anxiety, pain unendurable. *Acon.* 3, 4h. Pain < sitting, relieved somewhat by walking, entirely by lying down; sensation as if hamstring muscles were too short. *Am. mur.* 3x, 2h. Recent from cold and damp, sensitiveness of the part (right side especially), *Coloc.* med. Intense pain in the nerve, accompanied by cramps or alternating with numbness, *Gnaphal.* 3, 2h. Pain < in bed at night, or when at rest, *Rhus t.* 3, 2h. Right-sided, pain < in afternoon, < by lying on affected side or least touch, *Lyc.* 6—30, 4h. Tearing pains in r. leg, from point of exit of sciatic nerve, only felt when moving or sitting up, *Diosc.* 1—3, 2h. In the old and debilitated; purely neuralgic; paralysis, *Ars.* 3, 2h. After influenza; frequently left-sided, symptoms of both *Sulphur* and *Arsenicum* present, *Ars. sul. rub.,* 6—30, 2—4h. Drawing and lameness as if l. hip wrenched, *Iris v.* 1—3, 2h. Sycotic cases, *Glon.* 30, night and morning. Intractable cases, either side, chronic or acute, *Carb. sul.* 3, 2—4h. Exquisite sensitiveness, especially in lower extremities, general painfulness of the part, especially along the tract of

the great nerve, drawing, tearing, paralytic pain, *Tereb.* 3,
2h. Shooting, tearing, from hip to knee and foot, especially
when coughing, *Caps.* 3, 4h. Similar pain, especially if
aggravated, about 3 a.m., *Kali c.* 6, 8h. Lightning-like
pains, right side, > by warmth, *Mag. ph.* 3x, gr. v.—30, 2h.
Pains < at rest, and particularly when beginning to walk;
burning pains < at night, preventing sleep, anterior crural
neuralgia, *Gels.* 3x—30, 2h. Pain in region of hips, *Apocy.
can.* 3, 4h. Pain as if beaten, excited by touch, limbs give
way, *Ruta* 1, 2h. Pain only when stooping or rising from a
seat, *Nat. sul.* 6, 2h.

Scirrhus. *See* Cancer.

Scleroderma. *See* Morphœa.

Sclerotitis. *See under* Eyes.

Screaming of Children.—Night screaming, *Kali brom.* 1x, 8h.
Weeps all night; sopor interrupted by screaming; incessant
screaming; *Phos.* 3, 2h. During sleep cries and starts,
anxiety continues after waking, *Calc. c.* 30, 8h. In puny children, in boys with ill-developed testes, *Aur. bro.* 3, gr. v.—30,
8h. Piteous crying; continual crying and whining, gets only
short sleeps, *Ant. t.* 6, 2h. Wakes screaming from anxious
dreams and cries out, *Bry.* 3, 2h. Piteous moaning and
crying, *Cham.* 6, 2h. Weeping, moaning, howling, *Cicuta v.*
3, 2h. Before urine passes, *Borax* 3x, 2h.

Scrivener's Palsy. *See* Paralysis, LOCAL.

Scrofulous Affections. *See* Glands, Hip-joint Disease. Eyes
(OPHTHALMIA), etc.

Scrotum, DROPSY OF. *See* Hydrocele.

Scurf. *See* **Dandruff** and **Pityriasis.**

Scurvy.—[The diet must be corrected or no medicine will be of use; milk, fresh meat and vegetables, and lime-juice must be given. When it follows excessive feeding with sugar in infants, sugar must be discontinued. The expressed juice of raw beef is of great use in the scurvy-rickets of children.] Internally, *Merc. sol.* 2x, gr. v. 4h. Locally on open sores, compresses of a weak *Hamamelis* lotion (ten drops to the pint); as a wash for the mouth, a solution of *Kali chlor.* (two to ten grains to the half-pint). Scurvy-rickets, (1) *Bry.* 3—30, 2h.; (2) *Phos.* 3—30, 2h.; (3) *Rhus t.* 3—30, 2h.

Sea-sickness.—In general, give for two days before going on board, *Petr.* 3, 8h., and 1—2h. when the ship starts. When there is vertigo and empty feeling in head with nausea and vomiting, give for a few days before the voyage *Cocc. i.* 3. 6h., and every hour or two during the voyage. Vertigo remaining after the voyage; Constipation at sea, *Cocc. i.* 3, 2h. When there is tendency to bring up blood with straining; bruised and sore feeling, *Arn.* 3x—30, 6h. before, and 1h. during the voyage. (I have found this very generally effective.) In sea-fright, *Aco.* 1, 1—2h. With profound prostration and cold sweat, *Tab.* 30, 6h. and 1h. When the downward motion is most felt, *Borax* 30, 1h. If sickness comes on during the voyage, *Apom.* 3x, 2h.

Seborrhœa.—Smutty brown, mottled skin; yellow colour of face, *Ars.* 3, 8h. Greenish, dirty-looking, oily skin, *Bufo* 6, 8h. Back of head and behind ears most affected, *Graph.* 6, 8h. On chin, *Lyc.* 6, 8h. Earthy complexion, seborrhœa of face; severe itching of scalp; hair falls out; constipation, *Nat. m.* 6, 8h. Skin of face shines and feels oily, *Plumb.* 30, 8h. Skin greasy, makes hands greasy to touch it, *Staph.* 30,

3h. Of genitals. *Sep.* 6, 8h. Upper lip and base of nose, *Vinca m.* 1, 8h. Scales adhering firmly, leaving skin red and painful on removal, *Iod.* 3x, 4h. Of scalp, *Sul.* 30, 4h. An ointment of Sulphur ¼ the B.P. strength applied to the scalp twice a week is very effective.

Self-abuse.—[Moral treatment is required for this. In children, where the moral element of the disease is small, kind watchfulness is needed on the part of the nurse; in severe cases mechanical restraint must be adopted.] The following medicines will assist in allaying the irritability:—Lascivious ideas with sexual irritation; unconquerable impulse to abuse, *Origan.* 4, 4h. In females especially, *Grat.* 3—30, 8h. Masturbation; desire for solitude, *Bufo* 6, 4h. With priapism, *Picr. ac.* 3, 4h. In young children. *Durum* 1 m, once a week. (One of Burnett's cancer nosodes.) Excitement of desire with lascivious dreams; debility consequent on the habit. *Cina* 3, 4h. Nymphomania and satyriasis, *Calc. phos.* 3, gr. v. 8h. Where there is coldness, constipation, loss of power, *Nat. mur.* 6, 8h. Sinking at the epigastrium, flushing, pain in occiput, *Sul.* 30, 8h. Cold, clammy hands and feet, *Calc. c.* 30, 4h. Brain exhaustion and irritability with genital weakness, *Staph.* 3, 4h. Loss of confidence, *Anacard,* 3, 4h. Should these not suffice, give in addition one grain of *Kali brom.* at bed-time. For consequent debility, a carefully regulated, unstimulating diet; and *Phos. ac.* 1x, gtt. v. may be given in a tumbler of water for a drink at meals. *See also* **Emissions, Erotomania,** and **Spermatorrhœa.**

Sensitiveness.—Peevish; intolerance of pain. *Cham.* 6, 4h. Nervous, hysterical, *Ign.* 3, 4h. Great intolerance of light and noise, *Bell.* 3, 4h. Over-sensitiveness to all impressions; over-sensitive to the action of medicines, *Nux v.* 30, 4h.

Septicæmia. *See* **Pyæmia.**

Serpent-bites. *See under* **Stings:** OF SNAKES.

Sewer Gas Poisoning.—Foul tongue; diarrhœa, *Bapt.* 3. 1h.
Sore throat. *Phyt.* 3, 1h. *See also* **Pyæmia,** etc.

Shingles. *See* **Herpes Zoster.**

Shiverings (*Rigors*).—[Remedies are to be repeated frequently
until reaction sets in, and then given less often or suspended
altogether.] Immediately after a chill has been taken, *Camph.*
3, ¼h. Continued shivering; rigor beginning in limbs and
going over whole body, *Acon.* 3, ¼h. Shuddering when in
the open air, *Ars.* 3, ¼h. Shivering with blueness of extremities and signs of collapse, *Carb. v.* 6, ¼h. Chill; effects of
wet cold when heated, or cold drinks, *Bellis* 3, 1h. Shivering
in the evening, without thirst, *Phos.* 3, ¼h. Internal chills,
Astacus fluviat. 3, ¼h. [When rigors take place in the course
of illness, or without traceable cause, in all probability there
is suppuration going on, and this should always be definitely
ascertained.] *See also* **Cold, Fever, Intermittent Fever.**

Shock.—Cold sweat on forehead and body, *Ver. a.* 3, ½h. Icy
cold but will not be covered, *Camph.* 3, ½h. From fear or
fright with collapse or fever, *Aco.* 3, ½h. Especially from
sudden joy, *Coff.* 3, ½h.

Sick-headache. *See* **Headache.**

Sickness. *See* **Vomiting** *and* **Sea-sickness.**

Side, PAIN IN.—Pain in left side, in young girls, with digestive
troubles, anæmia or amenorrhœa, *Puls.* 3, 4h. Pain in left
side, in nervous women with uterine affections, *Act. r.* 3,

4h. Pain through base of left lung, *Oxal. ac.* 3, 4h. Pain in left side with enlargement of spleen, *Ceanothus* 1, 4h. Pain in right side, sharp, < by movement, *Bry.* 3, 4h. Sharp cutting pain below right free ribs, *Berb.* 3, 4h. Pain in the same region, > by moving about, *Diosc.* 3, 4h.

Sighing.—Long, sighing respirations, *Op.* 3, 4h. Sighing, desire to take a long breath as if in a close room, during menses, *Nat. phos.* 6, 4h. Involuntary sighing, *Calc. ph.* 30, 4h. Frequent sighing; sighing and sobbing continue long after crying, *Ign.* 30, 4h.

Sight. *See* **Eyes:** SIGHT.

Sinking, SENSATION OF.—Connected with uterine affections, *Act. r.* 3, 4h. After stool, *Ambra* 3, 4h. Weak, empty feeling at pit of stomach, not > by eating; involuntary sighing, *Ignat.* 3, 4h. Constant sinking sensation, *Hydrast,* 3, 4h. Sinking < at 11 a.m., *Sulph.* 6, 8h.

Skin, UNHEALTHY.—Chaps and becomes sore at the least provocation, *Hep. s.* 6, 6h. Slight injuries fester, *Petr.* 3, 8h. When the skin is irritable and there is tendency to itching eruptions, *Sul.* 3, 8h. Sensation of something alive creeping under the skin. *Selen.* 6, 8h. *See also* **Fester.**

Sleep and Dreams.—[Remedies for disorders of sleep should be given at intervals during the day, one dose being given at bed-time; this may be followed by another in an hour's time if necessary.]—Sleep too heavy; sleepiness during the day, *Op.* 3, 4h. Irresistible sleepiness, dreamy condition, closed eyes, pale face, *Nux mosch.* 3, 4h. Sleepiness after dinner, *Lyc.* 6, 4h. Sleepiness during the day, sleeplessness at night, *Cinnabar.* 3, gr. ii. 4h. Sleepy during the day and after eating; sleeplessness at night, sleep dreamful, restless; erotic dreams; confused dreams, *Phos.* 3, 4h. Simple sleeplessness from nervous excitement, *Camph.* φ in pilules, 1, ½h. Sleeplessness and restlessness in nervous persons: with depression, accompanying uterine affections, *Act. r.* 3, 4h. Sleeplessness from thoughts crowding into the mind; agitation, *Coff.* 3, 4h. Nervous, restlessness, sleepless; drowsy at first sleepless after, *Op.* 3, 1h. Sleeplessness, anxious dreams, hot, restless, tossing about; sleeplessness in the aged, *Aco.* 3, 4h. Starts in affright just when falling asleep; anxious and frightful dreams; sleepy but cannot sleep, *Bell.* 3, 4h. Restless, tosses off the clothes, cannot remain in bed, anxious dreams of business; frightful dreams with palpitation, *Rhus t.* 3, 4h. Sleepiness in the evening, wakeful after midnight, heaviness in the morning; sleepiness only in the morning; sleeplessness from abuse of coffee, *Nux v.* 3, 4h. Sleeplessness with nervousness, twitchings, restlessness, *Scutel.* φ, gtt. v. 4h. Wakes 3 a.m. and cannot get to sleep again, *Bellis* 3, 8h. Excessively frequent yawning; light sleep, hearing everything; restless dreamful sleep, *Ign.* 3, 4h. Sleeplessness with restlessness of eyeballs; sleep too dreamful, from the least excitement, *Hyo.* 3, 4h. Sleeplessness from emotional disturbance following the slightest excitement of the brain in the evening, *Gels.* 3, 4h. Sleeplessness with nervous exhaustion and restlessness, *Avena sat.* φ, gtt. v. 4h. Dreams of water, *Verat. v.* 3, 4h. Cannot fall asleep for a long time from the blood mounting to the head; violent starting on falling asleep; sleep restless, tossing, disagreeable dreams, *Sul.* 3, 4h. Anxious dreams of business transacted during the day, *Bry.* 3, 4h. Sleeplessness with bounding pulse, *Ver. v.* 3x, 2h. Sufferings from loss of sleep, *Cocc. ind.* 3, 4h. Whining in sleep, *Verat. a.* 3, 4h.

Weeps on being wakened; weeps in sleep; starting in sleep;
biting tongue; anxious starting out of sleep; moaning in
sleep, *Carb. v.* 3, 4h. *See also* **Nightmare, Screaming of
Children, Somnambulism, Starting, Yawning.**

Sleeping Sickness.—(*Trypanosomiasis*), *Antim. tart.* in the form
of *Atoxyl*, and *Arsenic* injected intravenously have cured
cases in the early stages. These two remedies should be
tried in the homœopathic preparations, low and high.
Antim. tart. corresponds to the lethargy. It may be given
3x—30, 2h. Lethargy, waking up with fear and anxiety,
Opium 1—30, 2h. Depression, weariness of life, wants to
die, *Ars.* 3x—30, 2h. Lethargic somnolency, *Chloral* 3, 2h.
Modern orthodox methods of treatment should be sought
wherever possible.

Sleepy Sickness.—*see* **Encephalitis Lethargica.**

Small-Pox.—In general, *Variol,* 6—200, 4h. (The same may
be given once or twice daily as prophylactic to those who
are brought within the range of the infection. As an alternative *Maland.* 30 may be given in the same way.) Coated
tongue, depression, prostration, back pain, nausea, *Ant. t.*
6, 1h. When maturation has commenced, *Merc. sol.* 6, 3h.;
locally, the patient's body may be sponged with a solution
of *Carbolic acid* (1 to 60). When hæmorrhages occur, *Ham.*
1, ½h. In small-pox which is malignant from the outset,
Crotal. h. 3, ½h.

For complications and sequelæ, *see* **Throat, Eyes, Ears, etc.**

Smell, SENSITIVENESS OF.—Great sensitiveness, bad smells have
a powerful effect, *Aco.* 3, 4h. Great sensitiveness; faintest
odours, especially of tobacco, unbearable, *Bell.* 3, 4h. Smell

abnormally acute; cannot tolerate flowers, *Graph.* 6, 4h. All
odours too strong; disgusting, *Carbol. ac.* 3, 4h. Everything
smells too strong, *Aur. met.* 3, gr. v. 8h.

ILLUSIONS OF.—Offensive smell as of old catarrh, *Puls.* 3, 4h.
Of old offensive mucus; of burnt bone: of soap suds; of
boiled peas, *Sul.* 3, 4h. Putrid smell, *Kali bichr.* 3x, gr. ii.
4h. Putrid smell in nose when blowing it, *Aur. met.* 3, gr.
ii. 8h. Of rotten eggs, *Bell.* 3, 4h. Very offensive smell,
Calc. c. 6, 4h. Bad smell like bilious fæces; an offensive
smell remains a long time, *Diosc.* 3, 4h. Of roasted onions,
Sang. 3, 4h. Constant smell before the nose of pigeon's dung,
or of burning tinder, *Anac.* 30, 8h.

LOSS OF.—During catarrh, with loss of taste, *Sang.* 3, 4h.
Loss of taste and smell after catarrh or influenza, *Mag. m.*
6, 4h. Loss of smell with cough, and stoppage of the nose,
Am. mur. 3x, 4h.

Smoking. *See* **Tobacco Habit.**

Snake-bites. *See* **Stings.**

Sneezing. *See* **Cold.**

Softening of the Brain. *See* **Brain.**

Somnambulism.—After a fright, in plethoric subjects, anxiety,
Acon. 3—30, 4h. With night terrors; drowsiness and
imbecility, *Kali brom.* 1x, gtt. v. 8h. From fright, or over-
exertion, *Artemisia vulg.* 3x, 8h. Drowsy condition, after a
fright, *Op.* 30, 4h. From sexual excitement, *Con.* 30, 4h.
Dreams of quarrels, murders, fire, thieves, *Nat. m.* 30, 8h.

Soreness of Infants. *See* **Excoriations.**

Spasms. *See* **Flatulence, Colic, Cramps.**

Speech.—Hesitating, *Kali brom*, 3x, 4h. Omits words, *Cham.* 6, 4h. Omits words and syllables, *Nux v.* 3, 4h. Uses wrong words and wrong syllables, *Lyc.* 6, 4h. *See also* **Stammering.**

Spermatorrhœa.—(Weakness of sexual organs resulting in passive losses of seminal fluid with urine, or whilst at stool or on the slighest irritation; often the result of self-abuse; different from **Emissions,** *which see.*) Passive losses during sleep, vertigo on rising in the morning, *Selenium* 30, 8h. When there is constipation, *Nux v.* 3. 6h. With much nervous irritability, *Potass. bromid.* gr. ss. 6h. Irritability and brain exhaustion; from irritation of mucous membrance of prostatic portion of the urethra, *Staphisagria*, 3, 4h. When this is the result of gonorrhœa, *Canth.* 3, 4h. Weakness after, *China* 3, 4h. Great weakness and palpitation of the heart, *Dign.* 3x, gr. i, in the morning on rising. Flaccidity of the parts, great weakness of the back and spine, *Con.* 3, gtt. ii. half an hour before meals. Chilliness, constipation, *Nat. m.* 6, 8h. Loss of prostatic fluid at stool when the stool is large and difficult, *Sil.* 6—30, 4h. Great weakness, *Calc. phos.* 3, gr. v. 8h. [In nearly all cases a beverage of *Phos. ac.* 1x, five drops to a tumbler of water, may be taken with the meals.] Kindly and judicious moral treatment is of paramount importance in these cases. Also the most careful attention to diet and regimen should be enjoined. No stimulating food or drink of any kind should be allowed. Three meals a day at intervals of not less than five hours, and nothing between the meals; avoidance of rich food, sweets, pastry, and starchy food should be enjoined. Patients should be counselled never to eat to repletion; to take exercise moderately, but not to over-exert themselves. A morning cold or tepid bath and brisk rub-down with a rough towel is of great advantage. Too long lying in bed must be strictly forbidden; eight hours at the outside is all that should be allowed. Hard beds are a necessity. Dyspepsia in connection with spermatorrhœa must be treated according to symptoms. *See* Dyspepsia, Emissions, Self-Abuse.

Spina Bifida.—(1) *Bacil.* 30—200, gtt. iv. once a week; (2) *Bry.* 3, 4h.; (3) *Calc. phos.* 3, gr. v. 4h. [Surgical measures must be adopted if the tumour increases. In all cases the tumour must be supported and protected from external irritation.]

Spinal Irritation.—[The treatment of this disease must be largely moral and physical, but the possibility of injury must be borne in mind. In that case a skilled osteologist must be consulted. The patient must be encouraged to ignore her sufferings as much as possible, to take open-air exercise whilst avoiding fatigue, and on no account to let her pains get the mastery of her. Generous diet must also be insisted on. These cases are often also Neurasthenic, and it will be well to compare the heading Neurasthenia. The following medicines will greatly assist the treatment.] In patients with tubercular history, *Bacil.* 30—200, gl. iv. once a week. In general; brow headache, numbness of limbs, pains in the stomach, flatulence, constipation, *Arg. n.* 6, 4h. In persons who have been much vaccinated and in those who have over-indulged in tea, *Thuj.* 6, 4h. In weakly women of low and feeble habit of body, with weak pulse, tenderness over cervical and dorsal spines, with headache, constriction across the chest, and flatulent eructations, *Agar.* 3, 4h. Burning along spine, with weakness of legs; pain shooting from spine into head, *Pic. ac.* 30, 4h. When there is a tendency to skin eruptions, sinking sensation worst about 11 a.m. *Sul.* 3, 8h. In chilly subjects, great sensitiveness to cold, headaches in back of head, coming forward, compelling patient to wrap up head, *Sil.* 30, 4h. In nervous, impressionable subjects, easily worried, *Ignat.* 3, 4h. Aching in the back; restlessness and sleeplessness, accompanied with uterine irritation; profound depression and gloom, *Act. r.* 3, 4h. Sensitiveness from last cervical to fifth dorsal vertebra, dread of having the part touched or approached, worse by fatigue, only partially relieved by repose, *Tellur.* 6, 4h. Burning and aching about the upper part of the spine, with difficulty of swallowing and constriction of the larynx, *Guaco* 3, 4h. With cramps and disorders of sensation, *Secale* 3, 4h.

Spine, CONCUSSION OF. *See* **Bruises.**

CURVATURE OF.—*Lateral Curvature.*—[The same general treatment as advised for Rickets. In addition, prolonged rest in horizontal position, so that the body-weight is kept off the spine as much as possible. Graduated exercises on the Swedish principle for developing the spine muscles.] In thin subjects, *Silic.* 30, 8h. In thin, narrow-chested, dark-eyed patients, *Phos.* 30, 8h. In pale, chilly, fat subjects, *Calc. c.* 30, 8h. *Pott's curvature, Calc. ph.* 3x, gr. v. 8h. and *Bacill.* 30—200, gl. v. once a week. Abscess formed, hectic fever, *Pyro.* 6—30, 8h. Abscess discharging, *Calc. sul.* 3, gr. v. 8h.

INFLAMMATION OF. *See* **Myelitis.**

INFLAMMATION OF MEMBRANES OF. *See* **Meningitis,** SPINAL.

IRRITATION OF. *See* **Spinal Irritation.**

PAIN IN EXTREMITY OF. *See* **Coccygodynia.**

Spitting of Blood. *See* **Hæmoptysis.**

Spleen.—Pain in, and enlargement of, *Ceanothus* 1, 4h. Pricking in spleen region, stitch in side, *Agaric.* 3, 4h. After abuse of quinine, *Nat. mur.* 6, 4h. Spleen pain in gouty subjects; "stored gout"; after intermittent fevers, *Urt. ur.* φ, gtt. v.—x. 8h. Spleen affections accompanied with giddiness, *Quercus* 3x, 4h. Cough with pain in spleen, *Scill. acet.* φ, gtt v. 4h.

Sprain.—In severe sprains, let the injured part be placed in water as hot as can well be borne, in which *Arnica* φ (a tea-spoonful to the pint) has been mixed; let this be repeated every three or four hours, and the part supported in the intervals by a light bandage (care being taken that it is not at all tight), and kept warm; internally, *Arn.* 3, every ten minutes for the first three hours, and then every hour and at increasing intervals. When the pain has ceased and the swelling subsided, external applications, except the light bandage, may be discarded, and the medicine alone given every four hours. Rest is necessary at first; but the joint must not be allowed to become stiff, and after all signs of inflammation have subsided movement must be encouraged. If after forty-eight hours there is not very decided improvement, *Bellis perennis* must be substituted for *Arnica*—*Bellis* φ for the hot bath, and *Bellis* 3 for internal administration. Rheumatic pain and stiffness remaining after a sprain, especially if the pain is < at night, and by rest, *Rhus t.* 3, 4h. Bruised pain in the bones, *Ruta* 3, 4h. In old sprains after above measures have been employed, and there is remaining weakness and or pain, a few doses of *Calc. carb.* 30, i.e. a dose three times daily for three or four days will often clear up remaining symptoms.

Sprue. *See* **Psilosis.**

Squint. *See* **Eyes:** SQUINT.

Stammering.—[This must be overcome by practice, under skilled teachers if possible, and determination on the part of patients. The cure may be assisted by the following medicines; they must be used perseveringly.] (1) *Stram.* 3, 6h.; (2) *Hyos.* 3, 6h. When it is a manifestation of chorea, the treatment recommended for that disease is available. *See* **Chorea.**

Starting.—At noise, *Carb.* v. 6, 4h. At noise, when lying awake, *Op.* 3, 4h. From sudden noise, *Borax* 30, 8h. Starts and twitches on falling asleep, *Agar* 3, 4h. Violent starting on falling asleep, *Sul.* 3, 4h. Starting out of sleep with anxiety, short breath, suffocating, trembling, *Samb.* 3, 4h. Starting in fright, *Stram.* 3, 4h.

Sterility.—IN THE FEMALE.—When due to some affection of the uterus or its appendages, this must be remedied. When not traceable to any organic defect:—With depression, tendency to suicide; menses scanty, late, or absent, *Aur.* 3, gr. iv.—30, 8h. When from excessive and premature menses, *Calc. c.* 30, 8h. From excessive sexual desire, *Phos.* 30, 8h. With depression, weeping mood, averse to consolation, earthy complexion, *Nat. m.* 6—30, 8h. With acrid leucorrhœa, *Bor.* 6, 8h. With scanty, insufficient menses, breasts painful, *Con.* 3, 8h. With dwindling of breasts and ovaries, *Iod.* 3x, 8h.

IN THE MALE. *See* **Impotency.**

Sternum. *See* **Chest.**

Stiff-neck.—From a draught or chill; tearing in the nape, painful stiff-neck, worse on moving the neck; pain extending down the neck into the shoulder, *Aco.* 3, 1h. Head and neck retracted; rheumatic pain and stiffness in muscles of neck and back, sensitiveness of the spine, *Act. r.* 3, 1h. Stiff-neck; neck stretched out, head bent back, *Ant. t.* 6, 2h. Stiff-neck, spraining on moving it, head twisted to one side, *Lachnan.* φ—30, 2h. Painful stiff-neck, < by touch or motion, *Bry.* 3, 1h. Paralysis; pains and stiffness, *Colch.* 3, 1h. From damp and cold; pain in the nape as if after lying with the head in an uncomfortable position, *Dulc.* 3, 1h. From dry cold, the pain < on the approach of stormy weather, *Rhod.* 3, 1h. Pain and stiffness in the right side, *Chel.* 1, 1h. [Locally the part may be ironed with a hot flatiron, a piece of flannel being placed over the part affected.]

Stings.—OF INSECTS.—Locally apply powder blue, or, if not at hand, *Ammonia* (*Sal Volatile* and smelling salts are convenient forms). Internally, *Ledum* 6, every ten minutes. (*Led.* φ may be painted on the part. It is sometimes more efficacious than *Ammonia.*) Bee stings, *Urt. ur.* φ, 2h. Symptoms of collapse in bee or wasp stings, *Apis* 30—200, every five minutes. In bee and wasp stings the application of freshly-sliced onion is very efficacious when *Ammonia* is not at hand. Should *Ledum* not prove successful, *Grindelia* 3, every ten minutes. Tarentula bite, *Lach.* 6, every ten minutes.

OF SNAKES.—Tie a handkerchief tightly above the part bitten. If possible, cause the patient to perspire, either by means of vapour or Turkish baths, or by wrapping in blankets and applying hot bricks or hot bottles. Administer stimulants freely, ammonia and whisky being the best, with hot water, as much as the patient can be made to swallow.

Medicinal Treatment.—For fainting and collapse; (1) *Hydrocy. ac.* 1, 10m.; (2) *Moschus* 3, 10m. For the swelling, ecchymosis, and pain of the bitten part, when reaction has set in, *Arn.* 3, 2h.; lotion of *Arn.* 3x, two teaspoonfuls to a pint of water, to be kept applied to the part.

Stomach: ACIDITY. *See* Acidity, Dyspepsia.

CANCER OF.—Burning at stomach; thirst for little and often; anguish, restlessness, wasting, *Ars.* 3, 4h. Balls of flatulence rolling about in upper abdomen, *Ornith. u. φ*, single doses at intervals of one, two, or three weeks. Constant sinking sensation; eructations of sour fluid; vomits all she eats except milk and water mixed; constipation, *Hydrast.* 3, 4h. Burning in stomach; cracks in corners of mouth, *Cundurango* 3, 6h. [These medicines may be given singly and persistently according to the general symptoms. Should the medicine that is being given appear to be losing its effect, one of the others should be substituted.] For the vomiting, *Kreas.* 3, 4h. Constant feeling as if the stomach were full of water, *Kali c.* 6, 4h. *See also* Cancer.

CATARRH.—Coldness, flatulence, cutting pains about the chest, vomiting of mucus, tongue clean or coated, *Carb. v.* 6, 3h. Vomiting, pain in pit of stomach spreading into the chest, flatulence, *Carbol. ac.* 3, 2h. Intense pain at the stomach, sharp or burning, vomiting of slimy matter; great prostration; coldness, *Oxal. ac.* 3x, 4h. Tongue milky white; eructations of wind and fluid tasting of food taken, *Ant. crud.* 6, 8h. Sodden-looking face, yellow slimy tongue, "goneness" after meals, alternate diarrhœa and constipation, *Hydrast.* 3, 3h. *See also* Duodenum and Dyspepsia.

Pain in. *See* **Gastrodynia.**

Ulcer of. *See* **Gastric Ulcer.**

Stomatitis. *See* **Mouth,** Inflammation of.

Stone. *See* **Calculus.**

Strabismus. *See* **Squint.**

Strain. *See* **Sprain.**

Straining at Stool. *See* **Tenesmus.**

Strangury.—Acute; also when due to Cantharides poisoning, *Camph.* 1x, gtt. 1, every five minutes. In less urgent cases, with burning and inflammatory symptoms, *Canth.* 3, ½h. With lumbago-like pain, *Tereb.* 3, ½h. In women especially, *Copaiba* 3, ½h. In purely nervous cases, *Bell.* 3, ½h.

Stricture. *See* **Urethra.**

Strophulus. *See* **Red-Gum.**

Struma. *See* **Scrofula.**

Stye.—At the beginning, *Puls.* 3, 2h. After *Puls.*, *Staph.* 3, 2h. Chronic cases, and for tendency, *Hep. s.* 6, 4h.

Sunburn. *See* **Ephelis.**

Sunstroke.—Dull, Stupid; pressure outwards, < sitting up; with anxiety and fear of death, *Acon.* 1—30, 15m.—1h. Giddy, as if intoxicated on trying to move; band-like pain; pain in occiput, *Gels.* 3—30, 15m.—1h. Violent throbbing, bursting pains; unconscious, limbs relaxed; tremors, jerks, involuntary evacuations, *Glon.* 3 every five minutes at first, the intervals being gradually increased. For the after-effects it may be given every four hours. Congestion to head and fever; vomiting, *Cactus* 3, in the same way. Late effects, *Nat. m.* 30, 8h. *Nat. c.* is most useful in the chronic effects of sun-stroke and in headaches or migraine attacks which return in hot weather. Debility and headache from the sun. Give one dose three times daily for two days of the 30 or 200 potency and await results.

Suppuration.—Impending; inguinal glands, *Merc. viv.* 6, 4h. Impending or inevitable; axillary glands, *Hep. s.* 6, 2h. In cases which do not readily yield, *Gunp.* 3x, gr. iv., 4h. Chronic, cold abscess, fistular abscess, *Silic.* 6, 6h. With erysipelas, *Ars.* 3, 1h. With hectic and signs of blood-poisoning, *Arn.* 3, 1h.; locally, *Arn.* 3x, ℥ii. distilled water, half a pint, as a lotion. As a local application in all cases of free suppuration, without blood infection, *Calend.* φ, ℥ii. to the half-pint of boiled or distilled water. *See also* **Abscess, Bubo, Glands, Pyæmia.**

Swallowing, DIFFICULT. *See under* **Throat**: SORE.

Sweat. *See* **Perspiration, Hands, Feet.**

Sweating Fever. *See* **Miliaria.**

Swellings. *See* **Abscess, Glands, Gumboil, Dropsy.**

Swimming in the Head. *See* **Fainting.**

Sycosis. *See under* **Beard.**

Sycosis (*Hahnemanni*). *See* **Condylomata.**

Syncope. *See* **Fainting.**

Synovitis. *See under* **Joints.**

Syphilis.—PRIMARY.—Modern methods of treatment with *Penicillin* etc. should always be obtained whenever available. No

authenticated instances of syphilis being resistant to penicillin have been reported, though some cases require higher
dosage than others. [In all syphilitic cases alcohol in every
form should be forbidden. Smoking also should be pro-
hibited. In inveterate cases a purely vegetable diet will often
be of service.] Throughout all stages of syphilis occasional
doses (once in three, four, eight, or ten days) of *Luet*. 30—
200 will be serviceable, especially if there is night aggravation. If the patient has already had full mercurial treatment
without good effect, and especially if warty growths appear
about the original sore, *Nit. ac.* 6—30, 4h.; locally, lotion
of *Nit. ac.* 1 (ʒii.—ʒviii.) When the original sore takes long
to heal; hard, long-lasting œdema of prepuce, *Guaiac*, 3x,
gtt. v. 8h. *See also* **Chancre, Condylomata.**

SECONDARY—*See Primary.*—Modern methods of treatment.
Sore throat and mouth, *Merc. cor.* 3, gtt. iii. 6h.; locally,
Phytol. φ, (ʒi.—ʒviii.), for wash, thrice daily. For the eruption, it is often useful to administer mercurial vapour baths.
[A cradle being placed over the patient in bed, the bedclothes are accurately fitted round the patient's neck, a few
grains of calomel are placed in a vaporizer over a spirit-
lamp, and the fumes conducted by a funnel under the
cradle. A bath may be given every third day, three will
usually be sufficient—sometimes a single one.]. Where the
bath is not available, *Merc. i. fl.* 5, 6h. When the sore throat
and rash are out together, the *Phytol.* lotion recommended
for the former may be used whilst *Merc. i. fl.* is being given
internally, or the bath employed. When mercury has been
already fully given, *Kali iod.* gr. iii.—30, 6h. [This should be
continued for two or three months, when the mercurials
may again be resumed if indicated.] If the symptoms are

condylomatous, instead of the *Kali iod.* the treatment recommended for **Condylomata** should take the place of mercurials. Pains in the bones and nodes, ulceration of mouth and throat, *Stilling, syl.* 1x, 4h. [Medicines for special developments of the disease may be given as indicated intercurrently with the remedy which is being given for the general syphilitic poisoning.] Where there is debility, *Berb. aq. φ,* gtt. v. 8h. Nightly bone pains, *Mez.* 3, 2h. Nodes on the bones of the cranium, *Kali bich.* 3x, gr. iii. 8h. Nodes on the face, *Phyt.* 1x, gtt. ii. 4h.

LATER SECONDARIES.—Vegetations and mucous patches, *Cinnabar.* 3x, gr. v.—30, 6h. locally, *Thuja φ* as a paint. Syphilitic psoriasis, foul and indolent ulcerations, *Graph.* 6, 6h.; locally (for the ulcerations), lotion of *Nit. ac.* 1, ʒii.—ʒviii. Psoriasis and ulceration of the tongue, *Kali bich.* 3x, gr. iii. 6h.; locally to be painted with a solution of *Kali bich.,* one grain to three ounces. Ulcerations in the rectum; constipation *Nit. ac.* 6, 6h. *See also* **Condylomata.**

TERTIARY.—Syphilitic tumours of internal organs, *Kali iodat.* gr. v.—30, 8h. Ulceration of bone, *Kali iodat.* gr. v.—30, 8h. Rupia, *see* **Rupia.** Cachexia, depression; pains or ulceration of bones, enlargement of testicles, *Aur. met.* 30, 8h. Tertiary affections of tongue and throat, *Fluor. ac.* 3, gtt. ii. 6h. Syphilitic phthisis, *Ars. i.* 3x, gr. ii. 8h., after food. Syphilitic ulceration of the rectum, *Nit. ac.* 6, 4h.

CONGENITAL.—During pregnancy and nursing the mother should take *Merc. sol.* 6, night and morning, and *Leut.* 30, once a week. If in spite of this the child manifests signs of syphilitic marasmus, it should have *Merc. s.* 6, night and morning.

Syringomyelia. *See* **Paralysis,** SYRINGOMYELIA.

Tabes Dorsalis. *See* **Locomotor Ataxy.**

Tabes Mesenterica.—In general, *Bacil.* 100, gr, v. once or
twice a week. Premonitory diarrhœa, *Merc. cor.* 6, 2h. Great
wasting, *Iod.* 3x, 3h. In scrofulous children of soft fibre,
Calc. c. 6, 4h. Obstinate constipation, *Plumb. acet.* 3. gr. iv.
8h. Large hard abdomen with excessive emaciation and loss
of appetite or sickness, *Abrot.* 30, 4h.

Tape-worm. *See* **Worms.**

Taste.—ACUTE.—Increased taste of all food, *Camph.* 3, 4h.

DEPRAVED.—Food tastes bitter—(1) *Nat. m.* 6, 4h.; (2) *Camph.*
3, 4h.; (3) *China.* 3, 4h.; (4) *Puls.* 3, 4h. Bread tastes sweet,
Merc. sol. 6, 4h. Slimy, sweetish metallic, *Cupr.* 6, 4h. Sour,
metallic, greasy, *Rhust.* 3, 4h. Food and drink have a sour
taste; milk tastes disgusting as if spoiled, *Nux v.* 3, 4h.
Everything tastes salt, *Bell.* 3, 4h. Food tastes strangely,
Hydrast. 3, 4h. Taste of food remains long after eating—(1)
Nat. m. 6, 4h.; (2) *Nit. ac.* 6, 4h.

DIMINISHED AND LOST.—Taste blunted, *Calc. c.* 6, 4h. Food
seems tasteless; milky-coated tongue, *Ant. t.* 6, 4h.
Diminished taste, moist, coated tongue, *Puls.* 3, 4h. Taste
flat and insipid, sore aphthous mouth, *Bor.* 3, 4h. Taste
lost, with loss of smell, after a cold, *Mag. m.* 6, 4h. Complete loss of taste—(1) *Nat. m.* 6, 4h.; (2) *Mag. c.* 6, 4h.; (3)
Sul. 3, 4h. Loss of taste, with tongue thickly coated white,
Ant. c. 6, 4h.

ILLUSIONS.—TASTES IN THE MOUTH.—Bad taste in the mouth
in the morning; food and drink taste sour; bad odour from
the mouth; sour, bitter taste, *Nux v.* 3, 4h. Bad taste after

sleeping, *Rheum*. 3, 4h. Bad taste in the morning; food tastes strangely; peppery; acid peppery taste, *Hydr*. 3, 4h. Bitter taste in the mouth, *China*. 3, 4h. Bitter taste, but natural whilst eating and drinking; sweetish taste of blood, *Chel*. 3, 4h. Taste of blood, *Alumina* 3, 4h. Taste of blood whilst coughing, *Nit. ac.* 6, 4h. Bitter; slimy; metallic, *Merc. cor.* 6, 4h. Salty; sweet; bread tastes sweet; taste of bad eggs, *Merc. sol.* 6, 4h. Coppery, metallic, *Æsc. h.* 3, 4h. Bitter; pasty; bilious; metallic; like vinegar; taste of blood, *Sul.* 3, 4h. Offensive; sour, *Calc. c.* 6, 4h. Sour; sour dry taste; sour taste to all food, *Lyc.* 6, 4h. Slimy; disgusting; bilious, *Puls.* 3, 4h. Flat taste, *Borax* 3, 4h. Clayey taste, *Arg. n.* 6, 4h. Putrid taste; putrid smell from mouth—(1) *Arn.* 3, 4h.; (2) *Aur. mur.* 3x, 4h. Dyspepsia, *Ab. n.* 3x, 8h.

Tea.—EFFECTS OF.—Cramp-like pain in stomach, least food disagrees, *Ferr.* 6, 4h. Flatulence and nervous debility in excessive tea-drinkers, *China.* 3, 4h. Neuralgia from drinking tea, *Thuj.* 6—30, 4h. Chronic effects of over-indulgence in tea. *Thuj.* 30—200, once or twice a week.

Teeth.—CARIES—To *prevent* caries, live on simple food; too rich, too sweet, or too exclusively animal a diet, each tends to produce such a condition of the digestion and secretions of the mouth as favours the destruction of the teeth. A quill toothpick, or dental silk, should be used after each meal, especially each meat meal, to remove all particles of food that lodge between the teeth. Vegetarians say that their teeth are easily kept clean. The next most important point is to clean the teeth thoroughly and regularly. The formation of tartar on the teeth is by no means preservative of them, as is vulgarly imagined; it tends simply to destroy the gum and rob the teeth of support. When it has formed it should be taken off by a dentist, if necessary, by the process of scaling. It should never be allowed to reform. The best dentifrices are the simplest. A tooth-brush should be tolerably hard. It is as important to brush the gums well as it is the teeth. The first teeth of children should be most scrupulously cared for. If they are allowed to decay and come out, the jaws fail to expand properly, and the seeds are laid of future trouble with the second set. Besides, the first set give evidence of depraved conditions of constitution when present which by proper treatment may be in large measure or wholly counteracted before the second set appear. For all reasons then, the temporary teeth demand the careful attention of both parents and physicians. It is quite necessary that carious temporary teeth should be stopped, whenever possible, as it is that the permanent should. The following medicinal treatment will be found effective when combined with proper dieting and proper cleansing:—

IN CHILDREN.—If the teeth are pegged, *Merc. viv.* 6, 8h.; this should be given persistently for three months at a time, omitting every fourth month, and then resuming. In rickety children, if thin, *Silic.* 6, 8h.; in fat scrofulous children, *Calc. c.* 6, 8h. If the teeth turn black and decay, *Kreas.* 6, 8h. Teeth with pits or holes in them, from defective enamel, *Bacil.* 100, a few globules once in ten days. [In all cases where it is tolerated cod-liver oil may be given with advantage. If possible, residence in the country should be advised, with abundance of milk and cream, and milk foods (*see under* Diet, INFANTS; *also* Dentition), and fresh meat and green vegetables. A chalk country is best.] For toothache, *see* Toothache.

IN ADULTS.—Where the teeth rapidly become black, and, when decay has commenced, rapidly break down, sensitiveness of the teeth to the least touch, aching after eating or drinking, *Staph.* 3, 8h. Decay; loosening; turning black; bleeding gums, *Merc. v.* 6, 8h. Rapid decay and falling out; sordes; teeth sore, sore, bleeding gums, *Plant.* 3, 4h. Teeth become discoloured, grey, hollow; bleeding of gums, discharges from teeth sockets; necrosis of jaw, *Phos.* 3, 4h. Rapid decay, blunt, elongated feeling in the teeth, *Mez.* 3, 4h.

EXTRACTION OF.—After extraction of teeth, *Calend.* φ, gtt. xxx. to one tablespoon of warm water to be used as a wash. If bleeding is persistent, *Arn.* φ, gtt. v. to one tablespoon of cold or tepid water may be used in the same way. Failing this *Ham.* φ, gtt. xx. to one tablespoon. Internally *Hyperic.* 1x, 1h.

FALLING OUT.—*Merc. v.* 6, 4h. With suppuration of the gums, *Phos.* 3, 4h. *See also* Gums, Pyorrhœa, Toothache, Neuralgia.

Tenesmus (*Straining at Stool*).—Incessant tenesmus most distressing, nothing but mucus and blood pass, *Merc. c.* 3, ½h. Burning in the rectum, much urging to stool, and with it passage of urine; involuntary stool; feeling of unsafeness, *Aloe* 3, 9h. Urging without result or with it passage of scanty, hard motion, *Bell.* 3, 2h. Much urging and difficult expulsion of stool, which is yet not hard, *Hep. s.* 6, 4h. Great urgency, no stool, rectum protrudes, *Ign.* 3, 2h. Frequent, ineffectual urging, especially if there is vesical urging at the same time, *Nux v.* 3, 2h. Urging and easy protrusion of rectum, *Pod.* 6, 2h. Pressive urging, only mucus passes, or else hard motion like clay-stones, with great difficulty, *Sil.* 6, 4h. Straining before and after stool; constant bearing down towards anus; stool loose, slimy, purulent, bloody, or constipated, *Sul.* 3, 2h.

Testicles.—INFLAMMATION AND ENLARGEMENT OF.—Acute orchitis, *Puls.* 3, 1h. If there is much fever and restlessness, *Acon.* 3, 1h. When there is great sensitiveness of the nervous system and intolerance of pain, *Bell.* 3, 1h. [Locally, compresses of *Hamamelis* φ (ʒi.—ʒviii.) to be kept applied.] If there is excessive local sensitiveness, *Ham.* 1, 1h. Chronic inflammation, with aching and swelling of testicles and cord, *Spong.* 3, 2h. Chronic inflammation following mismanaged gonorrhœa, *Clemat.* 3, 2h. Chronic enlargement, with pain in cord and testicles, *Aur. met.* 30, 4h. Syphilitic enlargement, *Merc. bin.* 3x, gr. iii. 4h.

NEURALGIA.—*Aur. met.* 30, 4h. With nocturnal emissions, depression, irritability, hypochondriasis, *Ham.* 3, 2h. Deficient virility from previous engorgement; feeble erethism, *Con.* 3, 4h.

UNDEVELOPED.—In puny boys, *Aur.* 3, gr. v. once or twice daily.

Tetanus.—Idiopathic, arising from exposure to cold, *Acon.* 3, 1h. Opisthotonus; head bent back or twisted to one side; jerkings and spasms, *Cicut.* 3x—30, ½h.—2h. From injury to nerves or punctured wounds, great tenderness of injured part, *Hyper.* 1x—200, 1h. Opisthotonus, risus sardonicus, turgid, livid face, *Œnanth.* 3x—30, 1h. Following injury, *Strychnia* $\frac{1}{200}$, ½h.—1h. If this fails to arrest the disease, *Hydrocy. ac.* (Scheele's), gtt. i. ½h.—1h. Locally, the wound to be dressed with *Calendula* lotion (ʒiv.—ʒviii.). *Trismus* *neonatorum :* Restless, crying, feverish, *Aco.* 3, 1h. Convulsions, tremors, side-to-side movement of jaw, *Gels.* 3, 1h. Dress the umbilical cord with *Calendula.*

Tetany.—(1) *Aco.* 3, 1h.; (2) *Thyr.* gr. ii.—30, 4h.

Tetter.—BRANNY, *see* **Pityriasis.** DRY, *see* **Psoriasis.** MOIST, *see* **Herpes.**

Thecal Abscess. *See* **Whitlow.**

Thirst.—ABSENCE OF.—Complete, *Ant. t.* 6, 4h. Absence of thirst during heat; no thirst when eating, *China.* 3, 4h. Thirstless during heat; in dropsy, *Apis* 3x, 4h. No thirst during the day, but returning in the evening; loss of appetite, *Cyc.* 3, 4h. Loss of thirst, *Puls.* 30, 4h.

INCREASED.—During fever, *Aco.* 3, 2h. Unquenchable thirst; drinks much, but little at a time; drinking does not refresh; prefers it very cold and often vomits it as soon as swallowed; dry mouth, *Ars.* 3, 2h. Excessive thirst for cold water, with dryness of mouth and throat and difficulty in swallowing, *Bell.* 3, 2h. Great thirst with burning in throat and stomach, *Canth.* 3, 2h. Unquenchable burning thirst, *Crot. h.* 3, 2h. Unquenchable burning thirst, great desire for cold water in large quantities; *Merc. c.* 6, 4h. Great thirst; must drink large quantities; during internal fever, *Bry.* 3, 2h. Violent thirst, but drink immediately vomited, *Dulc.* 3, 2h. Violent thirst; unallayed by water; desire for sour drinks; dry throat, *Stram.* 3, 2h. Great thirst with hunger; much thirst for cold drinks; excessive thirst with perspiration, *Verat.* 3, 2h. Great thirst with loss of appetite, *Sul.* 3, 2h. Thirst for cold water, followed in some hours by chill, *Eup. perf.* 3, 2h. Unquenchable thirst during chill, *Nat. m.* 6, 2h.

Thread-worms. *See* **Worms.**

Throat. *See also* **Aphthæ, Quinsy, Scarlatina, Syphilis, Tonsils, Trachea, Uvula.**

MUCUS IN.—Increased secretion of mucus and hawking; dropping from posterior nares; rawness and soreness: *Hydrast.* 3, 4h. Dropping of mucus down back of throat; in psoric, chilly subjects, *Psor.* 30, 4h. Constant hawking and sensation as of a lump in the throat; thick mucus, *Alumina* 6, 4h. Thick, tenacious mucus in the throat, obliging to hawk; in the morning, *Arg. n.* 6, 4h. Tough mucus in the throat, as though a lump was there which cannot be swallowed, *Carb. v.* 6, 4h. Constant hawking and clearing of the throat; mucus grey and salty; or sour, acrid, or rancid, *Phos.* 3, 4h. Hawking of blood; accumulation of mucus on waking from sleep, *Sul.* 3, 4h. Spitting of frothy saliva streaked with blood, *Canth.* 3, 4h. Hawking of bloody mucus; yellow, purulent; granular, *Lyc.* 6, 4h. Violent hawking up of thick mucus, which continually collects again, *Nat. c.* 6, 4h. Hawking of mucus with dryness in the throat, after a nap in the daytime, *Lach.* 6, 4h.

SORE, ACUTE (*Acute Inflammation or Catarrh of the Mucous Membrane of the Throat*). Simple, from cold, accompanied with fever, *Aco.* 3, 1h. Dryness and burning, bright red swelling, feeling of constriction, difficulty in swallowing, face flushed and hot; erysipelatous sore throat, *Bell.* 3, 1h. Bluish, dark livid, *Gymnoclad. canad.* 3, 1h. Subacute, pale, or bluish, red swelling, *Merc. v.* 6, 2h. Dark red, larynx involved, *Naja* 6, 1h. Much œdema of mucous membrane; appearance as if stung with a bee; swallowing painful or difficult; inability to swallow a single drop, *Apis* 3x, 1h. Rawness; difficulty in swallowing, *Iod.* 3x, 2h. Constant secretion of mucus in the throat, difficult to discharge and causing retching; mucus descends from the back of the nose to the throat; sore throat with difficulty in swallowing and frequent empty swallowing; sore throat with pain on swallowing saliva, *Merc. i. fl.* 6, 2h. Tenacious mucus in throat; sensation as of a hair in the throat, *Kali bich.* 3x, 2h. Dark red, swollen mucous membrane, great soreness and difficulty of swallowing; pustular spots (herpes of the pharynx), swelling and tenderness of glands externally at the angle of the jaw, *Phytolacca*, 3, 1h. Locally, *Phyt.* φ (gtt. xx. to the tumbler of water), to be used every two hours as a gargle. Septic sore throat—(1) *Gunp.* 3x, gr. iv. 2h; (2) *Ecchin.* φ, 2h; (3) *Pyro.* 6, 2h. Gangrenous or phagedenic sore throat, *Merc. cy.* 6, 1h.; locally, *Phytolacca* gargle every hour. For inflammation of the tonsils *see* **Quinsy.** [Medicines recommended below under CHRONIC SORE THROAT are equally applicable to ACUTE, if the particular indications correspond.]

SORE, CHRONIC (*Chronic Inflammation or Catarrh of the Mucous Membrane of the Throat, or Relaxed Throat; with Clergyman's Sore Throat, or Follicular or Granular Sore Throat*). Rawness, soreness, and swelling; dropping of mucus from back of nose, Eustachian tubes involved; granular sore throat, *Hydrast.* 3, 4h. Chronic relaxed condition of throat; general debility; especially if tonsils are chronically enlarged, *Calc. phos.* 3, gr. v. 4h. Burning pain; dark red swelling; ulceration; difficult and painful swallowing, even of fluids; spasm of the glottis on attempting to swallow; swelling of glands, *Merc. cor.* 3, 4h. Mucous membrane dry, glazed, and red, with cough, *Alumina* 6, 4h. Chronic catarrh; common chronic ulcer; syphilitic sore throat; tenacious mucus; sensation as of a hair in the throat, *Kali bichr.* 3x, gr. ii. 4h. Dryness, burning, sensation of constriction, difficult swallowing, burning thirst, *Ars.* 3, 4h. Scraping sensation, with deep, hoarse voice, *Brom.* 3x, 4h. Smarting pain in the throat when swallowing, though most on empty swallowing, *Baryta carb.* 6, 4h. Pain in the upper parts of fauces between the acts of deglutition, as if the parts were sore and being spasmodically drawn together as in water-brash; burning with constriction; spasmodic contraction of throat; difficult swallowing, *Caps.* 3, 4h. Nervous sore throat; sore pain on swallowing; feeling of "lump" in the throat; throat symptoms < when not swallowing, and when swallowing liquids; > when swallowing food, *Ign.* 2, 2h. Nervous sore throat, when the aching is out of proportion to the inflammation; chronic irritation of the throat, always uneasy, choking, hawking, coughing; dry spot or general dryness on waking; sensation of a "lump," or of two lumps, closing in the throat, on empty swallowing; pain or difficulty swallowing, not on swallowing food, *Lach.* 6, 1h. Clergy-man's sore throat from over-exertion of the voice, *Arn.* 3, 4h. Granular sore throat, especially in persons with tendency to piles, mucous membrane dark red, *Æsc. h.* 1, 4h. Chronic granular sore throat, *Phyt.* 1x—3, 4h. [Medicines recommended above under ACUTE SORE THROAT, are equally applicable to CHRONIC, if the particular indications correspond.]

ULCERS.—Simple, *Kali bichr.* 3x, gr. ii. 4h.; locally, *Phyt.* φ (gtt. xx. to the tumbler of water), for a gargle three times a day. Syphilitic, *see* **Syphilis.**

Throat-deafness.—(1) *Hydrast.* 3, 2h.; (2) *Merc. sol.* 6, 4h. *See* **Ear,** DEAFNESS.

Thrush. *See* **Aphthæ.**

Tic Douloureux. *See* **Neuralgia.**

Tinea. *See* **Favus, Ringworm.**

Tinnitus Aurium. *See* **Noises in the Head.**

Tobacco Habit, or Nicotism.—[All those who suffer from the effects of tobacco, whether in the eye, the heart, the nerves, the stomach, or the throat, should abstain from its use. Homœopathic medicines are of great assistance to those who wish to break themselves of the habit.] In leaving off tobacco, *Nux v.* 3 should be taken every four hours; and when the craving comes on, a *Camphor* pilule should be chewed. Tobacco heart, *Stroph.* 1, 2h. Tobacco blindness: dim sight, photophobia unable to read by candlelight, *Phos.* 3, 2h. Diplopia; cloudy vision; optic neuritis, *Plumb. acet.* 3, gr. v. 4h. For the dyspepsia, *Nux v.* 3, 2h. For the heart distress, *Spig.* 3, 2h. Granular sore throat, *Calc. phos.* 3, gr. v. 2h. To destroy the desire for tobacco; in nervous, flatulent, dyspeptic persons, *China.* 3, 4h. In chilly, restless persons, thirst for cold things, nausea, vomiting, *Ars.* 3, 4h.

Toe-nails.—AFFECTIONS OF. *See* **Nails.**

Tongue.—CANCER.—*Kali cyan.* 1—3, 8h. Stony hard nodules, *Aur. met.* 3x, gr. iv. 8h. Tongue dry; burning; sour feeling; stitches worse at tip, *Alumen.* 30, 12h. Painful pustules r. side of tip on upper surface; pain in l. half of tongue, *Cund.* φ—3, 8n. Of r. side of tongue, *Kali cy.* gr. $\frac{1}{100}$ once in four days. Tongue as if burned or raw, dark red appearance and raised papillæ, *Hydrast.* 1—30, 8h. *See also* **Cancer.**

CRACKS.—Cracked, dry, parched, *Bell.* 3, 2h. Peeling and cracking, *Ran. s.* 3, 2h. Cracked, painful, bleeding, *Arum. t.* 12, 2h. Cracked down the centre, *Rhus v.* 3, 2h.

ENLARGEMENT AND INFLAMMATION OF.—Great swelling and
protrusion, *Merc. viv.* 6, ½h. If there is much fever, *Aco.* 3,
½h.—4h., to be followed by *Merc. v.* 6, ½h.—1h. If the
inflammation arises from a burn or scald, *Canth.* 3, ¼h.
Acute œdema, *Apis* 3x, ¼h. Tongue swollen, sore; excori-
ated, desquamated, *Oxal. ac.* 6, 4h. [As soon as the swelling
is checked the intervals between the doses may be increased.]
Subacute inflammation of the mucous membrane, thick
yellow mucous coat; sweet taste in mouth, *Merc. viv.* 6, 2h.

PARALYSIS OF.—*Caust.* 6, 2h. Swollen and stiff, seems paralysed; cannot be protruded, *Dulc.* 3, 2h. Feels very thick,
can hardly speak, *Gels.* 3, 2h.

SURFACE AND SENSATIONS.—Numb; burning; red; dry; white
furred, *Aco.* 3, 2h. Dry, cracked, parched; papillæ deep
red, swollen, *Bell.* 3, 2h. Red with silvery coat; clean, red,
furred, with red streak down the middle and red tip; dry;
dry and brown coated; burning, as if covered with burning
vesicles, *Ars.* 3, 2h. Red with blackish coat; much coated,
moist, edges red; white coat in front, yellow behind; dry,
hot, *Merc. c.* 6, 2h. Swollen and red; prominent papillæ on
white ground; burning extending to stomach, *Mez.* 3, 2h.
Pippy strawberry-like tongue, (1) *Fragar. vesc,* φ—3, 4h. (2)
Bacil. 30, once a week. Red in streaks; red, dry in middle;
thinly coated white with reddened papillæ and raw edges;
thick white or bilious fur; brown, dry, *Ant. t.* 6, 2h. Swollen;
thick white coat; patched red and white spots; aphthous;
thick white dry coat in patches; tongue and fauces whitened,
Oxal. ac. 6, 6h. White patches, *Arg. n.* 6, 6h. Tongue thick,
darkened, and, together with mouth and fauces, covered
with greyish white coat; bluish; blistered and burning,
Mur. acid. 1, 2h. Bluish-white coat, *Gymnocl. c.* 3, 2h. Thick,

white, milky coat; dirty tongue in children, *Ant. c.* 6, 2h. White coat; thick white coat, *Bry.* 3, 2h. White; yellow, *Æsc. h.* 3, 2h. Yellow coat; broad yellow stripe; large, indented, feels scalded, *Hydrast.* 3, 2h. Swollen, thickly coated white, indented, *Merc. sol.* 6, 2h. Black, with red edges, pale, tremulous, *Merc. v.* 6, 2h. Black tongue, *Carb. v.* 6, 4h. Dry, with blackish-brown coating, *Phos.* 3, 4h. Swollen, thick, white-coated, yellowish-white; thick fur; baked appearance in the middle, *Bapt.* 3, 2h. Dry in the morning; covered with tenacious mucus as if with a membrane; tongue broad, *Puls.* 3, 2h. White, with prominent papillæ; white coat; yellow blisters; burning, *Lyc.* 6, 2h. White; clean at front part, yellow behind, *Nux v.* 3, 2h. Thick, dirty yellow fur, *Sul.* 3, 2h. Feels very thick, can hardly speak; red, white, or yellow, *Gels.* 3, 2h. Red at apex, *Rhus t.* 3, 2h. White in middle, back and edges red; red tip; cracks in middle; distress at root, *Rhus v.* 3, 2h. White at both sides, red in the middle, *Caust.* 6, 2h. Skin of tongue peeling off, *Tarax. φ*—3, 2h. Skin peeling, cracking, *Ran. s.* 3, 2h. Blisters with burning; white or yellow coat; mapped tongue, *Nat. m.* 6, 2h. Mapped tongue, *Tarax. φ*, gtt. v. 8h. Blisters; burning at tip, and rawness of mouth, *Carb. an.* 6, 2h. Cracked, painful, bleeding, root of tongue and palate feel raw, *Arum t.* 12, 2h. Sore, blistered, bad breath, *Nit. ac.* 6, 2h.

SYPHILIS.—*Fluor. ac.* 3, 4h. *See also under* **Syphilis.**

ULCERATION.—Recurring ulcers; fungous; swelling; induration, "psoriasis of the tongue," *Mur. ac.* 1x, or 30, 4h. Ulcers under the tongue, *Lyc.* 6, 4h. Sublingual ulcer in whooping-cough, *Nit. ac.* 6, 2h. Syphilitic ulcers, *see under* **Syphilis.**

Tonics.—There are very few medicines which act as "tonics" to persons in good health; and the very common habit of taking a "tonic"—no matter what—whenever a pimple appears on the face is not merely ridiculous, it is pernicious. Medicines in general only have a strengthening action when there is lack of strength in the patient; and the same strengthening medicine is not suitable for every kind of debility. The best "tonic" in any case is that medicine which has produced in the healthy a similar kind of weakness to that experienced by the patient. For special indications, *see* Debility.

Tonsils.—ACUTE INFLAMMATION OF. *See* Quinsy.

CHRONIC ENLARGEMENT OF.—Scrofulous subjects, pain on swallowing, feeling of plug in throat, (1) *Baryt. mur.* 5—30, 8h. [A dose of *Bacil.* 100, gl. v. once a week is often of great assistance in these cases.] (2) *Baryt. c.* 6, 6h. Chronic suppuration, *Gunp.* 3x, gr. iv. 4h. Pale large swelling, *Calc. phos.* 3, gr. v. 6h. Pale swelling; urine dark-coloured and strong-smelling, *Benz. ac.* 1x, Tab. ii., 8h.

Toothache.—Begin in most cases, if the indications for another drug are not clear, with *Plantago* 3, every ten minutes. *Plantago* φ may also be rubbed on the gum, or applied externally on the face over the painful nerve; or inserted, on cotton wool, into the ear of the side affected. [If this fails to relieve or cure within a few hours, the following should be given as indicated.] Where there is inflammation at the root of a decayed tooth, *Merc. sol.* 6, 1h. When there is much swelling as well as inflammation, *Apis* 3x, 1h., and afterwards *Merc. sol.* 6, 1h. When the teeth are carious, but no signs of inflammation or gumboil are present, *Kreas.* 3, 1h. [*Kreas.* cures a large number of cases and may be given as a routine remedy to start with.] Black, crumbling, carious, exfoliating teeth, very sensitive to touch and to cold drinks,

Staph. 30, 1h. Toothache > by cold water, *Coff.* 3—30, 1h.
When the teeth are sound, *Spigel.* 3, 1h. Toothache when
eating, *Kali carb.* 6, 4h. Toothache from cold air or cold
drink; teeth cannot endure air or any coldness; toothache
only when eating, *Calc. c.* 6, 4h. Pain when eating; from
drinking warm things; from motion; > when lying down;
or when lying on painful side; arising from cold; teeth feel
too long; molars on right side chiefly affected, *Bry.* 3, 4h.
Toothache on taking anything warm into the mouth, > by
cold water, > in the open air and from uncovering, < by
warmth, *Puls.* 3, 1h. Toothache made < by warm food or
drink; when warm in bed at night; pain intolerable, *Cham.*
6, 1h. [*Chloroform* on cotton wool inserted into a hollow
tooth, or into the ear on the same side, will give temporary
relief. *Kreasote* inserted into a hollow tooth in the same way
as chloroform, and *Friar's balsam*, or *Spirit of Camphor*
rubbed on the gum, are useful local measures.] Toothache
of pregnancy—(1) *Calc. c.* 6, 2h.; (2) *Sep.* 6, 2h. When the
pain is intolerable during repose, *Mag. c.* 6, 2h. *See also*
Neuralgia.

[I have adapted from Hering's *Domestic Medicine* and partly
rearranged his *Repertory of Remedies for Toothache*, which will be
found below with Hering's prefatory remarks. One or two addi-
tions of my own will be found in brackets.]

"It should be taken into consideration that not all the symptoms mentioned under a remedy are necessarily to be found in
the patient, but that all, or at least the greater part, of the symptoms of the patient must be found under the remedy selected.

"To explain this, we will give the following example:—A
patient has violent tearing or drawing pains in different places,
and tearing in the gums (*a*); sometimes tearing pain extending

into the head (*b*); cold air causes it and makes it worse (*c*); it is
mostly worst in the morning (*d*); accompanied by determination
of blood to the head (*e*).

"Among the different symptoms we find for—

"(*a*) Pains in the gums: Mercurius, Pulsatilla, Staphisagria,
Hepar, Arsenicum, Carbo vegetabilis, Hyoscyamus, Calcarea.

"(*b*) Which extend to the head: Mercurius, Staphisagria, Nux
vomica, Chamomilla, Sulphur, Arsenicum, Antimonium crudum,
Rhus, Hyoscyamus.

"(*c*) Worse in cold air: Belladonna, Mercurius, Staphisagria,
Sulphur, Hyoscyamus.

"(*d*) Worse in the morning: Ignatia, Mercurius, Pulsatilla,
Phosphoric acid, Staphisagria, Bryonia, Nuc vomica, Cinchona,
Sulphur, Arsenicum, Hyoscyamus.

"(*e*) Determination of blood to the head: Aconite, Pulsatilla,
Cinchona, Hyoscyamus, Calcarea.

"After striking out all the remedies that occur here only once
or twice you will find that Pulsatilla, Staphisagria, Sulphur,
Arsenicum, occur three times; Mercurius, four times; Hyoscyamus, five times; now, examine the symptoms under Hyoscyamus,
and you will find that Hyoscyamus or Mercurius answers best.

"The remedies in italics are more frequently indicated than
the others and are therefore of more importance."

REPERTORY OF REMEDIES FOR TOOTHACHE

LOCALITIES

MOST IN FRONT TEETH.—Bell., Caust., Carb. v., Cham., Chi.,
Coff., Ign., Merc., *Nat. m., Nux mos., Nux v.,* Pho., Pho.
ac., *Rhs.,* Sil., Staph., *Sul.*

——— EYE and STOMACH-TEETH.—Aco., Calc., Hyo., *Rhs.,*
Staph.

Most in Molars.—Arn., Bell., *Bry.*, Calc., *Carb. v.*, Caust., Cham., Chi., Coff., Hyo., Ign., Merc., Nux m., Nux v., *Pho.*, Pho. ac., Puls., Rhs., Sil., *Staph.*, Sul.

———— Upper Teeth.—*Bell.*, Bry., *Calc.*, *Carb. v.*, *Chi.*, *Nat. m.*, Pho.

———— Lower Teeth.—*Arn.*, *Bell.*, Bry., Carb v., *Caust.*, *Cham.*, Chi., Hyo., Ign., Merc., Nux v., Puls., *Rhs.*, *Sil.*, Staph.

One-Sided.—Aco., Bell., Cham., Merc., Nux v., Puls.

Left Side.—Aco., Apis, Arn., Carb, v., Caust., *Cham.*, Chi., Hyo., Merc., *Nux mos.*, *Pho.*, Rhs., Sil., *Sul.*

Right Side.—*Bell.* Bry., Calc., Coff., Lach., Nat. m., Nux v., Pho. ac., Staph.

A Whole Row.—Cham., Merc., Rhs., Staph.

In Decayed Teeth.—Ant. c. Arn., *Bell.*, Bry., *Calc.*, *Carb v.*, Caust., *Cham.*, Chi., Coff., Hep., *Hyo.*, *Lach.*, *Merc.*, Nux m. Nux v., Pho., Pho. ac., *Puls.*, *Rhs.*, Sil., *Staph.*, Sul.

In the Gums.—Ant. c., Arn., *Bell.*, Bry., *Calc.*, *Carb. v.*, Cham., Chi., Hep., Hyo., Lach., *Merc.*, *Nat. m.*, Nux m., *Nux v.*, Pho., Pho. ac., Puls., Rhs., Silic., *Staph.*, Sul.

———— Upper.—Bell., *Calc.*, Nat. m.

———— Lower.—Caust., Phos., *Staph.*, Sul.

———— Interior of.—Arn., Nat. m., Pho. ac., Puls., Rhs., *Staph.*

Gums Swollen.—Aco., Bell., Calc., Cham., Carb. v., Caust., Chi., Hep., Lach., Nat. m., Nux v., Pho., Puls., Rhs., Sul.

———— Painful.—Apis, Ars., Calc., Carb. v., Caust., Lach., Merc., Nux m., Nux v., Pho., Staph., Sul.

Gums Bleeding.—Bell., Calc., Carb. v., Caust., Lach., Merc., Nux m., Nux v., Pho., Staph., Sul.

—— Ulcerated.—Bell., Calc., Carb. v., Caust., Hep., Lach., Merc., Nat. m., Nux v., Pho., Staph., Sil.

Character of Pains and Sensations

Beating or Pulsating.—*Aco.*, Arn., Ars., *Bell.*, Calc., Caust., Cham., Chi., Coff., Glon., *Hyo.*, Lach., Merc., Nat. m., Pho., Puls., Rhs., *Staph.*, Sul.

Blunt, or Without Feeling.—Aco., Chi., Dulc., Ign., Lach., Merc., Nat, m., *Nux m.*, Pho., Pho. ac., *Puls.*, Sil., Staph., Sul.

Boring.—Bell., Calc., Lach., Merc., Nat. m. Pho., Pho. ac., Nux v., *Sil.*, *Sul.*

Bruised or Ulcerated, as if.—Arn., Ars., Bell., Bry., Calc., Carb. v., Caust.; *Ign.*, Nat, m., Nux v., Pho., *Puls.*, Rhs.

Burning.—Cham., Merc., Nat. m., Nux v., Pho., Puls., Rhs., Sil., Sul.

Digging.—Ant. c., Bry., Calc., Chi., Ign.

Drawing, Tearing.—Ant. c., Bell., Bry., Carb. v., Calc., Cepa, Cham., Chi., Glo., Hyo., Lach., Merc., Nux v., Pho. ac., Rhs., Staph.

Gnawing, Scraping, Scratching on the Nerves.—Cham., Nux v., Rhs., Staph.

Jerking, Twitching.—Apis, Ant. c., Ars., Bry., Bell., Calc., *Caust.*, Cepa., Cham., Coff., Hep., Hyo., Lach., *Merc.*, *Nux v.*, *Puls.*, *Rhs.*, *Sul.*

Long, as if too.—Arn., Ars., Bell., *Bry.*, Calc., Carb. v., *Caust.*, Cham., Hyo., Lach., Nat. m., Nux v., Rhs., Sil., *Sul.*

Loose.—Arn., Ars., Bry., Carb. v., Caust., Cham., Chi., Hep., *Hyo.*, Ignat., Merc., Nat. m., Nux m., Nux v., Pho., Puls., Rhs., Staph., Sul.

Loose Sensation as if.—Ars., Bry., *Hyo.*, Merc., Rhs.

Piercing.—Aco., Ant. c., Bell., *Bry.*, Calc., Caust., *Cham.*, *Chi.*, Lach., *Merc.*, Nux v., Nux m., Pho., Pho. ac., *Puls.*, Rhs., Sil., Staph.

Pressing.—Aco., *Arn.*, Bry., Carb. v., Caust., Chi., Hyo., Ign., Nat. m., Nux m., Nux v., Pho., *Rhs.*, Sil., *Staph.*, Sul.

———— Inwards.—Rhs., Staph.

———— Outwards.—Pho.

———— Asunder.—Pho. ac.

———— As if from Congestion of Blood, as if the Teeth were too Close.—Aco., Arn., Bell., Cham., Calc., Chi., *Coff.*, Hep., Hyo., *Nux v.*, *Puls.* (Tuberc. k.).

Pulled, or Lifted out, or Wrenched, as if.—Arn., Caust. (Ipec.), Nux v., Pho. ac., Rhs.

Time

Intermittent.—Bell., Bry., Cham., Coff., Calc., Chi., Merc., Nux v., Puls., Rhs., Sil., Staph., Sul.

Constant, Day and Night.—Bell., Calc., Nat. m., Sil., Sul.

During the Day, Better at Night.—Merc.

———— None in the Night.—Bell., Calc., Merc., Nux v.

———— Worse in bed.—Ant. c., Merc.

Night, worse in.—Aco., Ant. c., Ars., *Bell.*, Bry., *Carb. v.*, *Cham.*, Chi., Coff., Hep., Hyo., Merc., Nat. m., Nux m., Nux v., Pho., Pho. ac., *Puls.*, *Rhs.*, Sil., *Staph.*, Sul.

———— Only, not during day.—*Bell.*, Pho.

NIGHT, MOST BEFORE MIDNIGHT.—Bry., Cham., Chi., Nat. m., Rhs., Sul.

——— MOST AFTER MIDNIGHT.—Ars., Bell., Bry., Carb. v., Cham., Chi., *Merc.*, Nat. m., Pho. ac., Puls., Rhs., *Staph.*, Sul.

AWAKING, ON.—Bell., Carb. v., Lach., Nux v. (*See under* SLEEP in Ameliorations and Aggravations.)

MORNING, IN THE.—Ars., Bell., Bry., Caust., Carb. v., Chi., *Hyo.*, Ign., Nat. m., *Nux v.*, Pho., Pho. ac., Puls., *Rhs.*, *Staph.*, Sul.

FORENOON.—Carbo v., Caust., Nat. m., Nux v., Staph., Puls., Sul.

NOON.—Coccul., Rhs.

AFTERNOON.—Calc., Caust., Lyc. (4 to 6), Merc., *Nux v.*, Phos., *Puls.*, Sul.

TOWARDS EVENING.—Puls.

NIGHT.—Ant. c., *Bell.*, Bry., Calc., Caust., Hep., *Hyo.*, Ign., *Merc.*, Nux m., Nux v., *Pho.*, *Puls.*, *Rhs.*, Staph., Sul.

EVERY OTHER DAY.—Cham., Nat. m.

——— SEVENTH DAY.—Ars., Pho., Sul.

——— SPRING.—Aco., Bell., Bry., Calc., Carb. v., Dulc., Lach., Nat. m., Nux v., *Puls.*, Rhs., Sil., Sul.

IN SUMMER.—Ant. c., Bell., Bry., Calc., Carb. v., Cham., Lach., Nat. m., Nux v., Puls.

——— AUTUMN.—Bry., Chi., Merc., Nux v., Nux m., Rhs.

IN WINTER.—Aco., Ars., Bell., Bry., Calc., Carb. v., Caust., Cham., Dulc., Hep., Hyo., Ign., Merc., Nux m., *Nux v.*, Pho., Pho. ac., Puls., *Rhs.*, Sil., Sul.

Causation

Damp air.—Merc.

—— Night air.—Nux m.

—— Cold weather.—Cepa, Nux m., Rhs.

Draught.—Bell., Calc., *Chi.*, Sul.

Wind.—Aco., Puls., Rhs., Sil.

—— Keen, cutting.—Aco., Sil.

Taking cold.—Aco., *Bell.*, *Bry.*, Calc., Caust., Cham., Chi., Coff., *Dulc.*, Ign., *Hyo.*, *Merc.*, Nux v., *Nux m.*, *Pho.*, *Puls.*, *Rhs.*, Staph., Sul.

—— When overheated.—Glo., Rhs.

—— By getting wet.—Bell., Calc., Caust., Hep., Lach., Nux m., Pho., Pul., Rhs., Sul.

Suppressed perspiration.—Cham., Rhus.

Persons and Temperament

For children.—Aco., *Ant. c.*, Bell., Calc., Cham., Coff., Ign., Merc., Nux m., Puls., Sil.

For women.—Aco., Apis., Bell., Calc., Cham., Chi., Coff., Hyo., Ign., Nux m., Puls.

For sensitive nervous persons.—Aco., Bell., Cham., Chi., Coff., Hyo., Nux m.

For persons who have taken much Mercury.—Carb. v., Bell., Hep., Lach., Staph.

For those who drink much Coffee.—Bell., Carb. v., Cham., Coccul., Merc., Nux v., Puls., Sil.

Conditions of Aggravation

Air, from Cold.—Bell., Calc., Hyo., Merc., Nux m., Nux v., Sil., Staph., Sul.

—— In the Mouth.—Aco., *Bell.*, Bry., Calc., Caust., Hyo., *Merc.*, Nux m., Nux v., Pho., Puls., Sil., Staph., Sul.

Air, Drawing into Mouth.—Ant. c., Bell., Bry., Calc., Caust., Hep., Merc., Nat. m., Nux m., Pho., Sil., Staph., Sul.

—— Opening of the Mouth to.—Bry., Cham., Caust., Hep., Nux v., Pho., Puls.

—— In open.—*Bell.*, Calc., Caust., *Cham.*, *Chi.*, Hyo., Merc., *Nux m.*, *Nux v.*, *Pho.*, Puls., *Rhs.*, *Staph.*, Sul.

Air, Staying in.—Bell., Bry., Cham., Hyo., Merc., Nux v., Pho. ac., Staph., Sul.

—— Walking in.—Nux v., Pho., *Staph.*

Bed, in.—Ant. c., Bell., Bry., *Cham.*, *Merc.*, Nux v., *Puls.*

Breathing.—Puls.

—— Deep.—Nux v.

Cold in General.—*Ars.*, Ant. c., Calc., Carb. v., Merc., Nat, m., *Nux m.*, Nux v., *Puls.*, *Pho. ac.*, *Rhs.*, Sil., Staph., Sul.

—— Washing.—Ant. c., Bry., *Calc.*, Cham., *Merc.*, *Nux m.*, Nux v., Puls., Rhs., Sil., Staph., Sul.

—— Water, rinsing mouth with.—Sul.

—— Food.—Bry., Calc., Cham., Nux v., Puls., Rhs., Staph., Sul.

—— Drink.—Bry., Calc., Cham., Caust., Hep., Lach., Merc., Nat. m., Nux m., *Nux v.*, Puls., Sil., Staph., Sul.

Concussion.—Nux m.

DRINKING.—Cham., Calc., Caust., *Lach.*, Merc., Puls., Rhs., Sil.

DRINKING, COLD OR WARM.—Lach.

—— COFFEE.—Bell., Carb. v., Cham., Coccul., Ign., Merc., Nux v., Puls., Rhs.

—— MALT LIQUORS.—Nux v., Rhs.

—— TEA.—Chi., Coff., Ign., Lach.

DRINKING WATER.—Bry., Calc., Carb. v., Cham., Merc., Nux v., Puls., Sil., Staph., Sul.

—— WINE.—Aco., Ign.; (Nux v. for wine-drinkers).

EATING.—Ant. c., Arn., Bell., Bry., Calc., *Carb. v.*, *Caust.*, *Cham.*, Coccul., Hep., Hyo., Lach., *Merc.*, Nux m., Nux v., Pho., Pho. ac., *Puls.*, Rhs., Sil., *Staph.*, Sul.

—— ONLY WHILE.—Coccul.

EATING, AFTER.—Ant. c., *Bell.*, *Bry.*, Calc., Cham., Chi., Coff., Ign., Lach., *Merc.*, *Nat. m.*, *Nux v.*, Rhs., *Staph.*, *Sul.*

—— SOME TIME AFTER.—Bell.

—— SALTY THINGS.—Carb. v.

—— BITING.—Ars., Bell., Bry., Calc., Carb. v., Caust., Chi., Coff., *Hep.*, Hyo., Lach., *Merc.*, Nux v., Pho., Pho. ac., Puls., Rhs., Sil., Staph., Sul.

—— —— HARD FOOD.—Merc.

—— —— SOMETHING SOFT.—Verat.

—— —— SOFT FOOD.—Coccul.

—— CHEWING.—Arn., Ars., Bell., Bry., Carb. v., Caust., *Chi.*, Coccul., Coff., *Hyo.*, *Ign.*, *Merc.*, *Nat. m.*, *Nux v.*, Pho., *Pho. ac.*, *Puls.*, Sil., Staph., Sul.

—— —— ONLY WHEN.—Chi.

EATING, SWALLOWING, WHEN.—Staph.

———— MOVING THE MOUTH.—Caust., Cham., Merc., Nux v.

GUMS, FROM SUCKING THE.—Bell., Carb. v., Nux m., Nux v., Sil.

LYING DOWN, WHEN.—*Ars.*, Bell., Bry., *Cham.*, Hyo., Ign., Merc., Nux v., Phos., Puls., *Rhs.*, Staph., Sul.

LYING ON THE PAINFUL SIDE.—Ars., Nux v.

———— ———— PAINLESS SIDE.—Bry., Cham., Ign., Puls.

———— IN BED.—Bry., Cham., Nux v., *Puls.*

MENSTRUATION, BEFORE.—Ars.

MENSTRUATION, DURING.—Calc., *Cham.*, Carb. v., Nat. m., Lach., Pho.

———— AFTER.—Calc., Bry., Cham., Pho.

MENTAL EMOTIONS.—Acon.

———— ANGER.—Nux v.

———— VEXATION.—Aco., Cham., Rhs., Staph.

MENTAL EXERTION.—Bell., Ign., Nux v.

MOTION.—Arn., *Bell.*, *Bry.*, Chi., *Merc.*, Nux v., Pho., Staph.

NOISE.—Calc.

NURSING, WHILE.—Aco., Ars., Bell., Calc., Chi., Dulc., Merc., Nux v., Phos., Staph., Sul.

PREGNANCY, DURING.—Apis, Bell., Bry., Calc., Hyo., Merc., Nux m., Nux v., Puls., Rhs., Staph.

READING.—Ign., Nux v.

RISING.—Ign., Merc., Plat.

ROOM, IN A.—Apis, Ant. c., *Cham.*, Hep., Nux v., *Puls.*, Sul.

———— ON ENTERING FROM THE OPEN AIR.—Phos.

Sitting.—Ant. c., Merc., *Puls.*, *Rhs.*

———— Too Much.—Aco.

Sleep, During.—Merc.

———— With Yawning.—Staph.

———— When Going to.—Ant. c., Ars., Merc., Sul.

———— When Awaking from.—Bell., Bry., Calc., Carb. v., Lach., Nux v., *Pho.*, Sil., *Sul.*

Talked to by others, being.—Ars., Bry.

Talking.—Nux mos.

Teeth, Cleaning the.—Carb. v., Lach., Pho. ac., *Staph.*

———— When feeling the.—Hep.

Teeth, Picking the.—Puls.

———— Pressing on the.—Caust., Chi., Hyo., Nat. m., Staph., Sul.

———— Sucking them with the Tongue.—Nux v.

———— Touched by Food.—Bell., Ign., Nux v., Pho., Staph.

Teeth Touched by a Crumb.—Nux v., Staph.

———— Touching the.—Ant. c., Arn., Ars., *Bell.*, *Bry.*, Calc., *Carb. v.*, Caust., *Chi.*, Coff., *Hep.*, Ign., *Merc.*, Nat. m., Nux m., *Nux v.*, Pho., *Puls.*, Rhs., *Staph.*, Sul.

Teeth Touching with the Tongue.—Carb. v., Chi., Ign., Merc., Pho., Rhs.

———— ———— Even very Softly.—*Bell.*, Ign., Nux v., Staph.

Tobacco, Smoking.—Bry., Cham., Chi., *Ign.*, Merc., Nux v.

Travelling, when.—Ars., Bry., Cham., Puls., Rhs., Staph., Sul.

WARMTH.—Bry., *Calc.*, Carb. v., Cham., Coff., Lach., Merc., Nat. m., Nux m., Nux v., Pho. ac., *Puls.*, Sil., Sul.

—— EXTERNAL.—Bry., Cham., Hep., Merc., Nux m., Nux v., Pho., Pho. ac., Puls., Rhs., Staph., Sul.

—— OF ROOM.—Bry., Cepa, Cham., Hep., Nux v., Pho. ac., *Puls.*

—— OF STOVE.—Ars., Puls.

—— OF BED.—Bell., Bry., Cham., Merc., Nux v., Pho., Pho. ac., *Puls.*, Rhs.

—— BECOMING WARM IN BED.—*Cham.*, Merc., Pho., Pho. ac., Puls.

—— DRINKING WARM THINGS.—*Bry.*, Cham., Lach., Merc., Nux m., Nux v., Puls., Rhs., Sil.

—— EATING WARM THINGS.—Bry., Calc., Cham., Nux v., Pho., Puls., Sil.

—— —— SOMETHING HOT.—Bell., *Calc.*, Pho. ac.

CONDITION OF AMELIORATION

AIR, COLD.—Nux v., Puls.

AIR, DRAWING INTO MOUTH.—Nux v., *Puls.*

AIR, IN OPEN.—Ant. c., Bry., Cepa, Hep., Nux v., Puls.

BED, IN.—Sul.

BLOWING UPON IT.—Puls.

COLD, EXTERNAL.—Bell., Bry., Cham., Chi., Merc., Nux v., Pho., *Puls.*, Staph., Sul.

COLD HAND, BY APPLYING.—Rhs.

—— WASHING.—Bell., Bry., Cham., Puls.

—— WATER, BY APPLYING FINGER WET WITH.—Cham.

—— —— HOLDING IN MOUTH.—Bry., Cepa, *Coff.*

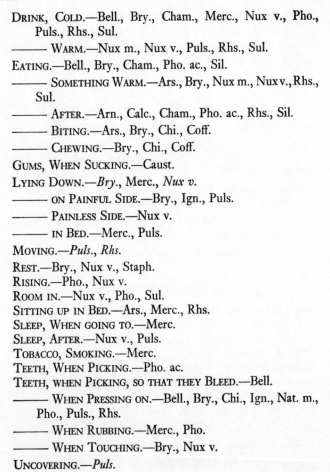

DRINK, COLD.—Bell., Bry., Cham., Merc., Nux v., Pho., Puls., Rhs., Sul.

—— WARM.—Nux m., Nux v., Puls., Rhs., Sul.

EATING.—Bell., Bry., Cham., Pho. ac., Sil.

—— SOMETHING WARM.—Ars., Bry., Nux m., Nux v., Rhs., Sul.

—— AFTER.—Arn., Calc., Cham., Pho. ac., Rhs., Sil.

—— BITING.—Ars., Bry., Chi., Coff.

—— CHEWING.—Bry., Chi., Coff.

GUMS, WHEN SUCKING.—Caust.

LYING DOWN.—*Bry.*, Merc., *Nux v.*

—— ON PAINFUL SIDE.—Bry., Ign., Puls.

—— PAINLESS SIDE.—Nux v.

—— IN BED.—Merc., Puls.

MOVING.—*Puls., Rhs.*

REST.—Bry., Nux v., Staph.

RISING.—Pho., Nux v.

ROOM IN.—Nux v., Pho., Sul.

SITTING UP IN BED.—Ars., Merc., Rhs.

SLEEP, WHEN GOING TO.—Merc.

SLEEP, AFTER.—Nux v., Puls.

TOBACCO, SMOKING.—Merc.

TEETH, WHEN PICKING.—Pho. ac.

TEETH, WHEN PICKING, SO THAT THEY BLEED.—Bell.

—— WHEN PRESSING ON.—Bell., Bry., Chi., Ign., Nat. m., Pho., Puls., Rhs.

—— WHEN RUBBING.—Merc., Pho.

—— WHEN TOUCHING.—Bry., Nux v.

UNCOVERING.—*Puls.*

WALKING.—Puls., Rhs.

WARM IN BED, ON GETTING.—Bry., Nux v.

WARMTH, EXTERNAL.—Ars., Bell., Calc., Cham. Chi., Hyo.,
Lach., Merc., Nux m., Puls., *Rhs.*, Staph., Sul.

———— OF ROOM.—Nux v., Pho., Sul.

WRAPPING UP HEAD.—Nux v., Pho., Sil.

EXTENSION OF PAINS

PAINS EXTEND TO HEAD.—Ant. c., Ars., Cham., Hyo., Merc.,
Nux v., Rhs., Staph., Sul.

———— TO EYES,—Caust., Cham., Merc., Puls., Staph., Sul.

———— TO EARS.—Ars., Bry., Calc., Cham., Hep., Lach.,
Merc., Staph., Sul.

———— TO CHEEKS.—Bry., Caust., Cham., Merc., Sil., Staph.,
Sul.

———— TO JAW-BONES AND FACE.—Hyo., Lach., Merc., Nux
v., Rhs., Sul.

CONCOMITANTS

HEAD, ACHING.—Apis, Glo., Lach.

———— HEAT IN.—Aco., Hyo., Puls.

———— RUSH OF BLOOD TO.—Aco., Calc., Chi., Hyo., Lach.,
Puls.

———— SWOLLEN VEINS OF FOREHEAD AND HANDS.—Chi.

EYES, BURNING OF.—Bell.

FACE, PALE.—Aco., Ars., Ign., Puls., Staph., Sul.

FACE, FLUSHED CHEEKS.—Aco., Arn., Bell., Cham., Merc.,
Nux m., Pho., Puls., Rhs., Sul.

———— SWELLING OF CHEEK.—Arn., Ars., Bell., Bry., *Cham.*,
Lach,. *Merc.*, Nat, m., Nux v., Puls., Pho., Pho. ac.,
Staph., Sul.

Mouth, Dry with Thirst.—Chi.

——— Without Thirst.—Puls.

Mouth, Salivation.—Bell., Dulc., Merc.

Throat, Dry with Thirst.—Bell.

Constipation.—Bry., Merc., Nux v., Staph.

Diarrhœa.—Cham., Coff., Dulc., Rhus.

Chilliness.—Puls., Rhus.

——— Heat, Thirst.—Lach.

Heat.—Hyo., Rhs.

Tooth-rash. *See* **Red Gum.**

Torticollis. *See* **Stiff-neck.**

Trachea.—Dryness in trachea; crawling in upper parts, as if something were there provoking cough; hoarseness; < in damp, cold weather, in the evening, and from speaking, *Carb. v.* 6, 2h. Adherent mucus high up in trachea, causing cough; upper parts feels constricted; tickling and itching in trachea, in the middle of sternum, causing cough, < on expiration, *Nux v.* 3, 2h. Tickling irritation in trachea, as if from feather-down; cough provoked by this or by eating; sensation as if something loose in trachea; difficult loosening of phlegm, especially at episternal notch; wheezing in trachea; sensation as if a lump of phlegm moving up and down trachea, *Calc. c.* 6, 2h. Dryness and burning in larynx and trachea; irritation at bifurcation of trachea, formation of mucus there which is difficult to expel, *Ars.* 3, 2h. Rawness of larynx and trachea with frequent hacking cough and hawking; irritability of lower part of trachea with suffocative pressing; coughing up of much purulent phlegm, constant tickling-scratching sensation at bifurcation of trachea, *Phos.* 3, 2h. In the morning, tough mucus in lower part of trachea, which cannot be dislodged by hawking or coughing;

after hawking and coughing trachea is raw and sore; finally the mucus loosens itself and he must hawk constantly, *Cann. sat.* 3, 2h. Irritation to cough in trachea, as from mucus; sore sensation low down in trachea after every cough; expectoration of yellow mucus from trachea, of foul taste or sweet, *Stan.* 6, 4h. Constant irritation in trachea; deep down; cough dry and spasmodic; or with copious mucus; < at night, *Sul.* 3, 2h. Rawness and soreness in the morning after rising, with dry cough, *Carb. a.* 6, 2h. Pain in trachea, < by smoking or talking; soreness after coughing; sensation of vapour in trachea; < on going into warm out of cold air, *Bry.* 3, 2h. Crawling and tickling in larynx and trachea after lying down in the evening; tickling in trachea causing violent sneezing, *Caps.* 3, 2h. Pain in larynx and trachea extending to middle of sternum as if raw and sore, cough very violent, *Osmium* 3, 2h. Expectoration of mucus from trachea immediately after eating, *Sil.* 6, 2h. Tickling in trachea; causing cough; contractive feeling as if the pit of the throat pressed on the trachea; formation of membrane in trachea; < on inspiration. *Brom.* 3x—20, 2h. (must be freshly prepared if given in the lower strength). Feeling as if something swollen in throat, but that cannot be swallowed; stitch through trachea; pain from pit of throat to root of tongue; trachea tender to touch, tickling at throat-pit, < after sleep and by touch, *Lach.* 6, 2h. Sensation in trachea as if swelled up; scraping, irritation, *Apis* 3x, 2h. Raw scraped sensation all down centre of chest and throat; paroxysmal cough provoked by tickling in trachea, and induced by pressure upon it; < in cold air, *Rum. c.* 6, 2h. Irritation of nose, larynx, and trachea, cough with difficult expectoration of tough white stringy mucus, *Kali bichr.* 3x, gtt. i. 2h. *See also* **Cold, Cough, Larynx, Bronchitis.**

Traumatic Fever (including CATHETERISM).—When simple continued, *Aco.* 3, 1h. When typhoid in character, *Ars.* 3, 2x. When pyæmic—(1) *Lach.* 6, 2h.; (2) *Arn.* 3, 2h. When hectic, *China.* 3, 2h. *See also* **Fever, Hectic, Pyæmia.**

Tremors.—Nervous from emotional disturbance, *Ign.* 3, 1h. From fright, *Stram.* 3, 1h. Of drunkards; jactitation; internal trembling; trembling of head and paralytic trembling of hands on every motion, *Ant. t.* 6, 2h. Tremors; never master of himself; tremors of tongue; stammering; unable to lift, write or eat; nervousness; tremors commencing in the fingers, *Merc. s.* 6, 4h. Weakness and trembling of the whole body; complete muscular relaxation, *Gels.* 3, 2h. Restlessness; inability to walk from trembling of the limbs; nervousness, *Act. r.* 3, 2h. Trembling of the limbs with blueness and coldness, *Agar.* 3, 2h. Tremors and weakness or faintness, *Thyr.* 3x, gr. ii.—30, 4h.

Trismus (*Lock-jaw and* **Trismus neonatorum**).—*See* **Tetanus.**

Tuberculosis.—ACUTE.—Fever, wasting, *Bacil.* 100, gl. iv. in half a tumbler of water, a teaspoonful 4h. To relieve the fever accompanying acute and subacute exacerbations, *Bapt.* φ—30, 2h. Delirium, typhoid condition, *Iodf.* 3x, 2h. Heat and perspiration of head, cold clammy hands and feet, *Calc. c.* 30, 1h. Flushed face, delirium, boring head into pillow, *Bell.* 3. 1h.

THREATENED. *See* **Consumption,** THREATENED. *See also* **Consumption, Meningitis, Mesenteric Disease, Peritonitis.**

Tumours.—Fatty, *Calc. c.* 30, once or twice a day. Fatty tumours, especially about the neck, *Baryt. c.* 6, 4h. *Carcin.* 100, once a week, is often helpful in these cases. General increase of fat, *Calc. ars.* 30, 6h. Encysted, *Calc. c.* 30, 6h. Vascular of urethra (Urethral Caruncle), (1) *Eucalypt.* 3x, 4h; locally, to be painted thrice daily with *Eucalypt. φ.* (2) *Rad. br.* 30, once or twice a week.

CANCER. *See* Cancer.

FIBROID. *See* Fibroma.

NODES. *See* Nodes.

OVARIAN. *See* Ovaries.

POLYPUS. *See* Polypus.

SEBACEOUS. *See* Wens.

VASCULAR. *See* Nævus.

WARTS *and* CONDYLOMATA. *See* Warts, Condylomata.

Tympanites.—Hysterical, *Asaf.* 3, 1h. In fevers and inflammation, *Tereb.* 3, 1h., locally, flannels wrung out of hot water, and a few drops of turpentine sprinkled on, to be applied to the abdomen every hour. *See* Enteric Fever, Peritonitis.

Typhlitis. *See* Appendicitis.

Typhoid Fever. *See* Enteric Fever.

Typhus Fever.—Uncomplicated, *Rhus t.* 1—3, 1h. Great restlessness, twitching, and tremor, *Agar.* 3x, 1h. Much drowsiness and delirium. *Bapt.* 1, 1h. Great vital depression, *Ars.* 3, 1h. Pneumonia, *Phos.* 3, 1h. Inflammation of salivary glands; accumulation of mucus, with nightly angina, increased saliva, *Chin. sulph.* 3x, gr. ii. 2h. Scorbutic gums, offensive odour, swollen glands, *Merc. sol.* 6, 2h. Bubo, *Merc. viv.* 6, 2h.

Ulceration and Ulcers.—[In all cases the constitutional state must be attended to, and the hygienic surroundings of the patient.]

PREVENTIVE TREATMENT.—When the skin is red and erysipe-latous-looking, and feels hard, *Bell.* 3, 2h. Skin about the ankle dark and painful, *Lach.* 6, 2h. Varicose patches, *Ham.* 3, 2h. Nodular swellings in syphilitic subjects, *Kali iod.* gr. ii. 4h. [In all cases the limb must be supported by suitable bandages, and rest enjoined.]

ULCERS.—Simple ulceration; perforating ulcers, *Sil.* 6, 4h.; locally, *Sil.* 6, ʒii. in ℥vi., to be kept applied as a lotion. In chronic cases, begin with *Sul.* 3, 4h., locally, *Calend.* φ, ʒii.—℥vi. for a lotion (or, ʒii.—℥i. of Cetacean ointment for an ointment). Atonic ulcer on legs, (1) *Hydrast.* 1, 3h.; locally, *Hydrast.* φ, ʒii. in ℥iv. for a lotion; or, ʒii.—℥i. of *Unguent cetac.* for ointment; (2) *Kali bichr.* 3x, gr. iii. 4h.; locally, *Kali bichr.* gr. i.—℥viii. for lotion. Ulcers bleed when touched; stinging pains; feeling of a splinter; hard, everted, irregular edges; fungating; carious, mercurial or syphilitic, *Nit. ac.* 3—30, 4h.; locally, *Nit. ac.* 1x, ʒii.—℥viii. for lotion. Chronic ulcers on the left side; ulcers with sensitive edges and fetid discharges, *Ast. rub.* 6, 4h.; locally, *Calend.* φ, ʒii.—℥vi. Irritable ulcer, *Lach.* 6, 2h.; locally, *Calend.* φ, ʒii.—℥vi. for lotion. Varicose ulcers with great sensitiveness of the part, *Ham.* 3, 3h.; locally, *Ham.* φ, gtt. xx.—℥vi. for lotion; or *Ham.* φ, ʒi.—℥i. of *Ung. cetac.* for ointment. Large varicose ulcers; with enlarged liver and spleen, *Card. m.* φ, 4h. Painful burning ulcers, *Ars.* 3, 4h.; locally, *Ars.* 3, ʒii.—℥vi. for lotion. Punched-out ulcers, ulcers that bleed readily, especially at catamenial periods; ulcers sur-rounded by smaller ulcers, *Phos.* 3, 3h.; locally, *Calendula* ointment or lotion. Ulcers with an areola, sensitive and easily bleeding, painful at, night; pus has tendency to form an adherent scab, under which more pus collects, *Mez.* 3, 3h.; locally, *Mez.* φ, ʒii.—ʒvi. for lotion; or ʒii.—ʒi. of *Ung. cetac.* for ointment. Weeping ulcers, *Merc. sol.* 6, 4h.; locally, *Calend.* Painful and fetid ulcers, *Pæon.* 3, 3h.; locally, *Pæon.* φ, ʒii.—ʒvi. for lotion; ʒii.—ʒi. of *Ung. cetac.* for ointment. Deep hard-edged ulcers, *Comocl.* 3, 3h.; locally, *Comocl.* φ, ʒii.—ʒvi.; or ʒii.—ʒi. of *Ung. cetac.* for ointment. "Constitutional" and syphilitic ulcers—(1) *Kali i.* gr. iii.—30, 4h.; locally, ointment of acid Nitrate of Mercury, dilute; (*Ung. hydrarg. nit.* B. P. ʒii., *Ung. cetac.* ʒi.). (2) *Nit. ac.* 6, 4h.; locally, *Nit. ac.* 1x, ʒii.—ʒviii. for a lotion. Sloughing or phagedænic ulcer, as from bed-sores—(1) *Crot. h.* 3, 2h.; to be kept constantly clean; if necessary, in a continual water-bath in which Condy's fluid (ʒi.—Oj.) has been mixed, the water being kept flowing through the bath in a constant stream. (2) *Nit. ac.* 6, 2h.; locally, *Nit. ac.* 1x, ʒii.—ʒvi. for a lotion (with frequent cleansing). (3) *Ars.* 3, 2h.; locally, *Ars.* 3, ʒii.—ʒvi. for a lotion. When there is much prostration, with coldness and vital depression, *Carb. v.* 6, 2h.; locally, *Nit. ac.* 1x, ʒii.—ʒvi. *See also* **Bed-sores.** [As an alternative for the Hydrastis or Calendula ointment, the *Resin ointment* of the B.P. is often of service; also *Boracic acid* ointment.]

Umbilical Hernia. *See* **Hernia.**

Uræmia.—[Put the patient in a hot pack, or give a vapour-bath.] For the coma give—(1) *Carbol. ac.* 2, ¼h.; (2) if there is no improvement within a few hours, *Op.* 3x, ¼h. (3) *Urt. ur.* φ, gtt. v. 2h. When there are convulsions, *Cupr. ac.* 3x, ¼h.

Urethra.—INFLAMMATION OF. *See* **Gleet, Gonorrhœa.**

CARUNCLE. *See under* **Tumours.**

SPASMODIC STRICTURE. Pure spasm, *Camph.* 1x, 10m. Fever as well as spasm, *Acon.* 3, 10m. (A dose of *Acon.* 3 given half an hour or fifteen minutes before the catheter is passed will frequently add greatly to the patient's comfort.) [These are well supplemented by a hot bath.] In more chronic cases, *Nux v.* 3, 1h. *See also* **Strangury.**

ORGANIC STRICTURE.—Commencing, *Clem. φ*, 2h. Established —(1) *Sil.* 3, gr. iv. 8h.; (2) *Phos.* 3, 4h. (3) *Thios.* 3x, 4h. When acute symptoms supervene, medicines recommended for **Strangury** must be given, and the necessity of catheterism must always be borne in mind.

Urine.—ABNORMAL CONDITIONS OF.—Strong-smelling, like horses', (1) *Benz. ac.* 3x, 4h. (2) *Nit. ac.* 4h. Smelling like violets, *Tereb.* 3, 4h. Fishy odour, *Uran. nit.*, 3x, gr. ii.—30, 8h. Pungent smell, *Borax* 6, 8h. Mucus; white sediment; incontinence in children, *Cina* 3, 8h. White deposit of oxalates, pain in the back. *Oxal. ac.* 5, 8h. Phosphatic (1) *Phos. ac.* 1x, 4h. (2) *Calc. ph.* 1—30, 8h. Red deposit, with constipation, *Lyc.* 3, gr. ii.—6, 4h. Red deposit, lithic acid dyspepsia, *Sep.* 6, 4h. Brown or white deposit, pain in groins, *Berb.* 6, 4h. Thick white deposit, ill-smelling, *Graph.* 6, 4h. White urine (with worms), *Cina* 3, 4h. Galacturia, or chylous, or milky urine, *Iod.* 3x, 4h. Bloody, *see* **Hæmaturia.** Pale and excessive in quantity, *Scill. acet.* 1, 4h. Sugar, *see* **Diabetes.**

MICTURITION, ABNORMAL.—Burning or scalding, painful emission, drop by drop, *Canth.* 3, 2h. Constant ineffectual desire; contraction of urethra; emission in drops, *Copaiva* 3, 2h. Urine scanty and high coloured; burning soreness when urinating; frequent desire, passes only a few drops, *Apis* 3x, 2h. Sudden and frequent urging to urinate, *Petrosel.* φ, 8h. Flow interrupted by sudden spasm of urethra. *Clem.* 1—30, 1h. Urine stops suddenly and does not begin to flow again for some moments, *Con.* 6, 2h. Difficult, *see* **Strangury.**

MICTURITION, FREQUENT.—At night in old people, *Caust.* 3x, 8h. Frequent at night; urging to urinate, but it is a long time before he is able, *Kali c.* 6, 8h. Urging after drinking water, *Carlsbad* 6, 8h. After drinking coffee, *Ign.* 3, 8h. Frequent urging with constipation, *Nux v.* 3, 2h. Violent urging with dragging pains, *Lil. t.* 30, once a day.

SUPPRESSION AND RETENTION OF URINE.—From cold, *Camph.* 1x, 10m. If it does not yield within one or two hours, *Tereb.* 3, ¼h. If there is fever, anxiety, restlessness, fear, *Aco.* 3, ¼h. Spasmodic, *Nux v.* 3, ¼h. Hysterical, *Ign.* 3, ¼h. Paralytic; after operations, *Op.* 3, ¼h. *See also* **Bladder, Kidneys,** INFLAMMATION OF, **Strangury, Urethra,** STRICTURE OF.

INCONTINENCE OF.—Simple nocturnal, in profound sleep, *Bell.* 3, 4h. In first sleep, *Sep.* 6, 8h. When the urine has a very strong odour, *Benz. ac.* 3x, 4h. In children of phthisical heredity or tendencies, *Bac. test.* 30, once a week. Incontinence, day or night, profuse emission, *Equiset.* φ—3x, gtt. v. 8h. From irritation from worms, *Cina* 3, 4h. In children when difficult to awaken, *Kreas.* 3, 8h. From too profound sleep, *Kali brom.* gr. ii. at bedtime. Dribbling whilst sitting and walking; on coughing; on emitting flatus; in bed at night, *Puls.* 3, 4h. Constant dribbling, *Verbasc. t.* 3, 4h. Incontinence during the day only, or chiefly, *Ferr. phos.* 3, gr. ii. 6h. Involuntary passage of water during coughing, laughing, sneezing, etc. (1) *Caust.* 6, 4h.; (2) *Ferr. met.* 6, or *Ferr. mur.* 3x, 4h.; (3) *Puls.* 3x, 4h.; (4) *Caps.* 3, 4h.

Urticaria. *See* **Nettle-rash.**

Uterus.—BEARING DOWN.—Frequent pressure and dragging from groin downwards, as if everything were being pressed out, with pressure on rectum and uterus, leaving soreness as after labour; leucorrhœa, *Til.* 6, 8h. Bearing down as if contents of pelvis would be pressed out; active congestion; offensive discharges, *Bell.* 3, 8h. Bearing down with heavy weight and pressure, as if whole contents of pelvis would pass through vagina; > by pressure of hand; dragging from navel; bladder affected, great nervous irritability, *Lil. tig.* 30, twice a day. Bearing down, must cross limbs to prevent protrusion of parts; oppressed breathing, *Sep.* 6, 8h. Bearing down, prolapse, *Fraxin. am.* φ, gtt. i.—v. 8h.

BLEEDING FROM.—Flow usually bright; intermittent; pain from sacrum to pubes, *Sabin.* 3, 2h. Metrorrhagia, bright red blood, bearing down in lower abdomen, *Ficus r.* 1x, 4h. Dark flow, passive, painless, *Ham.* 3, 2h. With forcing pains, flow dark, clotted, *Cham.* 6, 2h. Remaining long after cessation of menses, *Vinc. m.* 3, 2h. Intractable cases, *Thlaspi bursa pastoris,* 1x, 2h. Steady flow, bright arterial, persistent nausea, *Ipec.* 1—30, 2h, *See also* **Fibroma, Menstruation:** EXCESSIVE.

CANCER. *See* **Cancer.**

CONGESTIVE STATES AND DISPLACEMENTS.—Active congestion, with tendency to florid hæmorrhage, accompanied by irritation of bladder and bowels, *Sabin.* 3, 2h. Active congestion with down-pressing as if the contents of the pelvis would

be forced out; offensive discharges; congestion and tenderness of the cervix, *Bell.* 3, 2h. Active congestion or inflammation with fever, full, hard, bounding pulse, *Verat. v.* 3x,
4h. Active congestion or inflammation with severe, labour-
like pains in the region of the womb, extending to the back
and hips, *Gels.* 3, 4h. Prolapse, *Fraxin. am.* φ, gtt. i—v. 8h.
Active congestion, with great nervous irritability and local
pain and sensitiveness; prolapse or anteversion; bladder
affected, *Lil. t.* 30, 4h. Prolapse, pelvic distress; irritability;
fever; menses scanty, *Sep.* 6, 4h. Prolapse, pelvic distress,
menses profuse, *Murex p.* 6, 4h. Chronic congestion with
menses too early and too profuse. *Calc. c.* 6, 4h. Atonic
bodily condition, menorrhagia, leucorrhœa, sterility; an
uterine organ remedy, *Helonias d.* φ—6, 6h. Induration
from chronic congestion, great melancholy and depression,
Aur. met. 30, 8h. Follicular inflammation—(1) *Merc. sol.* 6,
8h.; (2) *Iod.* 3x, gtt. ii. 4h.; (3) *Hydrocot.* 1x, gtt. ii. 4h.;
A sitz-bath, 65°—75°F., for five to ten minutes every night
at bed-time, the body and limbs being kept warm, is sometimes helpful. [Pessaries may have to be resorted to in some
cases of displacement. The safest rule is not to apply a
pessary unless the displacement causes actual distress, and
not then if the distress can be removed, as is usually the
case, by medicines. *See also* **Leucorrhœa.**

HYDROMETRA (*Water in Uterus*).—*Sep.* 6, 4h.

PAIN IN.—Irritable uterus, pain rheumatic or neuralgic, restlessness, irritability, and sleeplessness, *Act. r.* 3x, 2h. Hysterical uterus, cramps, extending into the thighs and followed
by leucorrhœa, *Mag. mur.* 6, 2h.

PHYSOMETRA (*Air in the Uterus*).—(1) *Brom.* 3—30, 4h. (2)
Bell. 3, 4h.

Tumours. *See* Fibroma.

See also Labour, Menstruation, Parametritis, Pelvic Hæmatocele, Perimetritis.

Uvula.—Swollen, inflamed, or ulcerated, *Merc. c.* 6, 2h.; locally, to be touched with a brush charged with *Merc. c.* 3x, trit. Swollen, causes tickling cough, < lying down, *Hyo.* 3, 4h. Uvula elongated, relaxed; scraping in throat, *Alumen* 30, 4h. [This will also suffice to cure a troublesome tickling cough, depending on elongated uvula.]

Vaccination.—Effects of.—In the fever, *Acon.* 3, 2h.; there is much swelling, *Apis* 3x, 2h. When the vesicles are large and angry and the part becomes very red, *Bell.* 3, 1h. Erysipelas, *Vaccin.* 30, 2—4h. In the stage when pus has formed, *Merc. sol.* 6, 2h. Irritation during the healing process, *Sul.* 30, 2h.

Vaccinosis (Ill-health following Vaccination).—Neuralgia, debility; flatulent dyspepsia; eczema, *Thuja* 30, once a week. Chilliness, emaciation, rickety condition; abscesses; convulsions, *Silic.* 30, 4h. Nervous, impatient, irritable; red pimples or blotches on various parts, most evident when warm; languor; restlessness, *Vaccin.* 200 once a week. Unhealthy, dry, scurfy, or pustulating skins, *Maland* 30, once a week, *Gunp.* 3x, gr. iv. 4h., in the interim.

Vagina.—Spasm of.—Vaginismus, *Plumb.* 6, 4h. Hysteria, inflammation of vagina and vulva, *Ign.* 1, 4h. Weight or pressure in vagina, with painful bearing down, vagina being tender to touch, *Sil.* 6, 4h. Dysparunia, *Staph.* 6—30, 4h. Vagina very sensitive and narrowed by swellings of various size, *Alumen* 30, 4h. [Locally, a pledget of lint

charged with *Hamamelis* lotion (ϕ, ʒi.℥—vi.) may be
inserted at bed-time and removed in the morning.]

AIR IN.—*Brom.* 3—30, 4h.

DISCHARGE FROM. *See* **Gonorrhœa, Leucorrhœa.**

Varices. *See* **Veins.**

Varicocele. *See* **Veins.**

Variola. *See* **Small-pox.**

Veins.—INFLAMMATION (*Phlebitis.*)—Simple acute inflammation; much sensitiveness, *Ham.* 3, 1h.; locally, when possible, apply compresses of *Hamamelis* lotion (ϕ. ʒi.—Oj.).
After *Hamamelis;* when following childbirth, *Puls.* 3, 1h.;
locally, *Hamamelis* lotion. Septic phlebitis from putrid
absorption, (1) *Lach.* 6, 1h.; locally, compresses of *Lach.* 6,
lotion (ʒii.—Oj.). (2) *Gunp.* 3x. gr. iv. 4h. (3) *Pyro.* 6, 4h.

VARICOSE VEINS (including *Varicocele*).—As a preventative,
when an attack is feared, *Puls.* 3, 8h. When the veins have
become actually affected, *Ham.* 3, 3h.; locally, support, and
at night apply compresses of *Hamamelis* lotion (ʒi.—Oj.). If
there is much pain in the veins, *Puls.* 3, 2h. If there is
debility, *Formica* 3x, gtt. x. 8h. In old-standing cases,
Fluor. ac. 3, gtt. ii. 4h. After these (especially in varicocele)
—(1) *Ferr. phos.* 3, gr. iv. 4h.; (2) *Plumb.* 6, 4h. In cases of
rupture apply a pad saturated with tincture of *Hamamelis*
over the bleeding point and fix with a firm bandage.

Venereal Disease. *See* **Chancre, Gleet, Gonorrhœa,
Syphilis.**

Vertigo.—Simple giddiness, *Gels.* 3, 3h. With biliousness, tendency to pitch forward, *Bry.* 3, 2h. On going upstairs; on

looking up, *Calc. c.* 6. 8h. Dread of downward motion, *Borax* 6, 8h. When walking; after reading; when turning; as if from stomach; as if a hollow behind him, better in open air, *Kali c.* 6, 8h. *Vertigo a stomacho læso* (giddiness arising from stomach affection), with constipation, in persons of spare habit, *Nux v.* 3, 3h. After *Nux*, *Sul.* 3, 8h. Vertigo with sense of gyration; accompanying sea-sickness, *Cocc. ind.* 3, 2h. Congestive vertigo; vertigo on turning over in bed, or on rising from lying down, *Bell.* 3, 2h. Vertigo whilst lying down, *Con.* 3, 2h. Vertigo whilst lying down; unhealthy subjects; constipation, *Nat. m.* 6, 4h. When due to splenic affections; in old alcoholics, *Quercus* 3x, gtt. v. 4h. When due to heart disease, the heart conditions must be treated, *see* Heart. Accompanying deafness and noises in the head, *see* Ménière's Disease.

Vesicles. *See* Eczema, Herpes, Miliaria, Pemphigus.

Vicarious Menstruation. *See* Menstruation.

Vision. *See* Eyes: SIGHT, *also* Amaurosis, Amblyopia.

Voice.—LOSS OR WEAKNESS OF.—From over exertion, *Arn.* 3, 2h. From simple catarrh, *Caust.* 3, 2h. Hysterical, *Ignat.* 3, 2h.; locally, galvanism. Loss of voice at menstrual periods, *Gels.* 3, 2h. Loss of voice every time the patient is exposed to heat, *Ant. crud.* 3, 3h. Paralysis of vocal muscles, *Oxal. ac.* 3, 4h. With general weakness, wasting, *Iod.* 3x, 4h. Chronic hoarseness, *Baryt. c.* 6—30, 4h. Laryngeal phthisis. *See under* Laryngitis: CHRONIC.

Vomiting.—Vomiting of food or mucus, nausea, salivation, *Ipec.* 3, 1h. Nausea, vomiting coming on late, great prostration and complete muscular relaxation, white tongue; morning vomiting of drunkards; vomiting of liquids as soon as taken, *Ant. t.* 6, 1h. Red tongue, irritable state of stomach, inability to retain water, gastritis, *Ars.* 3, 2h. Cold water is vomited as soon as it becomes warm in the stomach, *Phos.* 6, 2h. Vomiting with flatulent dyspepsia; neuralgia over right eye, *Carbol. ac.* 3, 2h. With marasmus, indigestion of food, *Iod.* 3x, 2h. Vomiting of milk, *Æthus. c.* 3, 2h. Sudden vomiting of milk in infants, *Merc. sol.* 6, 2h. Vomiting of ingesta and lienteria, *Ferr. mur.* 3x, 4h. Acid or bilious vomiting, *Iris v.* 3, 2h. Nausea; vomiting of food, mucous, and bile; headache, *Petrol.* 3, 1h. Chronic vomiting, *Kreas.* 3, 4h. Hysterical vomiting, *Kreas.* 3, 1h. Cerebral or reflex vomiting; sudden, profuse, not preceded by nausea, followed by headache, *Apomorph.* 3x. 2h. From motion, as in sea-sickness, *Cocc. ind.* 3, 2h. *See also* **Dyspepsia, Pregnancy** (MORNING SICKNESS), **Sea-sickness,** etc.

Vulva.—PRURITUS OF. *See* **Irritation.**

Wakefulness. *See under* **Sleep.**

Waking.—Weeps on being aroused, *Cic. v.* 3, 8h. Starts from anxious dreams and screams out, *Bry.* 3, 8h. Wakes from nightmare uttering piercing screams, *Cham.* 6, 8h. Aggravation of symptoms on waking, *Lach.* 6, 4h. *See also* SCREAMING OF CHILDREN.

Walking.—DELAY IN.—If the child is fat, *Calc. c.* 6, 4h. If thin and puny, *Sil.* 6, 4h. In phthisical children, *Bacill.* 30, once a week. [Country air, and chalk soil for residence, with careful dieting, should if possible be secured.]

Warts.—In crops; wart-like excrescences on back of head, on chin, etc; flat black wart on left side of head; warts and condylomata, large, seedy, pedunculated; sometimes oozing moisture and bleeding readily, *Thuja* 3—30, 4h.; locally, to be painted with *Thuja* φ night and morning. Itching, sticking, and pricking in; large jagged, pedunculated, easily bleeding; cauliflower-like; on upper lip, *Nit. ac.* 12, 4h., numerous, small, horny; itching, stinging; inflamed; ulcerating, *Calc. c.* 6, 4h. Ulcerating, sensitive to touch, *Nat. c.* 6, 9h. Multiple, pedunculated lupoid warts, *Fer. picric.* 3x, gr. iv.—3, gtt. ii. 8h. Hard, painful, throbbing warts, *Sul.* 3, 4h. Many very small warts; warts soft at base, horny on surface; warts on arms and hands, warts on eyelids and face, *Caust.* 12, 8h. Warts back of glans penis, *Ant. t.* 12, 8h. Warts on the hands, *Kali mur.* 3, gr. v. 8h.; locally to be moistened once a day with a solution of *Kali mur.* 3x (as much as would lie on a sixpence, in a tablespoonful of water). Warts on the palm, *Nat. m.* 6, 4h. Warts on margin of prepuce; on the body; large hard black warts, *Sep.* 6, 8h.

LOCAL TREATMENT.—In general it is a dangerous thing to meddle with warts locally. Especially is this the case with mushroom warts (with short pedicle and flattened tops). Warts may be psoric or sycotic, or they may be closely allied to epithelial cancer. In the case of common warts, the same remedy that is being taken internally may be applied externally to the warts in a solution once a day. *Solid lunar caustic* is sometimes an effectual application. *Glacial acetic acid*, applied every three or four days, has the advantage of not discolouring the part. *Chromic acid* may be used also.

Wasting. *See* Atrophy.

Water-brash.—Everything tastes sour; sour eructations; acid gnawing stomach; flatulence, distension, *Lyc.* 6, 4h. Heartburn after eating; sour-smelling breath; difficult belching; eructations of water after eating; putrid in morning; heartburn < before breakfast; of drunkards, *Nux v.* 3, 4h. Risings, especially after having eaten, mostly bitter or sour with a taste of the food; pressure on stomach, *Bry.* 3, 4h. Heat rising from stomach to throat, *Mancinella* 3—30, 4h. With much pain after food and coldness of hands and feet, *Verat. a.* 3, 4h.

Water in the Head. *See* **Hydrocephalus.**

Weakness. *See* **Debility.**

Weaning.—MANAGEMENT OF THE CHILD. *See under* **Diet:** INFANTS.

MANAGEMENT OF THE BREASTS. *See under* **Breasts,** INFLAMMATION OF, and **Lactation.**

Wens.—On scalp; scalp sensitive and scurfy, *Baryt. c.* 6, 6h. Hordeola, recurrent, *Con.* 3—30, 6h. Suppurating, *Hep. s.* 6, 6h. In gouty subjects, with strong-smelling urine, *Benz. ac.* 3x, 8h. Ointment of *Benz. ac.* gr. v. to the ounce. If other things fail, inject a few drops of *Phyt. φ.*

Wetting the Bed. *See under* **Urine.**

Whites. *See* **Leucorrhœa.**

White Leg. *See* **Phlegmasia Alba Dolens.**

Whitlow.—If taken early, the formation may be cut short by *Silic.* 3x, gr. v. 2h. Pricking, sharp, agonising pain, *Diosc.* 3x—30, 1—2h. (Locally, paint with *Diosc. φ.* This will abort many cases.) Pricking, tingling; blue colour extending far around; felons with proud flesh, *Lach.* 6, 2h. Thumbs and fingers inflamed, acute throbbing pains, sensation as of a splinter under the nail, *Flu. ac.* 5, 2h. Heat throbbing, swelling, constitutional disturbance, worse at night, preventing sleep must hold the finger up, *Hep.* 6, 1h.

(Locally the finger may be painted with *Phos.* 3x,) When pus has formed, a deep incision is sometimes necessary; and afterwards *Sil.* 6, 2h.; locally *Calendula* lotion (ʒiv.—Oss.).

Whooping-cough.—*Prevention :* When whooping-cough breaks out in a family, all those members who have not had it should take *Dros.* 6, night and morning, [In giving medicine for whooping-cough it is a good plan to give a dose after each coughing fit.] To begin with, *Coquel.* 30, 4h. This will cut short a large proportion of cases. It may be given alone or in alternation with some other well-indicated remedy. When the stage of catarrh has set in, with teasing cough, *Aco.* 3, 2h. Spasmodic fits of coughing, *Ipec.* 3, 2h. Convulsive cough, with much eructation and hoarseness; deep cough with flow of water into the mouth; tough expectoration, *Ambra* 6, 2h. Spells of hacking cough, followed by vomiting if the mucus does not come up, < after midnight, *Dros.* 6, a dose after each paroxysm of the coughing. Vomiting of thick, viscid mucus; frequent passage of much pale urine with tenesmus, *Cocc. c.* 3, 2h. When the child begins to cry as soon as it feels the cough coming on; rupture of blood-vessels of the eye; bleeding from the nose or spitting of blood, *Arn.* 6, 2h. Cries after coughing, *Caps.* 3, 4h. With puffiness of upper eyelids, *Kali c.* 6, 2h. Where there is sublingual ulcer, *Nit. ac.* 6, 2h. Spasm very severe, convulsions threatening, *Hydrocy. ac.* 3x, 2h. Spasms, cramps, or convulsions, *Cupr. met.* 6, 1—2h. When there are symptoms of oppression of the brain between the convulsions, *Op.* 3, 1h. Convulsions and oppression of the brain in full-blooded children; cries before the cough, *Bell.* 3, 1h. When capillary bronchitis occurs, rattling on the chest, prostration, perspiration; cough brought on by fit of anger, *Ant. t.* 6, 1h. Spasmodic cough, rattling on the chest, child cannot bear the least draught, *Hep.* 6, 2h. When there is pneumonia, *see* **Pneumonia.**

Wind. *See* **Flatulence.**

Womb. *See* **Uterus.**

Woolsorter's Disease. *See* **Malignant Pustule.**

Worms.—*Hygienic Treatment.*—It often happens that the constitution is rendered more susceptible to the attacks of intestinal parasites and more tolerant of their presence, by faulty hygienic surroundings. In all cases this should be attended to, and the drainage especially; sewer gas has a strong tendency to predispose the system. The natural history of the parasite should be attended to as far as it is known. Uncooked or undercooked fish or meat should be avoided to guard against tape-worm and trichinæ. Sweets, sugar, pastry, raw fruit, and vegetables should be avoided. The thread-worm is always introduced into the mouth in the shape of eggs; the eggs hatch in the small intestine, and the worms lodge in the cæcum; they lay their eggs at the anus; and their whole life is only a fortnight. Children suffering from thread-worms should be prevented from putting their fingers into their mouth, as they are very apt to scratch the irritated parts in sleep. This caution may be necessary for older persons.

Constitutional Treatment.—As a return to healthy hygienic conditions will sometimes suffice to render a patient intolerant of intestinal parasites, and thus bring about their expulsion, so a return to a more healthy condition of body, when weakened by any other cause, will often produce the same effect. When the child is scrofulous fat, pale, lymphatic, head hot and perspiring at night, the perspiration not being offensive, feet cold and clammy, *Calc. c.* 12, 8h. Distension of abdomen, poor appetite, constipation, dark thick urine, pains in the body going from right to left, *Lyc.* 12, 8h. Scrofulous eruptive subjects, sinking sensation in epigastrium in forenoon, hot head, cold feet, *Sul.* 30, 8h. In strumous, feeble, precocious children, feverish, dry, hot skin, furred tongue, tumid abdomen, bowels confined, appetite rapacious, nervous irritability, *Spig.* 3, 8h. Fever, canine hunger, pale urine, picking nose, tendency to convulsions, *Cina* 30, 8h. Wakes screaming at night, cannot be pacified, wets bed, cheeks scarlet, other parts of the face, especially round mouth, white, eyes brilliant, skin dry, hot, violent rage when spoken to, *Bell.* 30, 4h. Indigestion with low feverish condition, *Bapt.* 3, 8h. Anæmia; passage of blood and mucus, *Ferr. mur.* 3x, 3h. Burnett noticed that when prescribing a course of *Scirrhinum* and other cancer nosodes for patients this was often followed by the expulsion of worms. This observation indicates that the liability to intestinal parasites may be one symptom of the cancerous diathesis, and it also suggests that *Scirrhinum* 30, once or twice a week should be included among the constitutional remedies for helminthiasis. The ringworm parasites are of the mould or vegetable order and one of the consumption nosodes, notably *Bacillinum*, is the basic remedy.

[If constitutional treatment does not suffice to remove all the symptoms of the parasites, *Direct Treatment* must be employed, as described below.]

ANKYLOSTOMA DUODENALE.—*Thymol* gr. v. 2h. till 20 grains are taken; followed by full dose of castor-oil, and turpentine. Diet to consist of milk and soup. Recently *Carbon tetrachloride* has been found very effective. The patient must not be constipated. The day before the dose liquid diet only for lunch and dinner. The dosage is three minims per years of age for children, and an adult dose of 46 to 60 minims. The dose is taken in a tablespoon or measure glass, and half an hour after an ounce of *Epsom salts*. Or, the drug may be given in the *Epsom salts* solution. Also Extract of male-fern (*Filix mas*) as for tape-worm.

ROUND WORMS (*Ascaris lumbricoides*).—When the presence of this parasite is made out, *Sant.* 1x, gr. v. every morning, fasting; there must be no solid food given during this time. This may be repeated three to six mornings. Its efficacy may be increased by combining with it *Merc. dulc.* 1x, gr. v., given for four mornings in succession and then followed with a castor-oil purge, If necessary the *Santonin* with *Merc. dulc.* may be given for three more mornings and followed with a further dose of *Castor-oil*. Or oil of *Chenopodium*, gtt. ii. 8h. for a day or two, followed by a dose of castor-oil. *See also* the use of *Filmaron* under **Tape-Worm**.

TAPE-WORM (*Tænia saginata* and *Tænia solium*).—After a twelve hours' fast, a draught of the fresh etherial extract of male fern (*Filix mas*) should be given. The best formula is: —*Filix mas* (liquid extract) gtt. xxx., syrup (not mucilage) ℨii., distilled water ℨi. Two hours after this an ounce of castor-oil should be taken. A new preparation of male fern is *Filmaron oil*—one part of Filmaron dissolved in 9 parts of castor-oil. The dose is 6 grammes (gr. 90) for a child of 10, 10 to 12 grammes (gr. 150 to 180) for adults, given in two divisions, half an hour apart and followed in one or two hours by a purge of castor oil. A glycerine and water enema should be given the day before. Oil of Filmaron in 1 to 3 grammes (gr. 15—45) doses in gelatine capsules is also useful in the case of ascarides. If this does not succeed in completely killing the worm, give *Filix mas* φ, gtt. v. 8h. persistently, for two or three months; or a strong infusion of *Kousso* taken in the morning, fasting, and followed in an hour by an ounce of castor-oil; or *Pumpkin seeds* (about 4 oz.) scalded and decorticated are crushed and made into a pottage with cream and eaten after a twenty-four hours' fast, as little drink as possible, also, being taken. The castor-oil purge to follow. It is best to take the seeds at bed-time, and early next morning a tablespoonful of castor-oil mixed with half a drachm of sulphuric ether. No breakfast to be taken, only a cup of tea or coffee. Or, *Carbon tetrachloride* may be given as advised for *Ankylostoma*.

THREAD-WORMS (*Oxyurides*, commonly but erroneously called *Ascarides*).—[Constitutional hygienic treatment, most applicable to sufferers from thread-worms.] All essential oils are poisonous to thread-worms. To give temporary relief, warm injections containing a few drops of oil of turpentine (five to the ounce of water) will destroy and bring away all that may be in the rectum. Internally, *Cina* 3, 4h. Where there is much irritation in the rectum, *Teucr*. φ, gtt. x.—1x, gtt. iii. 8h. When there is much acidity, *Nat. ph.* 1x. gr. v. 8h. Fever, dry skin, capricious appetite, swollen abdomen, constipation, nervous irritability, *Spigel.* 3, 4h. Low fever, with loaded tongue, loss of appetite, dull condition, *Bapt.* 3, 4h. An occasional dose of *Scirrh.* 200 will often bring them away. *See also* use of Filmaron *under Tape-worm.*

TRICHINÆ.—It is impossible to destroy these parasites when once they have commenced to migrate. As soon as it is known that infected pork has been eaten, if still in the

stomach, an emetic should be taken; if it has passed into
the intestines, a brisk castor-oil purge should be administered to expel what may remain. When the fever is once
established, all that remains is to support the patient's
strength, and administer such internal remedies as correspond to the general symptoms. In general, *Baptis.* 3x, 1h.,
or *Ars.* 3x, 1h., will prove suitable.

Wounds.—Contused, *Arn.* 3, 1h.; locally, *Arnica* lotion (φ,
ʒi.—ʒiii.). *See also* **Bruises,** and **Brain:** CONCUSSION OF.
Cuts, *Arn.* 3, 1h.; locally, *Calend.* lotion (φ, ʒi.—ʒi.).
Lacerated wounds, *Calend.* 3x, 2h. *Calend.* φ, (ʒi.—Oj.)
warm water for a lotion. *Hyperic.* 3, 1h.; locally, *Hyperic.*
lotion (φ, ʒi.—ʒi.) Punctured, *Led.* 6, 1h.; locally, *Ledum*
lotion, (φ, ʒi.—ʒi.). Poisoned, *Lach.* 6, 1h.; locally, *Lach.*
lotion (6, ʒi.—ʒiii.). *See also* **Pyæmia.**

Writers' Cramp. *See* **Paralysis,** LOCAL.

Wry-neck. *See* **Stiff-neck.**

Yawning.—Frequent yawning without sleepiness, *Aco.* 3, 2h.
Frequent yawning in the evening without sleepiness, *Arn.*
2, 3h. Yawning after dinner and supper, *Lyc.* 6, 2h. Yawning for hours after eating; immediately after waking, *Nux
v.* 2, 3h. Frequent yawning, after sleeping, with flow of
tears; excessive yawning, as if the jaw would be dislocated;
yawning whilst eating; yawning interrupted by spasmodic
rigidity of chest-walls, *Ign.* 1—30, 2h. Yawning so violent
and spasmodic that it threatens to dislocate the jaw, *Rhus t.*
3, 2h. Frequent yawning with eructations, during the day,
Sul. 3, 2h. Frequent yawning, stretching and sleepiness, as
after being awake all night, *Chel.* 3, 2h. Yawning with
internal chilliness, *Nat. mur.* 6, 4h.

Yellow Fever.—During the chill stage, *Camph.* (*Rubini's*) gtt.
ii. ¼h. When reaction sets in, fever, anxiety, restlessness,
vomiting, jaundice, *Aco.* 3, ½h. Where gastric symptoms
appear < by least movement, *Bry.* 3, ½h. Burning and cutting pain in stomach, intense retching, gagging, bringing up
tough mucus, intense nausea and vomiting; the least thing
touching the lips excites vomiting; black vomit, *Cadm. s.*
3—30, 1—2h. When the patient passes into a typhoid state,
Ars. 3, ½h. Exhaustion, hæmorrhages, jaundice, *Crotal.* 3,
¼h. (Preparations of the nosode must not be forgotten.)

Zona. *See* **Herpes Zoster.**